# RESEARCH IN
# HUMAN CAPITAL
# AND DEVELOPMENT

*Volume 5* ● 1988

## PUBLIC HEALTH AND DEVELOPMENT

Editorial correspondence pertaining to articles to be published should be sent to:

Professor Ismail Sirageldin, Series Editor
Department of Population Dynamics
The Johns Hopkins University
School of Hygiene and Public Health
615 N. Wolfe Street
Baltimore, Maryland 21205

All other correspondence should be sent to:

JAI PRESS INC.
55 Old Post Road, No. 2
Greenwich, Connecticut 06830

# RESEARCH IN HUMAN CAPITAL AND DEVELOPMENT

*A Research Annual*

## PUBLIC HEALTH AND DEVELOPMENT

*Editor:*  ISMAIL SIRAGELDIN
*Department of Population Dynamics*
*The Johns Hopkins University*

*Co-editor:*  ALAN SORKIN
*Department of Economics*
*University of Maryland*
*Baltimore*

VOLUME 5 • 1988

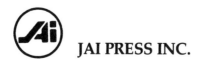

JAI PRESS INC.

*Greenwich, Connecticut*                    *London, England*

# CONTENTS

# LIST OF CONTRIBUTORS

*Joan L. Aron*

Department of Population Dynamics
The Johns Hopkins University

*Timothy Baker*

Department of International Health
The Johns Hopkins University

*Peter Berman*

Department of International Health
The Johns Hopkins University

*Dov Chernichovsky*

Health Sciences and Administration
Ben Gurion University of the Negev

*Jose deCodes*

Country Representative (Brazil)
The Pathfinder Fund

*David W. Dunlop*

ABT Associates
Boston

*Ronald H. Gray*

Department of Population Dynamics
The Johns Hopkins University

*Steven Jarrett*

UNICEF, Office of China

*Oey Astra Meesook*

The World Bank

*W. Henry Mosley*

Department of Population Dynamics
The Johns Hopkins University

*A. Mead Over*

Economist
The World Bank

*Barbara A. Ormond*              Research Assistant
                                 The Johns Hopkins University

*Robert L. Parker*               Program Health Officer
                                 UNICEF, Office for China

*William A. Reinke*              Department of International Health
                                 The Johns Hopkins University

*David S. Salkever*              Department of Health Policy and
                                     Management
                                 The Johns Hopkins University

*Debra Schumann*                 Department of Population Dynamics
                                 The Johns Hopkins University

*Ismail Sirageldin*              Department of Population Dynamics
                                 The Johns Hopkins University

*Alan L. Sorkin*                 Department of Economics
                                 University of Maryland
                                 Baltimore

*Carl E. Taylor*                 Department of International Health
                                 The Johns Hopkins University

*Seung-Hum Yu*                   Department of Preventive Medicine
                                     and Public Health
                                 Yonsei University College of Medicine

*Huda Zurayk*                    Department of Epidemiology and
                                     Biostatistics
                                 American University of Beirut

# INTRODUCTION

The associations between public health and national development are complex. The interaction is a two-way phenomenon, with health both being influenced by and affecting economic development. Traditionally improved health has been considered a byproduct of economic growth instead of one of its causes.

Much recent research on the relationship between public health and development has been based on the framework of human capital theory. In the most general sense, human capital is defined as any activity that renders human beings more productive. However, the term is usually used in relation to expenditures on education, health, on-the-job training, or migration. These expenditures are termed investments in human capital. To the extent that better health results in higher income, expenditures made by an individual or a community to improve health status can be considered as resulting in the acquisition of human capital. The investment generates revenues in future years and also may be subject to depreciation. Rates of return or cost-benefit ratios can thus be calculated for health investments in a similar manner to those computed for investments in physical capital.

Once the economic return to a particular health program has been determined, important information is available for evaluating the policies undertaken by ministries of health and other organizations such as planning agencies, whose activities affect the level of resources allocated to health. Moreover, the relative importance of health, in comparison to other social programs, can also be considered.

The first part of this volume includes papers that focus on conceptual issues concerning public health and development. The Sirageldin-Mosley paper explores the relationship between health and population activities. It identifies three types of mechanisms linking health and population policies and activities, namely programmatic, biological and indirect. One major theme is that these three mechanisms are not only dependent on the social environment but are also interdependent with each other. For example, they demonstrate that the efficiency of the health service delivery system will depend on the efficacy of the indirect mechanisms such as the allocative efficiency and equity of the labor market and the education system. Ultimately population and health policies should be specified subject to financial, technological and social limitations. Given these constraints it becomes possible to discuss and resolve the intra- and inter-generational allocation of the costs and benefits of population and health programs. Gray's paper focuses primarily on the changes in disease patterns and causes of death that have accompanied mortality declines. This process is termed the epidemiologic transition. As the nutritional and communicable diseases of childhood diminish, adult chronic degenerative and neoplastic diseases have become the major causes of death. Aron's paper discusses mortality and morbidity in Africa due to measles, malaria and AIDS. She argues that although activities targeted against specific diseases have made a noticeable demographic impact, such as in the case of malaria control in Sri Lanka, selective disease control is not a total substitute for other programs in public health. Her analysis provides a cautionary note to the present concern and strategic approaches dealing with AIDS. Zurayk discusses the role of health information systems in improving the planning and delivery of health services in developing countries. The development of computer technology and its capacities for data linkages and for complex data analysis have created a large gap in information handling potential between developed and developing countries. However, in many cases, simple systems may provide the necessary information base for planning and management purposes. Her analysis questions the cost-effectiveness of establishing a sophisticated system to satisfy the information needs for public health policies and services in developing countries.

Part II of the volume presents papers that provide an overview and commentary on a particular dimension of the relationship between public health and development. Sorkin reviews the literature on the relationship between water, sanitation, health and economic progress. A second focus of the paper concerns selected economic aspects of water supply and sanitation, including issues of financing. Dunlop and Over examine the relationship between health programs in developing countries and the availability of foreign exchange. They find that poor economic performance has resulted in insufficient foreign exchange earnings to finance the purchase of drugs and medical supplies. They argue that donor assistance is necessary in order for these nations to obtain the necessary foreign exchange. DeCodes, Baker and Schumann study the cost of illness in a poor rural Brazilian county. They find that the indirect cost of illness (lost productivity) accounts for the bulk of the total costs of illness as compared to its direct costs. Only in the case of respiratory disease was the direct cost larger than the indirect cost. The Berman-Ormand paper is an overview of the relationship between the demand for health and economic development. They conclude that as national incomes rise government expenditures on health services also tend to increase, often more rapidly than aggregate income. Except in countries where public sector care is dominant, private health care expenditures may rise at a faster rate than public expenditures.

Part III of the volume focuses on country case studies of the interaction of public health and development. Reinke's paper traces the development of Indonesia's health care system over the past twenty years. While efforts have been made to expand government services in the rural areas, much remains to be accomplished. He explores the role of incentives in the quality of health services in the public sector. For example, because of low salaries, most government physicians are simultaneously employed in private practice. This lowers the quality of government services. The study by Chernichovsky and Meesook compares expenditures and consumption of food between urban and rural dwellers in Indonesia. In spite of the relative affluence of the urban population, the latter does not fare better than the former in terms of diet. Price differentials between the urban and rural sections of the country appear to outweigh the income differentials as far as food consumption is concerned. The Taylor, Parker and Jarett paper discusses the evolution of health care in rural China since liberation. Apparently, the Chinese health gains result from concentrating first on rapid expansion of coverage for basic services and subsequently focusing on improvement in the quality of care. As the epidemiologic transition takes hold, i.e., the changing pattern of disease as the population ages, more attention is given to the fiscal viability of the program. But other social objectives of China's health policy may suffer. For example, the recent increased emphasis on fee for service financing has the danger of causing inequity in access to services and decreasing the emphasis on preventive medicine. Yu's paper points out that in Korea the health problems are rapidly becoming similar to those of Europe or the United States. However, as a percentage of its GNP Korea spends less than half of the level of U.S. expenditure on health care. But he indicates that Korea has developed a number of innovative health insurance plans in order to reduce cost and increase access to care by all segments of the population. For example, nearly 1,000 physicians are doing mandatory service as directors of health subcenters. Salkever's study seeks a more comprehensive measure of U.S. morbidity costs than previous research. He finds that debility cost is a major component of morbidity costs for noninstitutionalized males aged 17-64. These costs are at least as large as the costs associated with work-loss days.

Considerable effort has gone into the production of this volume. Ruth Levine and Pamela Burdell provided outstanding editorial assistance and support. Ruth Skarda did her usual excellent job in typing the entire manuscript and providing highly efficient secretarial and organizational assistance.

Ismail Sirageldin
Alan Sorkin
*Co-editors*

# PART I

# CONCEPTUAL ISSUES IN PUBLIC HEALTH AND DEVELOPMENT

# HEALTH SERVICES AND POPULATION PLANNING PROGRAMS:

## A REVIEW OF INTERRELATIONS

Ismail Sirageldin and W. Henry Mosley

## I. INTRODUCTION

Do population/family planning programs have a cost-saving effect on health delivery systems that increase their efficiency and/or their effectiveness? This is the central question of the current literature on the relationships between health and family planning activities. The question gained recent prominence for at least two reasons. The *first* has to do with the negative effect of reduced economic growth rates of the less developed countries during the decade of the 1980s, and the reduced aid commitments from the richer countries to the achievement of the "Health for All" goal that was launched in 1978. In that context, the policy problem is how to smooth out mortality and morbidity

**Research in Human Capital Development, Vol. 5, pages 3-23.**
**Copyright © 1988 by JAI Press Inc.**
**ISBN: 0-89232-508-9**

fluctuations in periods of economic adjustments and, more fundamentally, how to sustain in the longer term the social gains, including health improvements, that have been achieved or planned (cf. the contributions to the Second Takemi Symposium, 1986 and to Cornia, Jolly and Stewart, 1987). The *second* reason is more pragmatic. It is how to justify, in the face of changing political commitments for population programs and an increasingly constrained financial environment, a viable public role for family planning programs based on their potential contribution to improving the health status of mothers and children.

Both reasons mentioned above are important. How countries adjust, with minimum injury to their basic social programs, under crisis circumstances of rapidly changing technical environment, unfavorable fluctuations in the prices of the major export and import commodities, and a dramatic rise in the relative size and economic burden of the international debt and its service, should be at the forefront of any responsible public policy. Accordingly, more efficient and effective health programs become a policy imperative. And identifying the segments of society that suffer the most from these external shocks is an essential step for the design of more viable and targeted strategies.

On its face value, the truth of the second reason mentioned above is self-evident. The ultimate objective of population policies, or for that matter, other social policies, should be to improve the present and future well-being of individuals and families in which health status is a major element. In that context, population and health services programs should be viewed as coordinating parts of an overall socioeconomic policy—a necessary condition for a consistent social policy framework. And although each of these programs has its own specific goals and targets under this general welfare objective, they, as in the case of most social programs, overlap, directly or indirectly, in terms of their input-output relations. However, the implied relationships between health and population programs are neither simple nor necessarily positive. The main objective of the present paper is to provide a systematic discussion of these relationships.

On one level of generalization, the need for a coordinated health and population policy may not require a formal or an empirical proof. High levels of mortality and fertility are generally not acceptable as a foundation for a stable sociodemographic system. Lower levels of mortality (and morbidity) are socially desired by the less developed countries and accordingly targeted as a health policy objective. But in the longer-term, lower fertility becomes a necessary condition for the stability of this new sociodemographic solution. More pertinent to the present discussion is to seek an answer to the question of whether a more coordinated linkage between the desired paths of these two main elements of population dynamics is also necessary in the short-run in order to minimize the potential social and economic costs of that transition. Such coordinated linkage implies an adequate conceptual and empirical knowledge about the dynamic nature in general and the time-lag structure in particular of the implied interrelations. Indeed, the scope and generality of such analyses is limited by conceptual and empirical constraints.

Furthermore, the present discussion is also guided by the type of policy concerns being raised in the health-population field, and for which answers are being sought. These concerns are not void of unsettled controversies. Three main concerns may be identified and serve as the background for the present discussion. The first relates to questioning the significance of the influence of population programs on the demand for health. The second relates to the potential social cost of reinforcing an inefficient and inequitable health system. The third relates to questioning the role of family planning programs in contributing significantly to reducing the overall level of mortality, especially among children and mothers, in countries where the overall average is high, as opposed to just influencing its variance in the population.

## II. SOME POLICY ISSUES ON THE RELATIONSHIP BETWEEN HEALTH AND POPULATION

*On the Demand for Health*

In an intriguing paper, J. Caldwell (1986) examined various "routes to low mortality in developing countries." He identified 11 developing countries as "superior health achievers." Their per capita GNP level in 1982 varied between $190-1,430 and their infant mortality rates (per 1,000 live births per capita GNP) between 10-106. Achievement is defined by ranking the individual country based on the level of its infant mortality relative to that of the countries in its income group and independent of the level of mortality. In his analyses Caldwell highlights female education as the key factor related to the improvement of child health (Caldwell, 1981). Three explanations are usually given linking female education to child health. Educated mothers are more likely to break with tradition, become less "fatalistic" about illness, and more willing to adopt more modern and effective alternatives in child care and treatment of illness. An educated mother is more willing and able to assert herself in the modern world and demand and use treatment and facilities in a more effective way. Furthermore, educated women could break the balance in traditional familial roles and relationships. However, the alleged effect of education should most probably depend on the degree of equity in the distribution of educational opportunities and on the demand for its utilization. Furthermore, education should influence other demographic outcomes, more specifically the level and structure of fertility, that may in turn influence mortality. Nothing in Caldwell's analysis refers to levels or trends in fertility. Such omission introduces a bias in the specification of the underlying causal mechanisms. For example, when the level of the infant mortality rates (IMR)

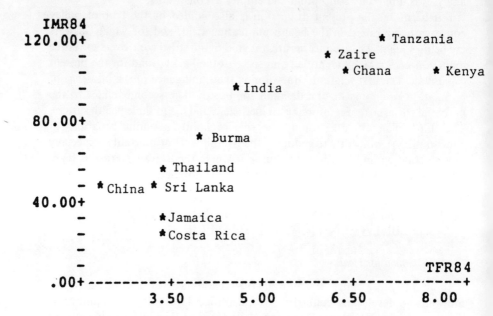

*Source:*  Based on J. Caldwell (1986, p. 174) and World Bank, *World Development Report, 1986.*

*Figure 1.*   Infant Mortality Rates (IMR) and Total Fertility Rates (TFR)
among 11 Superior Health Achievers Selected from
99 Third World Countries, 1984.

of these 11 superior health achievers is related to the level of their total fertility rates (TFR), a significant statistical association emerges ($\bar{R}^2 = .73$). Without inference about causation or sophisticated modelling, it is evident that lower fertility seems to be strongly associated with lower mortality levels among the "superior health achievers" identified by Caldwell. As Figure 1 illustrates, a decline of one child in TFR is associated with a 16 point reduction in IMR. It is possible that there are alternative routes leading to the observed mortality reduction (cf. Caldwell [1986], Mosley [1983, 1985], or Preston [1980, 1985]). These routes are probably much more complex than those implied in Caldwell's illustration. For example, it is equally plausible that there is a reinforcing mechanism between the activities and outputs of effective population and health programs.

*On Reinforcing Ineffectiveness and Inequity in Health Delivery Systems*

In a recent policy statement (Akin and Birdsall, World Bank, 1986) four main problems with health services in developing countries were indentified: insufficient resources available for public health programs; poor use of resources; low output; poor quality; and inequitable distribution of benefits. In 1982 total health expenditure per capita (among 12 countries representing the low, middle and the industrialized countries) varied between $3 for Ethiopia and $9-10 for China, Uganda and Sri Lanka among the low income group; and between $15 and $66 for Indonesia, Egypt, Zambia and Peru among the middle-income group; compared to $444 to $1,403 per capita expenditure for Italy, Japan, Sweden and the U.S. among the industrialized countries (Akin and Birdsall, 1986, Table 2, p.22). One would expect a positive correlation between performance and the level of per capita expenditure. However, achievement seems to be independent of per capita expenditures. For example, China and Sri Lanka achieved a very favorable cost-effectiveness ratio in their health system programs in spite of the relatively low level of per capita expenditure.

There is also evidence of inadequate resource allocation in the health systems of the developing countries as a whole. More than 75 percent of total expenditures seem to be devoted to curative activities where the cost per additional life saved is highest, while less than 10 percent of resources are devoted to community service (e.g., vector control programs, education programs and monitoring of disease patterns) where the cost-effectiveness ratio is lowest.

The apparent relative inefficiency and ineffectiveness of the health system are sometimes defended partly as a cost society has to pay in order to achieve and equity objective. Such objection is not necessarily supported by the available evidence. In an attempt to give equal access to everyone, very few governments charge for their health and educational services. In cases where they do, charges tend to be very low. However, the system is far from being equitable. For example, according to a review of the evidence by E. Jimenez (1986, p.112): "Despite these efforts at equity, the services do not benefit each income group equally, let alone progressively."

The findings of Jimenez on inequity in the educational system are relevant since, as discussed earlier, many view education, especially for females, as a major factor in improving infant and child health status (cf. Caldwell, 1986) as well as in reducing fertility. As Tables 1 and 2 (reproduced from Jimenez, 1986, pp.114-115) illustrate, there is a significantly unequal access to educational resources by occupational groups and to the receiving of public health subsidies by income groups. In 1980, farmers in Francophone Africa had access to 44 percent of public school resources although comprising 76 percent of the population. In the case of Latin America, the figures were 18

*Table 1.* Share of Public Resources for Education Appropriated by Different Socioeconomic Groups, by Region, 1980

| Region | Percentage in the population | | | Percentage of public school resources | | | Ratio between percentage of resources and of population | | |
|---|---|---|---|---|---|---|---|---|---|
| | *Farmers* | *Manual workers and traders* | *White-collar* | *Farmers* | *Manual workers and traders* | *White-collar* | *Farmers* | *Manual workers and traders* | *White-collar* |
| Africa | | | | | | | | | |
| Anglophone | 76 | 18 | 6 | 56 | 21 | 23 | 0.73 | 1.19 | 3.78 |
| Francophone | 76 | 18 | 6 | 44 | 21 | 36 | 0.58 | 1.15 | 5.93 |
| Asia | 58 | 32 | 10 | 34 | 38 | 28 | 0.59 | 1.19 | 2.79 |
| Latin America | 36 | 49 | 15 | 18 | 51 | 31 | 0.49 | 1.04 | 2.03 |
| Middle East and North Africa | 42 | 48 | 10 | 25 | 46 | 29 | 0.60 | 0.35 | 2.87 |
| OECD | 12 | 53 | 35 | 11 | 46 | 42 | 0.95 | 0.87 | 1.2 |

*Source:* Mingat and Tan (1986).

*Source:* Jimenez (1986)

Table 2.  Percentage Share of Public Health Subsidies by Income Group

| County and source | Year of data | Type of health subsidy | Income group | | | | |
|---|---|---|---|---|---|---|---|
| | | | Poorest 20% | 20-39% | 40-59% | 60-79% | 80-100% |
| Chile (Foxley, Animat, and Arellano 1979) | 1969 | Public Health | 31 (poorest 30%) | | 35 (31-60%) | 35 (61-100%) | |
| Colombia (Selowsky 1979) | 1974 | NHS hospitals[a] | 30 | 23 | 20 | 18 | 12 |
| | | SS hospitals[a] | 8 | 15 | 29 | 24 | 23 |
| | | Health center | 25 | 29 | 23 | 15 | 8 |
| | | Overall public | 20 | 21 | 20 | 20 | 20 |
| Indonsia (Meesook 1984) | 1980 | Overall public | 19 (poorest 40%) | | 36 (40-69%) | 45 (70-100%) | |
| Iran (Richards 1982) | 1977[b] | Overall public | 30 | 21 | 19 | 18 | 13 |
| Malaysia (Meerman 1979) | 1974 | Inpatient hospital | 19 | 27 | 10 | 24 | 20 |
| | | Outpatient hospital | 22 | 20 | 23 | 14 | 6 |
| | | Rural clinic | 28 | 27 | 19 | 19 | 8 |
| | | Overall public | 21 | 26 | 15 | 22 | 17 |
| Philippines (Richards 1982) | 1975[b] | Overall public | 14 | 13 | 15 | 18 | 40 |
| Sri Lanka (Richards 1982) | 19978[b] | Overall public | 25 | 21 | 20 | 19 | 14 |

Note: Rows may not sum to 100 percent because of rounding.
a. NHS = National Health Service; SS = social security.
b. These data are from restricted International Labor Organization (ILO) documents. The years quoted are the dates of the original studies.
Source: Jimenez (1986)

and 36 percent, respectively. If we also add that the labor markets in the less developed countries are not very efficient and mostly segmented, then we must be guarded when concluding about the educational effects on health status without defining the underlying social context.

In the case of public health, the poorest 40 percent of the population in Indonesia, for example, had access to 19 percent of public health subsidies in 1980; for the Philippines (1975) it was 40 percent and 27 percent, respectively. In most cases the final effect was either proportionate or regressive—but not progressive as intended by the equity criterion underlying the policy. Unequal access to health and other social services seems to manifest itself in terms of unequal health status. For example, in Turkey with an IMR of about 90, 41 percent of the population lives in areas with an IMR above 149 (UNICEF, 1985). Even in countries with relatively lower IMR, e.g., Venezuela (IMR =39), 44 percent of the population lived in areas with IMR above 50 (see Table 3 for more details). In such circumstances, the education and health systems interact to perpetuate and probably increase existing patterns of inequity. Jimenez's (1986, p,124) policy implications, based on his review of the evidence, are worth quoting in detail:

"The distribution of government subsidies for health and education is not progressive; for education it is strongly regressive. The reasons are:

- Free provision does not mean free consumption. Income still determines consumption, even if no charges are levied by the public sector.
- Costs are higher for poor people because they lack access to credit and insurance markets and because they live in remote areas.
- Subsidies are largest for the types of public services (higher education, private rooms in hospitals) consumed by richer groups.

"Public subsidies and controls contribute to the inefficiency of social services. The reasons are:

- There is underinvestment in social services as a whole, largely because of restrictions on the private sector.
- Resources are misallocated among types of education, and, perhaps, health services: too much is spent on higher education in relation to primary levels; health services favor high-cost, in-patient curative care over preventive care.
- Resources are misallocated within social services: the wrong students or patients may be chosen, and there are no incentives for administrators to minimize costs."

Various policy prescriptions are being advocated to improve the ability of the health system to deal more adequately with issues of equity and effectiveness. These include introducing a system of user charges to improve efficiency. In a review of patterns of paying for health services in developing countries, de Ferranti (1985) suggested that, for purposes of deciding on user charges policies that minimize inequity, health services may be categorized into (a) curative care; (b) preventive care/patient related; and (c) preventive care/

*Table 3.* IMR Internal Differentials by Country 1970-1980

In descending order of 1982 national IMR as estimated by the UN Population Division

| Country | IMR (1983) | Percentage of births in areas with an IMR more than 25% above or below the national average | | | Percentage of population areas with an IMR of | | | |
|---|---|---|---|---|---|---|---|---|
| | | More than 25% above | 25% below | Total | 150 and over | 100-149 | 50-99 | Less than 50 |
| Sierra Leone | 180 | — | — | — | 100 | 0 | 0 | 0 |
| Yemen | 135 | — | — | — | 57 | 43 | 0 | 0 |
| Benin | 120 | 25 | 26 | 51 | 25 | 49 | 26 | 0 |
| Nepal | 141 | — | — | — | 50 | 50 | 0 | 0 |
| Senegal | 140 | 21 | 17 | 38 | 21 | 50 | 29 | 0 |
| Mauritania | 135 | 20 | 15 | 35 | — | — | — | — |
| Swaziland | 130 | — | — | — | 27 | 73 | 0 | 0 |
| Bolivia | 125 | — | — | — | 45 | 55 | 0 | 0 |
| India | 110 | — | — | — | 23 | 54 | 19 | 4 |
| Ivory Coast | 110 | — | — | — | 20 | 63 | 17 | 0 |
| Sudan (North) | 120 | 0 | 13 | 13 | 0 | 0 | 100 | 0 |
| Cameroon, U. Rep. of | 100 | 5 | 14 | 19 | 0 | 58 | 42 | 0 |
| Egypt | 100 | — | — | — | 0 | 67 | 33 | 0 |
| Lesotho | 110 | — | — | — | 0 | 100 | 0 | 0 |
| Turkey | 90 | — | — | — | 41 | 59 | 0 | 0 |
| Haiti | 130 | — | — | — | 21 | 60 | 19 | 0 |
| Morocco | 95 | 12 | 0 | 12 | 0 | 43 | 57 | 0 |
| Ghana | 95 | 27 | 10 | 37 | 0 | 27 | 63 | 10 |
| Peru | 100 | — | — | — | 40 | 27 | 33 | 0 |
| Indonesia | 95 | 0 | 6 | 6 | 0 | 62 | 38 | 0 |
| Tunisia | 85 | 15 | 14 | 29 | 0 | 15 | 85 | 0 |
| Nicaragua | 75 | — | — | — | 0 | 14 | 86 | 0 |
| Kenya | 80 | 30 | 36 | 66 | 0 | 44 | 56 | 0 |
| Ecuador | 70 | — | — | — | 0 | 14 | 86 | 0 |
| El Salvador | 70 | — | — | — | 0 | 0 | 58 | 42 |
| Guatemala | 70 | — | — | — | 0 | 5 | 78 | 17 |
| Dominican Republic | 75 | — | — | — | 0 | 32 | 68 | 0 |
| Jordan | 55 | — | — | — | 0 | 0 | 100 | 0 |
| Syrian Arab Republic | 60 | 0 | 13 | 13 | 0 | 0 | 87 | 13 |
| Colombia | 50 | — | — | — | 0 | 0 | 91 | 9 |

*Table 3.    (continued)*

In descending order of 1982 national IMR as estimated by the UN Population Division

| Country | IMR (1983) | Percentage of births in areas with an IMR more than 25% above or below the national average | | | Percentage of population areas with an IMR of | | | |
|---|---|---|---|---|---|---|---|---|
| | | More than 25% above | 25% below | Total | 150 and over | 100-149 | 50-99 | Less than 50 |
| Mexico | 55 | 0 | 2 | 2 | 0 | 0 | 100 | 0 |
| Philippines | 50 | — | — | — | 0 | 0 | 90 | 10 |
| Thailand | 48 | — | — | — | 0 | 0 | 94 | 6 |
| Chile | 23 | — | — | — | 0 | 0 | 11 | 89 |
| Sri Lanka | 39 | 0 | 0 | 0 | 0 | 0 | 100 | 0 |
| Venezuela | 39 | 21 | 24 | 45 | 0 | 0 | 44 | 56 |
| Argentina | 36 | — | — | — | 0 | 0 | 6 | 94 |
| Korea, Republic of | 30 | 0 | 0 | 0 | 0 | 0 | 36 | 64 |
| Mauritius | 28 | — | — | — | 0 | 0 | 17 | 83 |
| Fiji | — | — | — | — | 0 | 0 | 42 | 58 |
| Malaysia (Peninsula) | 30 | — | — | — | 0 | 0 | 0 | 100 |
| Jamaica | 21 | 25 | 34 | 59 | 0 | 0 | 25 | 75 |
| Panama | 26 | — | — | — | 0 | 0 | 9 | 91 |
| Costa Rica | 19 | — | — | — | 0 | 0 | 0 | 100 |
| Cuba | 17 | — | — | — | 0 | 0 | 0 | 100 |

1.  *Source:*   World Fertility Surveys
2.  *Source:*   Population censuses, sample registration data and World Fertility Surveys
*Source:*   UNICEF (1985)


*Table 4.*   World Differentials and Trends in IMR

| | Range | Median | | IMR ÷ IMR | |
|---|---|---|---|---|---|
| | | IMR 1983 | IMR 1960 | 1983 | 1960 |
| Very High IMR | 101+ | 135 | 190 | .71 | |
| High IMR | 55-100 | 75 | 150 | .50 | |
| Middle IMR | 25-50 | 36 | 85 | .42 | |
| Low IMR | < 25 | 11 | 37 | .30 | |

*Source:*   UNICEF (1985)

nonpatient related. Fees for curative services should be increased. The case for introducing user charges for patient-related preventive services is not as strong and is clearly not desirable for nonpatient-related preventive care. It seems that a well designed health-family planning system could introduce equity without loss of efficiency into the health system. However, the structural problems of inadequate access to education, health, family planning and other social services, mentioned above, set limits on the generalization of such conclusion. Situations need to be examined more closely on a case-by-case basis.

*Fertility Decline and the Level of Mortality*

A more equitable distribution of social and economic resources evidently could have a positive effect on health status through its effect on intracountry differentials. Such effect could be trivial in high mortality settings, especially if the cause of such high levels is structural in nature. It is evident, from an international perspective, that the challenging policy problem is how to reduce inter-country disparity in average levels of mortality and morbidity. In 1983, 40 countries had an infant mortality rate above 100 (median = 135); 35 countries between 55-100 (median = 75); 21 countries between 25-50 (median =36); and 35 countries with low IMR rates below 25 (median = 11). Furthermore, the proportionate decline in IMR between 1960 and 1983 was much faster in the groups with the lowest levels in 1960. As indicated in Table 4, the 1983 median rate of the low IMR countries was 30 percent of the 1960 median, compared to 71 percent for the very high IMR group. A significant structural change seems to be required if such disparities are to be altered. To make present programs more efficient through the integration of family planning activities may provide a necessary but not a sufficient condition to achieve and sustain a significant reduction in overall mortality and morbidity levels in low income countries. What is required is a critical evaluation of the apparent socioeconomic limitations of current health and other social strategies.

## III.  FAMILY PLANNING AND HEALTH PROGRAMS: WHAT ARE THE LINKAGES?

What are the mechanisms through which a family planning program may influence the efficiency or effectiveness of health services? It is evident that the possible points of contact are numerous. As a starting point, we may begin with a familiar identity. Mortality behavior is part of the total social system. It cannot be altered independently. As is well known, it is related through an accounting identity to fertility, migration and income growth. For example:

$$CDR = CBR + NEMR + r(y) - r(Y) \; (\approx S/k)$$

where

r(y) = rate of per capita GNP growth,

r(Y) = rate of GNP growth ($\simeq$ S/k),

[where S = saving ratio and k = incremental

capital-output ratio]

r(P) = rate of population growth,

= CBR − CDR + net external migration rate (NEMR), and

r(y) = r(Y) − r(P) = r(Y) − CBR + CDR − NEMR

Changes in mortality must be accounted for by changes in fertility, migration or in income and poplation growth. As Figure 2 illustrates, differentials in infant mortality are associated with differentials in almost all the essential social parameters. For an elaboration, see Preston (1980).

Population policies in general and family planning programs in particular might have played an important role in this dynamic interaction between health and socioeconomic change. But the exact mechanism of this relationship is not adequately understood. And in the absence of such understanding it is difficult to provide evaluative statements about cause and effect. In the present discussion we will build upon a framework developed earlier by Mosley (1984). That framework is basically a proximate determinants approach to elucidate how the risk or morbidity and mortality is determined. That framework is based on the premises that reduction in the survival probability of newborn infants from an expected optimal level (over 97 percent) in any society is due to the operation of social, economic, biological and environmental forces, and that these socioeconomic determinants must operate through basic proximate determinants. Our purpose, however, is to identify the lines of influence between family planning and health; therefore, a more detailed account of the health system and family planning activities is needed. Figure 3 illustrates this expanded framework.

Family planning and health policies are determined by socioeconomic planning and by the socioeconomic factors at various social hierarchies. The health system is illustrated within an input-output framework. The mix of inputs depends on the types of health strategies and activities performed. Health inputs intervene at various levels: personal illnesses control either through treatment or prevention; primary health care based on the assessment of community health needs with emphasis on activities that are not necessarily physician-centered (e.g., health education, preventive activities, family health including family planning); and environmental health activities provided on a mass basis by engineers, sanitarians and others to control and improve the quality of the environment (e.g., water, food, air and housing). Finally, the health system includes important components of health information,

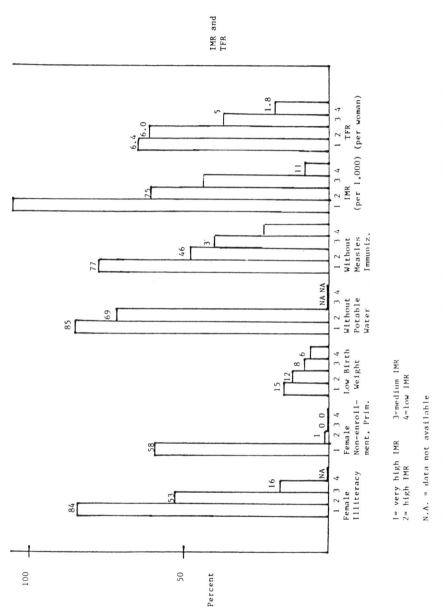

*Figure 2.* Socioeconomic Indicators Associated with Levels of Infant Mortality

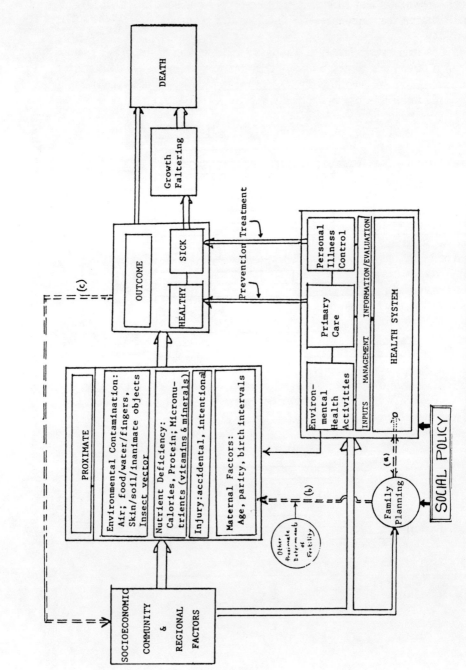

*Figure 3.* Family Planning-Health System Linkages

surveillance, research and evaluation. The outcome of the system is the health status of mothers and children. Its objective is to achieve a desired level of health status that minimizes the incidence of controllable morbidity and mortality.

In this framework, family planning activities influence the health system through three basic routes, namely programatic, sociobiological and indirect linkages. These are identified by the dashed lines a, b and c, respectively, in Figure 3, and will be examined below in turn.

## A.  Programatic Linkages

The programatic effects of family planning programs on health activities will depend on the level and degree of integration between the two systems. At the one extreme, family planning activities may have a large degree of administrative and financial autonomy. Its targets may be purely demographic, to the virtual exclusion of health objectives as illustrated, for example, by the case of Bangladesh. At the other extreme, family planning activities may be part of the health system with no identifiable demographic orientation. Its main objectives are health oriented (e.g., Chile). In the case of Chile, the high rate of unwanted pregnancies, especially in young ages, which is manifested in high abortion rates, is considered a major health risk. For example, between 1958 and 1960, abortions accounted for 8 percent of all admissions to National Service Hospitals and 27 percent of all blood transfusions, and were responsible for a sizable part of hospital care expenditures (World Bank, 1980). In 1983, the goverment of Chile did not identify a demographic policy objective. Its perception toward fertility policies was that intervention was not appropriate (U.N., Vol 2, 1985, p. 195). However, in the context of the health hazards and socioeconomic costs of the high rate of abortion, family planning is being promoted and viewed as part of a health-stabilization policy (i.e., to reduce the socioeconomic costs of unwanted children). Between these two programatic extremes (e.g., Bangladesh and Chile) lies the majority of the developing countries, some with a dual approach toward demographic and health objectives.

Is there a benefit to the health system through this programatic linkage? First, some terms need clarification and some assumptions need to be stated explicitly. Specifically we need to define conceptually and operationally the term "cost saving." Cost saving can only have an economic meaning when associated with a flow of output per unit of time. That flow of output per unit of time must be specified in terms of type and quality. In other words, the output of the health system must be operationally specified. As a cost saving device, the effect of family planning activities on the output of health should be evaluated through its impact on the input structure of the health system. For that purpose, the output of health should be clearly defined. In the case of Chile, for example, the additional family planning inputs (cost) may be evaluated in terms of the number of abortions averted. The cost saving to the health system is the difference between the cost of the family planning inputs and the cost of performing the abortion operations by the system if not averted. In this case, the situation may seem to be straightforward since there is no apparent jointness in the production process. It is not. There may be other outputs (externalities) resulting from the family planning activities. It is possible that not all women protected against abortion would have opted for abortion. Family planning activities may have the added effect of achieving a more desirable child spacing pattern between pregnancies. Adequate spacing may have the effect of improving child health and accordingly would reduce the need for health service utilization by mothers and children. It is also possible that averting an abortion through family planning services within the health system gives mothers and potential mothers more confidence in the system and increases their effective demand for better health. Each of the previous statements follows a chain of acceptable logic but needs adequate empirical quantification. How much is actually spent, how much "output" has been produced and how much cost has been saved are empirical as much as conceptual questions.

The other extreme of defining family planning objectives in terms of purely demographic objectives to the exclusion of health may not be to the best advantage of both systems. Such a conclusion is not without qualification, however. If the demographic objectives were achieved, they should have positive effects on the outcome of health. But, in most cases, family planning workers and personnel, even when separated administratively, utilize health facilities and may be drawn from the existing health manpower. If relatively low priority is given to health activities, the efficiency of the health system deteriorates. What causes even more harm is the shifting of priorities depending on funding availability, especially when dictated from outside the system and independently of the country's social objectives. There is no question that demographic objectives in Bangladesh are of the highest priority (cf. Sirageldin, 1987, and references cited therein). The issue is whether the health and demographic objectives are jointly specified in the context of a sustainable and achievable integrated socioeconomic policy, backed with political commitment.

Conceptually, programatic linkage will provide a cost-saving mechanism if there is an improvement in the efficiency or the effectiveness of the system. The following may be stated as conditions under which family planning could provide cost-saving to the health system on the programatic linkage side:

a.   health resources used by the family planning activities are underutilized;
b.   the family planning strategy is community-based and provides the infrastructure for primary health care;

c.  incentives provided for family planning workers and clients do not distort the reward system in the health manpower system;
d.  the family planning management, information, and input-output evaluation system is integrated in the health system without burdening its operational activities.

## B.  Sociobiological Linkages

Family planning activities may have a cost-saving effect through their influence on health output. This mechanism is illustrated by the (b) arrow of Figure 3. To the extent that family planning activities have an effect on fertility behavior (notice that the effect of the program is conditioned by other proximate determinants of fertility) it could influence infant, child and maternal mortalities. There is enough evidence indicating that childbearing at an early age (less than 18) or closely spaced (less than two years) increases the risk of infant mortality (e.g., John Cleland, 1983; also S. Hobcraft, 1987). Other evidence indicates an increase in maternal deaths with birth order (D. Maine, 1981) and low birth weight with insufficient birth spacing (J. Cleland, 1983). It must be emphasized, however, that the relative policy importance of this linkage will depend on the level of infant mortality, on the proportion of intervals with small duration, and on the offsetting effects of changes in other proximate determinants, e.g., lactation (for more details, see Bongaarts, 1987). Although our focus is on the consequences of family planning activities on health, it may be noted that once a significant and sustained decline in infant and child mortality has been initiated, it enhances the demand for family planning, e.g., the child survival-fertility linkage, and thus causes a reinforcing feedback mechanism between family planning activities and health.

## C.  Indirect Linkages

There are other health risks that derive from high fertility rates in developing countries. These are mainly indirect effects. They may influence health at the community level or at the family level (World Bank, 1980). However, the complexity of the underlying mechanism makes it difficult to provide clear-cut conclusions. For example, the argument that, in rural areas, population pressure leads to overcropping, soil degradation, and accordingly poor nutrition and poor health, is being debated, since population growth is only one element in a system that is probably distorted by many other elements (cf. Mosley, 1979). Accordingly, reducing fertility is not a sufficient condition to improved nutrition and health. However, the debate seems to continue.

Two decades ago, in 1968, Robin Barlow made a study of the economic effects of malaria eradication in Sri Lanka. His conclusion is that the malaria eradication campaign, although it raised per capita income in the short-run,

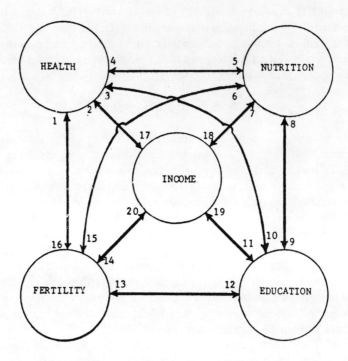

*Source:*   Barlow (1979)

*Figure 4.*   A General Model of Health and Development

lowered it in the long-run, mainly because of the net negative effects of the
accelerated rate of population growth on per capita income growth. These were
mainly indirect effects. Barlow's main policy conclusion was that it would have
been better to initiate a family planning program concurrently with the malaria
eradication program.

   Ten years later Barlow, in the first issue of the present annual on Research
in Human Capital and Development (1979), reviewed the conceptual and
empirical evidence linking health (H) to fertility (F), nutrition (N), education
(ED) and income (Y). His system is summarized in Figure 4 in terms of the
5 factors mentioned above. There are 20 direct relations linking the 5 factors.
For purpose of the present discussion, with the exception of relations (1) and
(16), the remaining relations are defined as indirect. They indicate the first-
order indirect effect of fertility on health through its effects on income (20 and
2), nutrition (6 and 4) or education (12 and 3). Although not elaborated by
Barlow, these indirect effects are conditioned by the specificity of the social
and economic system and include a complex time lag structure, especially when

second order effects are taken into account. Barlow then defined an individual or family utility function to include the five variables as endogenous in a constrained utility maximization system:

$$U = U(H, N{\bullet}H, E{\bullet}H, C{\bullet}H, L{\bullet}H).$$

The conclusions of Barlow's review seem to be valid today and worth quoting in detail:

"There is a continuing need for good empirical estimates of the twenty direct relationships in the general system. Many important diseases and populations remain unanalyzed. The analyses already conducted are for the most part of uncertain validity. Future work should aim at higher methodological standards. One might note again that a competent study of a particular disease in a particular locality does not then remove that disease from the research agenda. The same disease may have different economically relevant effects in some other locality, and also different effects in the same locality at a later time. So the empirical results from one study are not readily transferrable to another context. What should be transferrable, however, is a competent methodology. In order to allow for indirect relationships in the system, work should proceed on developing models which incorporate all five endogenous variables. Simulations with such models can then measure the net effects of whatever events are of interest, whether these be events that have already occurred, or others that are under consideration, such as the introduction of a new health care program. A model of this type will be usable in widely differing contexts, although it will normally be necessary to adopt new assumptions about parameter values when moving on to a different population.

## IV.  CONCLUDING REMARKS

The present discussion identified three types of mechanisms linking health and population policies and activities, namely, programatic, biological and indirect. The main thesis advanced is that these three mechanisms are not only dependent on the social context but are also interdependent with each other. For example, the efficiency of the service delivery system will depend on the efficiency of the indirect mechanisms such as the allocative efficiency and equity of the labor market and that of the education system. The issue is further complicated by the implied time lags in the dynamic nature of the system. Identifying some factor as key linkages, e.g., female education, may provide misleading conceptual and policy conclusions if other conditioning socioeconomic factors are not adequately specified. In the final analysis, population and health policies and programs should be specified with a constrained welfare criteria. The constraints should be indicated in terms of financial, technological and social elements. In such context it becomes possible to discuss and resolve the intra- and inter-generation allocation of the costs and benefits of population and health programs.

## ACKNOWLEDGMENT

This study is partly funded by a Population Council grant. The authors would like to thank Christina Russell and Ruth Levine for helpful research assistance.

## REFERENCES

Akin, John and Nancy Birdsall. (1987). "Financing of Health Services in LDCs," *Finance and Development* June.

Barlow, Robin. (1979a). *Malaria Eradication and Development in Ceylon,* Ann Arbor: University of Michigan Press.

Barlow, Robin. (1979b). "Health and Economic Development: A Theoretical and Empirical Review," in *Research in Human Capital and Developement,* Vol. 1, Ismail Sirageldin (ed.) Greenwich: JAI Press, Inc., pp. 45-76.

Bongaarts, J. (1987). "Will Family Planning Reduce Infant Mortality Rates." Background paper prepared for the International Conference on Better Health for Women and Children through Family Planning, October, 1987, Nairobi, Kenya, New York: The Population Council.

Caldwell, John C. (1986). "Routes to Low Mortality in Poor Countries," *Population and Developement Review* 12:2 June:171-220.

Caldwell, John C. (1981). "Maternal Education as a Factor in Child Mortality," *World Health Forum* Vol. 2, No. 1.

Cleland, John. (1983). "New WFS Findings Prove Spacing Benefits," *People* Vol. 10, No. 2.

Cornia, Giovanni, Richard Jolly, and Frances Stewart. (1987). Eds. *Adjustment with a Human Face,* Vol. I, Oxford: Clardendon Press.

de Ferranti, David. (1985). "Paying for Health Services in Developing Countries: An Overview," *World Bank Staff Working Paper No. 721,* Washington, DC: World Bank.

Jimenez, Emmanuel. (1986). "The Public Subsidization of Education and Health in Developing Countries: A Review of Equity and Efficiency," *The World Bank Research Observer* Vol. 1, No. 1, January.

Maine, Deborah. (1981). "Family Planning: Its impact on the health of women and children," *Center for Population and Family Health,* New York: Columbia University.

Mosley, W. Henry. (1983). "Will primary health care reduce infant and child mortality? A critique of some current strategies, with special reference to Africa and Asia." Paper prepared for the IUSSP seminar on Social Policy, Health Policy and Mortality Prospects, Paris.

Mosley, W. Henry and L.C. Chen. (1984). Eds. "Child Survivial: Strategies for Research," *Population and Development Review,* a Supplement to Vol. 10, New York: The Population Council.

Mosley W. Henry. (1984). "An analytical framework for the study of child survival in developing countries," in *Child Survival: Strategies for Research,* eds, W.H. Mosley and L.C. Chen, *Population and Development Review,* a Supplement to Vol. 10, New York: The Population Council.

Mosley, W.H. (1979). "Health, Nutrition, and Mortality in Bangladesh," in *Research in Human Capital and Development,* Vol. 1, Ismail Sirageldin (ed.), Greenwich: JAI Press, Inc., pp. 77-94.

Preston, Samuel H. (1980). "Causes and consequences of mortality declines in less developed countries during the twentieth century," in *Population and Economic Change in Developing Countries,* ed. Richard A. Easterlin, Chicago: University of Chicago Press, pp. 289-341.

Preston, Samuel H. (1985). "Resources, knowledge and child mortality: A comparison of the U.S. in the late nineteenth century and developing countries today," in *International Population Conference, Florence,* 1985, Vol. 4, International Union for the Scientific Study of Population, Liege: IUSSP, pp. 373-386.

Second Takemi Symposium. (1986). School of Public Health, Harvard University.

Sirageldin, I. (1986). "Demography and Policy: An Asia Experience," Paper prepared for the IUSSP Committee on the Utilization of Demographic Knowledge in Policy Formulation and Analysis, Liege: IUSSP.

United Nations. (1984). World Population Trends, Population and Development Interrelations and Population Policies: 1983 Monitoring Report, Vols. 1 & 2, New York: United Nations.

UNICEF. (1985) *The State of the World's Children 1986,* New York: Oxford University Press.

World Bank. (1980). *Health Sector Policy Paper,* Washington, D.C.: World Bank.

World Bank. (1986). *World Developement Report,* Oxford: Oxford University Press.

# FUNDAMENTALS OF THE EPIDEMIOLOGIC AND DEMOGRAPHIC TRANSITIONS

Ronald H. Gray

## THE DEMOGRAPHIC AND EPIDEMIOLOGIC TRANSITIONS

The demographic transition is the tempo and pattern of the decline of mortality and fertility that has occurred in all currently industrialized and many middle level developing countries over the past 200 years. In the majority of cases, death rates declined prior to birth rates, although there have been notable exceptions such as the experience in France where fertility reduction preceded changes in mortality. In contrast to this historic experience, most developing countries have had significant falls in death rates, particularly over the past three decades, without fully compensatory declines of birth rates. During the period of the demographic transition, the disparity between birth and death rates results in rapid population growth, and the rates of growth are largely determined by the magnitude and rapidity of the mortality declines and the

Research in Human Capital Development, Vol. 5, pages 25-42.
Copyright © 1988 by JAI Press Inc.
All rights of reproduction in any form reserved.
ISBN: 0-89232-508-9

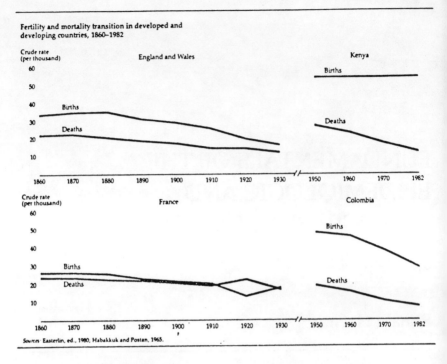

Fertility and mortality transition in developed and developing countries, 1860–1982

*Source:* World Development Report, 1984

*Figure 1.* The Demographic Transition in Developed
and Developing Countries

delay in responsiveness of the birth rates. The varying patterns of the demographic transition are illustrated in Figure 1.

The epidemiologic transition refers to the changes in disease patterns and causes of death which have accompanied mortality declines (Omran, 1982). A universal phenomenon has been the reduction of death rates from infectious and parasitic diseases and malnutrition, particularly in the most vulnerable age groups such as infants and children (Figure 2). As the communicable and nutritional diseases of childhood diminish, adult chronic degenerative and neoplastic diseases have become the major causes of death, and this pattern is frequently reinforced by lifestyle changes that increase the risk of such noncommunicable diseases (Figure 3). For example, smoking, consumption of high fat diets, sedentary lifestyles and stress have contributed to major increases in ischemic cardiovascular diseases and stroke in developed countries, and these disorders are now becoming more prominent causes of death in many developing countries (Harulinen et al., 1986). Similarly, trends in tobacco

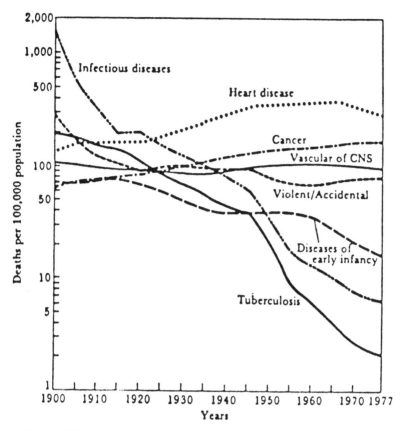

*Source:* Omran, 1980

*Figure 2.* Trends in major causes of death in the United States (1900-1977) (Semilogarithmic scale).

consumption have been responsible for the rising mortality from lung cancer, and alcohol consumption is linked to deaths from cirrhosis of the liver. There is also evidence that diets containing a high proportion of meat and dairy products and relatively little vegetable content account, in part, for the excess of cancers of the breast, uterus, and large intestine have been observed in many industrialized countries (excluding Japan). These chronic and neoplastic conditions have been termed the "diseases of affluence," as distinct from the infectious/parasitic disorders and malnutrition which are aptly described as the "diseases of poverty."

Another feature of the epidemiologic transition has been the marked declines in maternal mortality associated with improvements in obstetric care and

RONALD H. GRAY

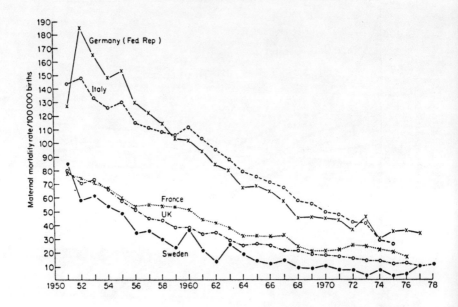

*Figure 3.* Maternal mortality for five European countries, 1951-1978.

*Table 1.* Estimated Range of Maternal Mortality

| Region | Range of Maternal Mortality Rates (deaths per 100,000 births) |
|---|---|
| Africa | 160 - 1100 |
| Asia South | 30 - 1000 |
| East | 7 - 180 |
| Europe | 6 - 129 |
| Latin America | 16 - 468 |
| North America | 7 - 15 |
| Oceania | 11 - 800 |
| World | 6 - 1100 |

*Source:* Petros-Barvazian, 1984.

changes in reproductive patterns (Russell, 1983, Figure 3). However, in less developed countries maternal mortality remains excessively high with rates frequently over 150 per 100,000 births (Table 1).

The epidemiologic transition has been accompanied by major improvements in expectation of life at birth, despite the increased mortality due to adult chronic degenerative and neoplastic diseases. Most of the improved life

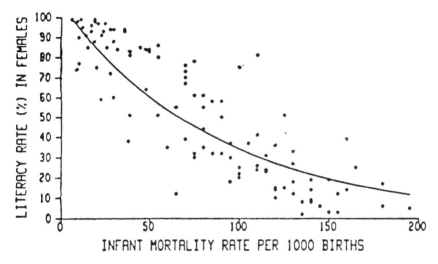

*Source:*   Foege and Henderson (1986)

*Figure 4.*   Relationship between female literacy rates and
infant mortality rates for 106 countries.

expectancy results from major reduction in infant and childhood mortality
(Figure 4). An analysis by Gwatkin (1980) suggests marked gains in life
expectancy particularly in the 1950s and 1960s, but over the most recent
decades the rate of improvement has diminished (Table 2), and in some
countries expectation of life has actually declined in the late 1970s and early
1980s. Hungary is an example of this latter disturbing trend.

    The temporal pattern of the epidemiologic transition has varied from country
to country. Omran (1982) describes three general patterns, a "classical or
Western" model, an "accelerated" transition, and a "contemporary or delayed"
model. In the classic Western model there was a gradual transition from high
to low mortality which commenced first in Western Europe, Scandinavia, and
North America during the eighteenth and nineteenth centuries. In most
countries it required more than a century for completion of the transition.
Socioeconomic development appears to be the major cause of the mortality
decline, augmented by the sanitary revolution of the late nineteenth century,
and contributions by modern preventive and therapeutic medicine in the
twentieth century. The "accelerated" transition observed in Japan, Eastern
Europe and the Soviet Union occurred later and more rapidly than the classical
transition. Improvements in mortality started during the first quarter of the
twentieth century, accompanied by socioeconomic development and the
widespread application of modern sanitary and medical advances. The third
model posited by Omran (1982), the "contemporary" or "delayed"

*Table 2.*    Levels and Rates of Increase in Life Expectancy by
Major World Regions, 1950/55-1970/75

*Life Expectancy at Birth (in years)*

| Region | 1950/55 | 1955/60 | 1960/65 | 1965/65 | 1965/70 |
|---|---|---|---|---|---|
| World | 47.4 | 50.2 | 52.7 | 54.5 | 56.2 |
| More Developed Regions | 65.2 | 68.3 | 69.8 | 70.4 | 71.2 |
| Less Developed Regions | 42.6 | 45.8 | 48.8 | 51.4 | 53.4 |
| Africa | 37.6 | 39.8 | 42.2 | 44.5 | 46.5 |
| Latin America | 52.0 | 55.0 | 57.3 | 59.4 | 61.3 |
| Asia | 43.3 | 46.9 | 50.4 | 53.4 | 56.0 |

*Average Annual Increase in Life Expectancy at Birth (in years)*

| Region | 1950/55-1955/60 | 1955/60-1960/65 | 1960/65-1965/70 | 1965/70-1970/75 |
|---|---|---|---|---|
| World | 0.56 | 0.50 | 0.36 | 0.34 |
| More Developed Regions | 0.62 | 0.30 | 0.12 | 0.16 |
| Less Developed Regions | 0.64 | 0.60 | 0.52 | 0.40 |
| Africa | 0.44 | 0.48 | 0.46 | 0.40 |
| Latin America | 0.60 | 0.46 | 0.42 | 0.38 |
| Asia | 0.70 | 0.70 | 0.60 | 0.52 |

*Source:*    Gwatkin (1980).

*Table 3.*    Infant Mortality Rates for 130 Countries

| Infant Mortality | No. of Countries in | |
|---|---|---|
| | 1960 | 1983 |
| > 200 | 14 | 0 |
| 150-199 | 45 | 11 |
| 100-149 | 25 | 33 |
| 50-99 | 22 | 32 |
| 25-49 | 16 | 19 |
| < 25 | 8 | 35 |

*Note:*    Date for number of deaths under one year of age per 1,000 live births
are from UNICEF (1986).

epidemiologic transition describes the situation in most developing countries.
Although there were some declines in death rates before World War II, most
gains have occurred since 1945, and appear to be closely associated with
complex socioeconomic and political factors as well as advances in public
health, medical technology and new strategies for the delivery of health care.
In 1960, 59 developing countries had an infant mortality rate in excess of 150

per 1,000, whereas in 1983 only 11 countries still experienced such high mortality (Table 3). There have been remarkable improvements in East Asian countries such as China, Taiwan, South Korea, Hong Kong and Singapore, in small island nations such as Sri Lanka, Mauritius, Cuba and Jamaica, as well as Latin American countries such as Costa Rica. However, mortality remains high in most of South Asia and Sub-Subharan Africa, and in the poorer countries of Latin America or the Middle East.

The remainder of this chapter will focus on the factors responsible for the "contemporary" transition in the less developed world, and the implications for future strategies in health and development.

## CAUSES OF DEATH AND DECLINES IN MORTALITY

Numerous studies have explored the factors responsible for mortality declines in both industrialized and nonindustrialized countries, but there is continuing controversy particularly with regard to the mortality impact of specific medical interventions. The confusion in literature arises in part from inadequacy of data or study designs, conceptual problems with the notion of "cause" of death, the complexity of socioeconomic and biomedical factors influencing health, and difficulties in quantifying the activities of health programs.

Data constraints present major problems in most developing countries where national or regional statistics on mortality and morbidity are often deficient and the quality or completeness of data varies over time. Problems arise with the enumeration of events due to inadequate vital registration and with the enumeration of the population at risk due to inadequate or infrequent censuses, or inaccuracy of reporting. Although special demographic methods have been developed to estimate mortality levels by indirect techniques using survey data, these methods are often unsatisfactory for the measurement of changes in mortality over time (UN, 1983). Furthermore, even if total mortality can be estimated, statistics on cause of death are deficient because the majority of deaths are not registered by medically qualified personnel and diagnoses are frequently inaccurate. A high proportion of deaths are ascribed to unknown or nonspecific causes, and even when a specific underlying cause is recorded, no information is available on the varying constellation of diseases that contribute to death. This is particularly a problem with children in whom death is often the end product of a cumulative series of infectious or parasitic illnesses and malnutrition, rather than the result of a single disease.

Studies of mortality decline largely employ observational or quasi-experimental designs. Social scientists have conducted many cross-sectional investigations which search for correlations between socioeconomic or health service characteristics and levels of mortality, often employing aggregate data. For example, numerous investigators have shown a correlation between

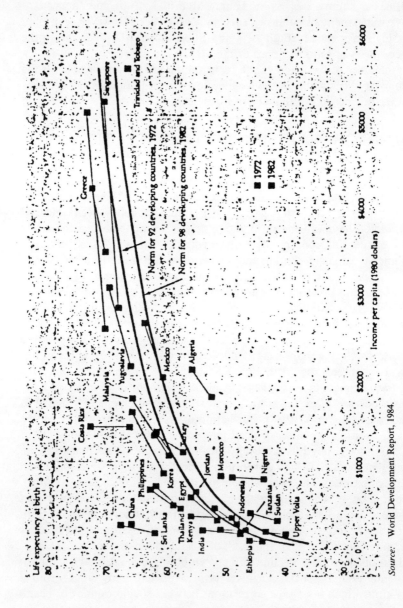

*Source:* World Development Report, 1984.

*Figure 5.* Life expectancy in relation to income in developing countries, 1972 and 1982.

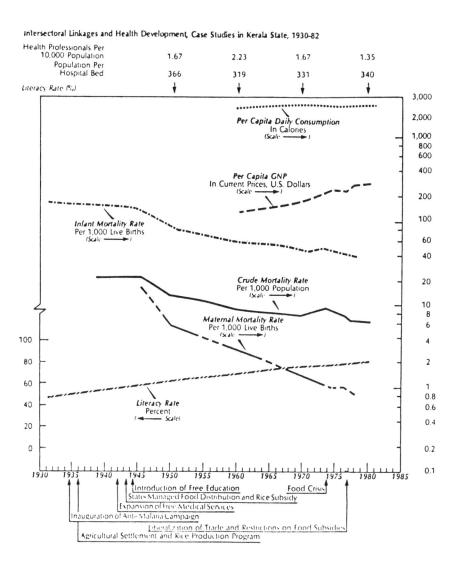

Intersectoral Linkages and Health Development, Case Studies in Kerala State, 1930-82

| Health Professionals Per 10,000 Population | 1.67 | 2.23 | 1.67 | 1.35 |
| Population Per Hospital Bed | 366 | 319 | 331 | 340 |

*Source:* Guatilleke, 1985

*Figure 6.*    Mortality trends in relation to changes in socioeconomic indicators. Kerala State, India 1930-82.

socioeconomic factors such as maternal education, national or household income or availability of health services, and levels of infant or child mortality using cross-sectional approaches (Figure 5). The problem with these studies is that causality cannot be inferred from correlation, and there is inadequate information on the proximate mechanisms through which socioeconomic factors modify mortality risk. A temporal sequence of cross-sectional studies can, however, reveal changing relationships over time. For example, Preston and others have shown that the relationship between income and life expectancy has shifted, and low levels of national income are now associated with substantially higher life expectancy as compared to previous time periods (Figure 6). Many countries have today achieved remarkably low levels of mortality despite continuing poverty. Another research approach has been to monitor both mortality and various socioeconomic or health changes in countries or regions over time. Such ecological studies have shown associations between mortality decline and progress in education, economic development or health expenditure (Figure 7 and 8), although the temporal relationships are not always clear cut, and multivariate analyses may yield only modest results in terms of explained variance (Rosero-Bixby, 1985). One problem with this approach is that many changes can occur simultaneously and it is difficult to disaggregate the contributions of specific factors, or of broad based programs such as education. A recent conference reviewed the experience of four countries which had achieved low mortality at relatively low levels of economic development as measured by GDP per capita (Halstead, Walsh and Warren, 1985). The countries were China, Kerala State in India, Sri Lanka and Costa Rica. These divergent countries shared some common characteristics; each had governments ideological committed to health and to equity in availability of services, and each devoted major economic and human resources to health. The four countries implemented a variety of special health programs such as nutritional supplementation, immunization, control of communicable diseases and family planning, and all provided comprehensive primary health care. Also, there was a long-standing investment in education with high levels of literacy for both sexes (Kunstadter, 1985)

Biomedical researchers have frequently employed prospective studies using experimental or quasi-expermental designs to evaluate the mortality or morbidity impact of specific health interventions (e.g., immunization) or integrated health programs. Emphasis has been placed on detailed studies of biological risk factors for specific diseases and socioeconomic factors have often been treated as confounding variables rather than major determinants of risk (Mosley and Chen, 1984). Despite considerable effort, unequivocal evidence of mortality reduction in response to health interventions has been difficult to obtain. Logistic constraints and costs limit such prospective investigations to relatively small populations in which it is difficult to convincingly measure declines in mortality. Unexpected crises or secular trends

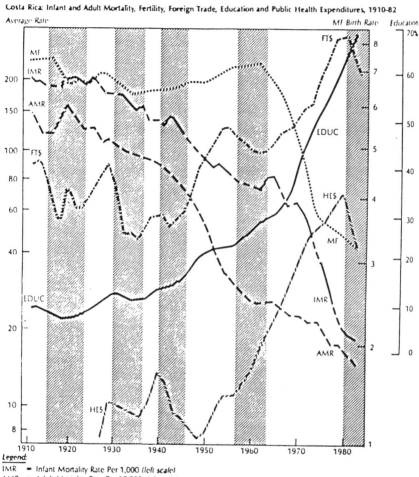

Costa Rica: Infant and Adult Mortality, Fertility, Foreign Trade, Education and Public Health Expenditures, 1910-82

Source: Rosero-Bixby, (1985)

*Figure 7.* Mortality trends in relation to changes in socioeconomic indicators, Costa Rica, 1910-82.

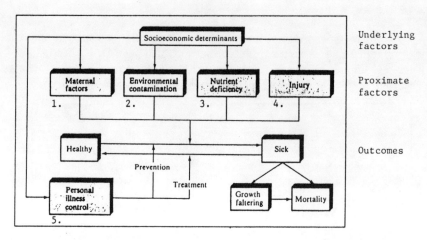

*Proximate determinants are number 1-5.

*Source:* Mosley and Chen, 1984

*Figure 8.*    Conceptual framework for studies of child survival.

due to factors beyond the investigators' control have also complicated findings. Moreover, the provision of health services is often a sequential process, and it is difficult to determine when an intervention program truly begins, matures and achieves optimal coverage (Chen et al., 1981). In order to link services to mortality change it is necessary to carefully monitor service coverage, utilization and efficacy over time, and to collect reliable data on disease rates and cause of death. There are only a few selected studies with such detailed information and these have mainly been conducted in special population surveillance areas such as Matlab in Bangladesh, Narangwal in Punjab, the Gambia, Kenya and Guatemala (Chen et al., 1981; Taylor and Faruqee, 1983; McGregor et al., 1970; Van Ginneken and Muller, 1984; Delgrado et al., 1986). However, due to extensive health inputs and the logistical infrastructure needed for detailed surveillance, these special populations may be atypical of the country as a whole, and this constrains the generalization of research findings.

   Mosley and Chen (1984) have suggested a framework for the study of determinants of child survival which attempts a synthesis of the social science and biomedical research approaches. This is summarized in the model shown in Figure 9. Socioeconomic factors are considered to be underlying determinants of child survival which operate through a series of proximate determinants to influence the risk of illness and subsequent death. The socioeconomic determinants may be individual level variables such as parental education, traditions/norms, etc.; household level variables such as income or wealth; and community level variables (e.g., the political economy, the environment or the health system). There are five proximate determinants. First, there are maternal factors such as reproductive patterns (age, parity, birth interval), and child care arrangements. Second, there are environmental risk factors or sources of exposure such as water supplies and sanitation; food preparation/storage, breastfeeding, supplementation and weaning; housing conditions (including overcrowding and construction materials); personal hygiene (use of soap, etc.). Third, nutritional risk factors comprise food availablity, types of foodstuffs and their relative contributions to the diet; food distribution in the family with particular emphasis on inequalities by sex, age, or bodysize. Breastfeeding, supplementation and weaning are clearly important nutritional risk factors as well as measures of exposure to environmental hazards for infants and children, and in this regard the age of the child at supplementation or weaning is of critical importance (Jason et al., 1984; Seward and Serdula, 1984). Fourth, risk factors for injury are patterns of maternal or surrogate child care, number of children under care, hazards such as cooking facilities (open fires) or unprotected water (e.g., canals or tanks), motor vehicles, domestic and other animals. Fifth, personal illness control includes preventive measures such as vaccination, contraceptive use, antenatal care, or malaria prophylaxis, as well as curative measures such as cultural practices in response to illness (e.g. traditional remedies, withholding of food), self-medication using modern technologies (e.g., use of oral rehydration therapy, malaria therapy), and care-seeking behavior (e.g., use of traditional practitioners or modern medical services). With regard to utilization of health services, it is necessary to consider knowledge, acceptability and availability of services per se, and accessibility in terms of distance or cost (Scrimshaw and Hurtado, 1984). Unfortunately, the less educated and poorer individuals in greatest need frequently underutilize available services, and it may be important to focus programs on these high risk groups.

Death, the dependent variable of this theoretical model, is seen not as an isolated event, but as the end result of a continuum of acute and chronic illnesses which cause growth faltering by undermining the child's nutritional status (Mosley and Chen, 1984). There is ample evidence that poor nutrition is associated with more severe and protracted illness, and an increased likelihood of child death, largely as a consequence of impaired immunity. Conversely, numerous studies have shown that infectious diseases erode children's nutritional reserves by the direct metabolic effects of infection, by reduced nutrient intake due to anorexia, vomiting and diarrhea, and by cultural practices such as the withholding of food or interruption of breastfeeding (Martorell and Ho, 1984). This interaction between infection and malnutrition is of fundamental importance to child health and survival in developing countries; only if the cycle is broken can one anticipate substantial declines in mortality or improvements in health. However, the situation is complex and it may be difficult to determine the optimal strategies for health interventions or to predict the potential impact of such interventions.

Measles provides an example of the problems of measuring health impact. Measles is a major cause of death with case fatality rates as high as 27 percent within 1 month of the illness. However, there is an excess delayed mortality for up to 9 months after the acute disease, and it is estimated that 1-5 percent of children born in the developing world die of acute measles or its delayed effects (Hull et al., 1983; Foster, 1984). Mortality from measles is highest for severely malnourished children and for infants under one year of age, it is also increased if other medical complications such as diarrhea or pneumonia are present (Foster, 1984). Finally, measles mortality is much higher among children living in more crowded households with several infected children, probably as a result of the higher infectious doses of the virus received under these circumstances (Aaby, 1984). Measles vaccine can be very efficacious if given around nine months of age, and several studies have shown declines in measles mortality as a result of immunization campaigns. However, the Kasongo study in Zaire found that although vaccinated children had better short-term (7-21 months) survival rates compared to unvaccinated groups, by three years of age there was no difference in net survival (Kasongo Project Team, 1981). This suggests that there is "replacement" mortality whereby children protected from measles are still subject to the competing risks of other causes of death.

Thus, an immunization campaign may be very effective in preventing short-term and delayed measles mortality, particularly if it covers high risk individuals such as infants, the undernourished, and the lower socioeconomic groups. However, in the absence of other health inputs, the net gain in survival may be minimal. Another example of a single disease-specific intervention is neonatal tetanus which is a major cause of death that can be prevented by maternal immunization, but which may not effect overall survival beyond the neonatal period (Stanfield and Galazka, 1984).

The problems of health impact evaluation are further compounded with the treatment of recurrent diseases such as diarrhea or acute respiratory infections in which the therapy may prevent death during one episode of illness but may not affect overall mortality unless used consistently for all or at least the majority of episodes. Moreover, curative care alone will not prevent the debilitating effects of recurrent illness on nutritional status or modify the circumstances that first led to illness (e.g., poor home environment), and it is possible that curative care alone can result in survivors with impaired resistance to subsequent disease (Mosley, 1986). The mortality impact of therapeutic programs has not been outstanding; for example, follow-up of children with diarrhea discharged from hospital in Bangladesh showed a 30 percent higher than expected mortality compared to nonhospitalized groups. This argues the case for integration of curative and preventive measures, and there is a growing body of evidence to suggest that environmental sanitation, improved water supplies and better personal hygiene, which reduce diarrhea incidence may have more substantial effects than a program that merely focuses on oral rehydration therapy (ORT) for each diarrhea episode (Feachem et al., 1983; Esrey et al., 1985; Esrey and Habicht, 1986).

Broad based indirect health inputs such as family planning can also be beneficial, particularly if targeted on high risk groups. For instance, substantial reductions of infant, child, and maternal mortality can potentially be achieved by reducing or eliminating closely spaced births under two years apart, confining reproduction to low risk age groups (20-34), and avoiding high order births (Trussel and Pebley, 1984).

In summary, the impact of isolated health interventions targeted at specific diseases is questionable, and there is a need to examine broader strategies for the improvement of child survival.

## STRATEGIES FOR CHILD SURVIVAL PROGRAMS

It is generally recognized that good health is an important societal goal in its own right, and that a healthy population is beneficial to socioeconomic development. This has led WHO to propose the goal of "health for all by the year 2000" as a major commitment, with an emphasis on broad based comprehensive primary health care as the means of achieving this goal. However, given the economic problems facing developing countries, and the limited resources available for, or allocated to, health, it is clear that there is a need to establish priorities since governments cannot simultaneously implement all components of primary health care programs, and the allocation of resources to one sector implies the scarcity of resources in another. One approach to establishing priorities has been to estimate morbidity and mortality from specific diseases, linked to a consideration of the technical possibilities for prevention or treatment and the related requirements in terms of skills, manpower, logistics, and costs (Walsh and Warren, 1980). This approach has led to an emphasis on disease-specific technologies such as immunization, oral rehydration therapy, nutritional monitoring, vitamin A supplementation, etc., but as previously argued, the evidence for the impact of these isolated interventions is limited, and assumptions about the number of deaths prevented by specific measures may be unwarranted. For example, WHO has estimated that 10 million preventable infant and child deaths occur annually, but this does not take into account the effects of competing risk or replacement mortality (Mosley, 1986).

There is no single strategy applicable to all countries, nor are there any prescriptions which can be guaranteed to work. Nevertheless a number of general principles appear to be valid. First, preventive measures such as immunization which reduce both morbidity and mortality warrant high priority, and ideally these should be combined with other measures such as improved nutrition which increase resistance to disease. Prevention of exposure to disease such as diarrhea through water or sanitation improvement are likely to be of considerable benefit, but because these are capital intensive and long-term, therapy with ORT provides a cost-effective interim alternative. Nondisease-specific interventions such as family planning or basic primary health care are also beneficial by improving health status and preventing debility (Foege and Henderson, 1986; Mosley, 1986). However, the social dimension cannot be ignored. High risk groups in particular need of services must be identified to ensure adequate coverage. Although education is beyond the control of the health sector, the strong and consistent link between maternal education and child survival argues the need for education as an integral part of health promotion. In particular, emphasis should be given to self-reliant behavior so that women have a greater sense of control over the health of their children (Mosley, 1986).

# REFERENCES

Aaby, P. (1984). Overcrowding and intensive exposure as determinants of measles mortality, *American Journal of Epidemiology*, 120:49.

Chen, L.C., Chakraborty, J., Sardar, A.M., and Yurus, M.D. (1981). Estimating and partitioning the mortality impact of several modern medical technologies in Basic Health Services. International Union for the Scientific Study of Population. International conference, Manila:2:113-139.

Delgrado, H.L., Valverde, V., and Hurtado, E. (1986). Effects of health and nutrition interventions on child mortality in rural Guatemala. In Determinants of Mortality Change and Differentials in Developing Countries. The Five-Country Case Study Project. United Nations. New York:145-170.

Esrey, S.A., Feachem, R.G., and Hughs, J.M. (1985). Interventions for the control of diarrheal diseases among young children: Improving water supply and excreta disposal facilities. *Bulletin of the World Health Organization*, Vol. 63(4):757-772.

Esrey, S.A., and Habicht, J.P. (1986). Epidemologic evidence for health benefits from improved water and sanitation in developing countries. *Epidemiologic Reviews*, 8:117-128.

Feachem, R.G., Hogan, R.C., and Merson, M.H. (1983). Diarrheal disease control: Reviews of potential interventions, *Bulletin of the World Health Organization*, 61:637-640.

Foege, W.H., and Henderson, D.A. (1986). Selective primary Health Care XXV. Management priorities. *Review of Infectious Diseases*, 8:467-475.

Foster, S.O. (1984). Immunizable and respiratory diseases and child mortality. In Mosley, W.H., and Chen, L.C., (eds.), Child Survival, Strategies for Research, *Population Development Review*, Vol. 10, Supplement, pp. 119-140.

Guatilleke, G. (1985). Health and development in Sri Lanka: An overview. In S.B. Halstead et al. (eds.), Good Health at Low Cost, Rockefeller Foundation, New York:111-124.

Gwatkin, D. (1980). Indications of change in developing country mortality trends. The end of an era? *Population Development Review*, 6:615-644.

Halstead, S.B., Walsh, J., and Warren, R. (1985). Good Health at Low Cost. Conference report. Rockefeller Foundation, New York.

Harulinen, T., Hansluwka, H., Lopez, A., and Nakada, T. (1986). Global and regional mortality patterns by cause of death in 1980. *International Journal of Epidemiology,* 15:227-233.

Hull, H.F., Pap, J.W., and Oldfield, F. (1983). Measles mortality and vaccine efficacy in rural West Africa. *Lancet* i:972-975.

Jason, J.M., Nieburg, P., and Marks, J.S. (1984). Mortality and infectious disease associated with infant-feeding practices in developing countries. *Pediatrics* supplement. Task Force on Infant-Feeding Practices, pp. 702-726.

Kasongo Project Team. (1981). Influence of measles vaccination on survival pattern of 7-35 month-old children in Kasongo, Zaire, *Lancet* i:764-767.

Kunstadter, P.L. (1985). Remarks. In S.B. Halstead et al. (eds.), Good Health at Low Cost, Rockefeller Foundation New York, pp. 223-238. MacMillan Publishing Co., New York. Vol. I pp. 172-183.

Martorell, R., and Ho, T.J. (1984). Malnutrition, morbidity and mortality. In Mosley, W.H., and Chen, L.C., (eds.), Child Survival, Strategies for Research, *Population Development Review,* Vol. 10, Supplement.

Mcgregor, A., Rahman, A.K., Thompson, A.M., Billewicz, W.Z., and Thompso,n B. (1970). The health of young children in a West African Gambian village. Transactions of the Royal Society of Tropical Medicine, 64:48-77.

Mosley, W.H. (1986). The demographic impact of child survival programs: implication for policy and program strategy. Unpublished paper presented at the international symposium on "New Avenues in Health Care Organzation." Center for Public Health Research, Ministry of Health, Mexico.

Mosley, W.H., and Chen, L.C. (1984). An analytical framework for the study of child survival in developing countries. In Mosley, W.H., and Chen, L.C., (eds.), Child Survival, Strategies for Research, *Population Development Review,* Vol. 10, Supplement, pp. 25-45

Omran, A.R. (1982). Epidemiologic Transition in the International Encyclopedia of Population, edited by J. Ross. the Free Press, MacMillan Publishing Co., New York. Vol. I, pp. 172-183.

Petros-Barvazian, A. (1984). World priorities and child health for the year 2000. *International Journal of Obstetrics,* 22:439-448.

Rosero-Bixby, L. (1985). Infant Mortality Decline in Costa Rica. In S.B. Halstead et al. (eds.), Good Health at Low Cost, Rockefeller Foundation, New York:125-138.

Russell, J.K. (1983). Maternal mortality. In S.L. Barron and A.M. Thomson (eds.), Obstetrical Epidemiology, London:399-416.

Scrimshaw, S.C.M, and Hurtado, E. (1984). Field guide for the study of health-seeking behavior at the household level. *Food and Nutrition Bulletin,* 6:27-45.

Seward, J., and Serdula, M.K. (1984). Infant feeding and growth. *Pediatrics* supplement. Task Force on Infant-Feeding Practices, pp. 728-762.

Sommer, A., Tarwotjo, I., Hussani, G., and Susanto, D. (1983). Increased mortality in children with mild vitamin A deficiency, *Lancet* ii:585-588.

Stanfield, J.P., and Galazka, A. (1984). Neonatal tetanus in the world today. *Bulletin of the World Health Organization,* 62:647-669.

Taylor, C.E., and Faruqee, R. (1983). Child and Maternal Service in Rural India. A World Bank Research Publication. The Johns Hopkins University Press, Baltimore, MD. Vol 1.

Trussel, J., and Pebley, A.R. (1984). The potential impact of changes in fertility and on infant child mortality. *Studies in Family Planning,* 15:267-280.

UNICEF. (1986). The State of the World's Children 1986. UNICEF, New York.

United Nations. (1983). Manual X, Indirect Techniques for Demographic Estimation. Department of International Economic and Social Affairs. Population studies No. 81. United Nations, New York.

Van Ginneken, J.K., and Muller, A.S., (eds.). (1984). Maternal and Child Health in Rural Kenya, An Epidemiological Study, Croom Helm, London and Sydney.

Walsh, J.A., and Warren, K.S. (1980). Selective primary health care: An interim strategy for disease control in developing countries. *Soc Sci and Med,* 14c:145-163.

World Development Report. (1984). New York. Oxford University Press. Published for the World Bank.

# DISEASE CONTROL AND MORTALITY REDUCTION

Joan L. Aron

## I. INTRODUCTION

In developing countries, only a few diseases may be responsible for a sizable mortality burden. Hence, selective disease control can be useful in an overall public health program to reduce mortality. An inexpensive means of prevention or treatment for a major disease may be a cost-effective way of utilizing scarce health resources.

This paper examines three candidate diseases for special emphasis in public health programs—measles, malaria and acquired immunodeficiency syndrome (AIDS). Currently available information strongly suggests that all three diseases have a great population impact, even though precise quantification of the effect is difficult. Measles is found worldwide and its lethal impact on young children in poor health has been documented. Malaria is widespread but varies regionally within countries because of its ecological dependence on the breeding of vector mosquitoes. In high-risk areas, it can add to the burden of mortality, particularly in children. The public perception of malaria risk

Research in Human Capital Development, Vol. 5, pages 43-56.
Copyright © 1988 by JAI Press Inc.
All rights of reproduction in any form reserved.
ISBN: 0-89232-508-9

may be even higher in areas where malaria has the capacity to recur in epidemic form affecting all ages. AIDS, a new disease, has not yet made the impact of measles and malaria. However, its invariably fatal course thus far and its rising incidence worldwide are sufficient cause for action.

## II.   THREE CASE STUDIES

### A.   Measles

Measles is an important cause of death in young children in developing countries. For example, in Matlab, Bangladesh from 1975 to 1977, the measles mortality rate among children ages 1 to 4 years was 4.46/1000, 16 percent of a total mortality rate of 28.43/1000. In the same population, infant measles deaths occurred at a substantial rate of 3.06/1000, although these deaths were only a small percentage of a total infant mortality rate of 129/1000 (D'Souza, 1986, p. 130). This represents a major mortality burden due to a single viral infection.

Measles is an excellent candidate for prevention by immunization. In the absence of a vaccination program, every child is at risk of measles infection. No strain variation has been observed in the measles virus so that a vaccine may be used worldwide (Black, 1982, p. 400). Currently, in developing countries, the World Health Organization Expanded Programme on Immunization (EPI) recommends that a single injection of a live, attenuated measles vaccine be provided at the age of 9 months. It is estimated that between 1981 and 1985, 32 percent of all children in developing countries were vaccinated against measles by the end of the first year of life (Population Information Program, 1986a, p. L-156).

However, precise estimation of the demographic effect of measles immunization is difficult. Mortality from measles often occurs as a result of secondary complications of pneumonia or diarrhea. Evidence that measles alone very rarely causes death is provided by the virtual disappearance of measles deaths in developed countries decades before vaccination became available to prevent infection (Anderson, 1982, p.3) (Vaccination was introduced primarily to prevent measles encephalitis.) Malnutrition and overcrowding appear to increase the case-fatality of measles. This line of argument would suggest that the impact of vaccination without modification of other factors might be minimal.

On the other hand, it is well known that measles itself can weaken a child. Thus, beneficial effects of measles prevention could actually be amplified and extend months or years beyond exposure to measles itself. A study of 6-12 month-old infants in Haiti shows that those who had had measles subsequently had indicators of poorer nutritional status (Halsey et al., 1985). Older studies from Britain indicate that measles may give rise to chronic pulmonary infection and collapse and possibly to permanent lung damage (Mercer, 1986, p. 137). Follow-up of a cohort of babies in Burkina Faso shows that a history of measles in the past four months is associated with elevated levels of measles as well as non-measles mortality in the following four months (Van de Walle, 1985).

The Kasongo Project in Zaire attempted to quantify the net demographic effect of measles immunization with a randomized trial (Kasongo Project, 1981). The data suggest that there is definitely an early improvement in survival of the vaccinated children. Whether or not the survival advantage persists is open to question. The authors of the study stress that the cumulative mortality difference at the age of 35 months is less than the difference observed at the age of 21 months. They conclude that the demographic benefits of measles immunization is low. Aaby et al. (1981) criticize this interpretation on the grounds that mortality between the ages of 21 and 35 months is so low in all groups that they cannot nullify the strong effects seen between the ages of 7 and 21 months. They also point out that the benefit of immunization may be even greater than reported because some deaths in the vaccinated group may have been measles deaths among vaccination failures.

From a statistical point of view, deaths are rare events subject to random fluctuation. The statistical problem in assessing mortality is illustrated by assuming that 30 percent (a generous estimate) of deaths are due to measles and that measles is eliminated with a vaccination program. If one observed 37 deaths among 1,000 unvaccinated children in a year, then vaccination in a comparable cohort would prevent around 11 deaths. The Z-statistic (Cox and Lewis, 1966) would equal $(37-26)/\sqrt{(37 + 26)}$ or 1.39 which has a marginally significant p-value of .08 in a one-tailed test. Nowadays this level of mortality among young children is considered extremely high (Cantrelle et al., 1986). If the mortality rate were only 16 deaths among 1,000 unvaccinated children, the difference of 5 deaths would be statistically insignificant. This lower level of mortality is characteristic of Coast Province in Kenya and is still considered moderately high (Ewbank et al., 1986). The statistical problem is coupled with an ethical one. Once vaccination has been shown to be beneficial, it is unethical to conduct large-scale randomized trials to clarify the degree of benefit.

Observational studies, while uncontrolled, can contribute important information on immunization programs. Fortunately, the individual benefit of measles immunization is amplified at the community level by an overall reduction of disease transmission which delays exposure to infection among the unvaccinated. Since case-fatality rates in young children decline with age, a rise in the typical age at infection will reduce measles mortality. A delay in infection will also widen the interval of opportunity for vaccination for many children. Vaccination must occur late enough to avoid interference by maternal antibodies but early enough to precede infection.

It is tempting to project further that a measles immunization program can eradicate measles. At initial glance, measles appears to be similar to smallpox. They are both caused by viruses which infect only humans and are spread person-to-person. Neither virus displays antigenic variation which would limit the applicablity of a vaccine. Surveillance is feasible because cases are easily identified. However, even the United States has not succeeded in eradicating measles and case reports have actually risen in the last two years (CDC, 1986a). A closer examination reveals that smallpox had some clear biological advantages for eradication. Transmission from smallpox cases could be eliminated because cases could be identified during the contagious period and the disease spread relatively slowly. Moreover, the vaccine was easy to transport, store, and administer (Population Information Program, 1986a). The greater contagiousness of measles means that the age distribution of measles cases is much younger than that of smallpox cases. It is difficult to reach the targeted population. The age of nine months is particularly awkward because a child is too big to be carried easily but too young to walk. (New formulations which may be administered earlier are being tested). Health personnel are also reluctant to administer a vaccine to an already sick child even if vaccination is safe and effective. This could be especially important if the child is going into a hospital ward which may contain other children with measles.

Realistic cost estimates of measles immunization should anticipate an ongoing program for the foreseeable future. Demand will grow with projected rises in world population. Using Africa as an illustration, a total of 37 million births is likely in the year 2000, as compared with an estimated 22 million births in 1980 (United Nations, 1985, pp. 13,19). International organizations may provide vaccination supplies and cold chain equipment but the bulk of the cost (health personnel, operating costs, capital costs) must be provided locally (Henderson, 1984). Training is essential because vaccines may lose their potency if handled improperly. However, the infrastructure required is similar for all vaccines of the World Health Organization's Expanded Program on Immunization (Population Information Program, 1986a). Cost-effectiveness of measles vaccination may be improved if the EPI structure is fully utilized.

An overall evaluation of measles immunization must consider a number of interactions with other health programs and other diseases. Although measles is universal, the complications and mortality depend on local epidemiological patterns. In one community, interaction between measles and diarrhea may be more important while, in another community, concurrent respiratory infections may pose the bigger problem. Improvements in nutrition and housing may contribute independently to mortality reduction. Even the age at which maternal antibodies are lost may rise. Loss of maternal antibodies occurs a few months earlier in developing countries as compared with developed countries. This phenomenon is not well understood, although nutritional status of the mother may play a role (Black et al., 1986). Measles immunization should be offered as a component of a larger health program. The impact of immunization is greatest when acting synergistically with other improvements in public health.

## B. Malaria

The World Health Organization estimates that the annual number of new clinical cases of malaria is roughly 92 million (WHO, 1986c, p. 9). The impact of malaria on mortality is difficult to assess, but it is clear that malaria can be a major contributor to mortality in certain areas. For example, in Saint-Louis, Senegal during the years from 1973 to 1980, malaria was responsible for 5.2 percent of mortality in children aged from 5 to 14 years (Cantrelle et al., 1986, p. 97).

Malaria control measures may be directed against the mosquito vector or the malaria parasite (Bruce-Chwatt, 1985, p. 265). Vector control may include environmental modification to reduce vector breeding habitats and the use of insecticides to reduce the density and longevity of the vector population. Individual protection, such as mosquito repellents and bednets, can also lessen the risk of infection via biting mosquitoes. Antimalarial drugs may be used in treatment of acute cases or in prophylaxis and suppression of malaria infection. At present, there are no vaccines to prevent malaria, although research has progressed to the point of clinical trials in humans for safety and immunogenicity.

Despite the variety of modes of control, the selection of an appropriate malaria control program is limited by the twin concerns of rising costs and decreasing effectiveness. The classic example is the use of the chlorinated hydrocarbon DDT to kill biting mosquitoes. It became widely used in malaria control programs after World War II because it is highly toxic to insects and is chemically stable. On nonabsorbent surfaces, it may remain active for up to a year. In many countries, the use of DDT contributed to the eradication of malaria. Once malaria is eradicated, mosquito control need not be continued, although careful surveillance for imported cases is necessary. However, where malaria was not eradicated, the continued use of DDT (for public health and agricultural purposes) eventually selected for mosquitoes resistant to DDT. Resistance may be physiological in that high doses of DDT are tolerated, or behavioral in that high doses of DDT are avoided. (If mosquitoes do not rest where the insecticide is applied, it has no effect.) Resistance to DDT may extend to HCH and dieldrin, other chlorinated hydrocarbons which are used as insecticides. Some substitutes may be biologically effective but economically infeasible. For example, malathion (an organophosphate) application is about five times as expensive as that of DDT. Moreover, applications of insecticide require specially trained teams and separate guidelines for each insecticide. The biological problem of resistance has combined with the financial problem of maintaining malaria-spraying operations to reduce spraying in many areas.

At the same time, drug-resistance of the parasite has emerged. Although the term is general, it more commonly refers to the resistance of a particular species of malaria, *Plasmodium falciparum,* to a particular drug, chloroquine, which has been used as a chemoprophylactic and as a mode of treatment. This drug-parasite interaction is especially important because *P. falciparum,* the most common species of malaria in many tropical countries, is the primary cause of malaria deaths. Treatment of malaria with chloroquine is the mainstay of malaria control in primary health care programs, particularly where spraying has been discontinued. Alternative drug regimens are more lengthy and expensive (WHO, 1986c, p. 27). At present, resistance fortunately appears to be a matter of degree in that chloroquine may still help to suppress parasites. In a recent cluster of *P. falciparum* cases among U.S. travelers to Kenya, symptoms did not appear until 1-6 days after the last dose of chloroquine (CDC, 1986b). Some partially resistant strains of malaria may still be treated with increased dosages of chloroquine. Drug resistance continues to spread and evolve. The ultimate consequences for malaria are not known.

The declining effectiveness of the most economical and effective of the current methods of malaria control has spurred great progress in the development of a malaria vaccine. Components of the malaria parasite that elicit immunity when injected have been synthesized using modern methods in biotechnology. Nevertheless, much work remains before a vaccine (or set of vaccines) may be used in a public health program (Schindler, 1985). One puzzle is the nature of naturally-acquired immunity to malaria. In areas of intense exposure, people eventually acquire partial immunity which delays or limits but does not prevent infection. Even this partial immunity appears to require boosting by continued re-exposure. Vaccine-induced immunity (produced by one or two doses) must be better than naturally-acquired immunity produced by repeated exposure.

Pre-existing levels of immunity may also affect the strategy of vaccination in malarious areas. In nonimmunes, absolute protection against sporozoites (the stage of parasite injected by the mosquito vector) may be most desirable. Protection of even limited duration could be useful for temporary laborers, tourists or soldiers. For residents of endemic areas, some protection against the cycle of red blood cell invasion (the phase associated with clinical illness) might be more useful. In this circumstance, the duration of effectiveness might be more important than the degree of effectiveness. Vaccination may also be directed against a stage of the parasite in the blood called gametocytes which continue the life cycle of the parasite when a case is bitten by a mosquito vector. This indirect effect of vaccination in reducing transmission is complex, but it might be an important component of a strategy of disease control. The development of a vaccine involves components directed against multiple stages and species of human malaria. Different vaccine strategies need to be worked out for different populations depending on their immune status and risk of exposure.

*Table 1.* Malaria and Mortality in Sri Lanka, 1945-1974

| Year | Number of Malaria Cases | Number of Malaria Deaths | Crude Death Rate (per 1,000) | Infant Mortality Rate (per 1,000) |
|------|------------------------|--------------------------|------------------------------|-----------------------------------|
| 1945 | 2,539,949 | 8,539 | 21.5 | 140 |
| 1946 | 2,768,385 | 12,587 | 19.8 | 141 |
| 1947 | 1,459,880 | 4,562 | 14.0 | 101 |
| 1948 | 775,276 | 3,349 | 13.0 | 92 |
| 1949 | 727,769 | 2,403 | 12.4 | 87 |
| 1950 | 610,781 | 1,903 | 12.6 | 82 |
| 1951 | 448,100 | 1,599 | 12.9 | 82 |
| 1952 | 269,024 | 1,049 | 12.0 | 78 |
| 1953 | 91,990 | 722 | 10.9 | 71 |
| 1954 | 29,650 | 477 | 10.4 | 72 |
| 1955 | 11,191 | 268 | 11.0 | 71 |
| 1956 | 7,906 | 144 | 9.8 | 67 |
| 1957 | 10,442 | 8 | 10.1 | 68 |
| 1958 | 1,037 | 1 | 9.7 | 64 |
| 1959 | 1,596 | NA | 9.1 | 58 |
| 1960 | 422 | NA | 8.6 | 57 |
| 1961 | 110 | NA | 8.0 | 52 |
| 1962 | 31 | NA | 8.5 | 53 |
| 1963 | 17 | 1 | 8.5 | 56 |
| 1964 | 150 | 1 | 8.8 | 57 |
| 1965 | 308 | 1 | 8.2 | 53 |
| 1966 | 499 | NA | 8.3 | 54 |
| 1967 | 3,466 | 1 | 7.5 | 48 |
| 1968 | 440,644 | 64 | 7.9 | 50 |
| 1969 | 537,705 | 49 | 8.1 | 53 |
| 1970 | 468,202 | 12 | 7.5 | 48 |
| 1971 | 145,368 | 7 | 7.7 | 47 |
| 1972 | 132,604 | 4 | 8.0 | 46 |
| 1973 | 227,713 | 2 | 7.7 | 46 |
| 1974 | 315,448 | 2 | 9.0 | 51 |

*Sources:* Meegama, 1986, p. 7
Fernando, 1985, p. 83

The current status of malaria control is an uneasy balance. The great reductions in malaria following World War II have been followed by a resurgence in the 1970s. However, the resurgence has not continued unabated and even its impact has not been comparable to earlier periods. The demographic and health statistics of Sri Lanka in Table 1 demonstrate that the resurgence of malaria was not accompanied by many deaths. During the period 1945-1974 shown in Table 1, crude death rates and infant mortality rates have steadily declined so that mortality during the period of resurgence has been even lower than that achieved during the dramatic improvements in the late 1940s.

Nevertheless, the situation may be slowly worsening. As indicated above, some traditional methods of control may be losing their effectiveness. New epidemiological problems of malaria are associated with the movement of rural populations to temporary labor camps and urban slums. Because of the variety of epidemiological patterns of malaria, it is necessary to monitor the impact of malaria in order to better utilize existing methods of control. Evaluation of the impact of malaria control must take into account the capacity of the vector population to transmit, the level of resistance in the vector population, the species composition of malaria, the drug resistance of the various species of malaria, the degree of immunity in the human population and the general availability of health care.

## C. AIDS

Acquired immunodeficiency syndrome (AIDS), a fatal disease with no effective treatment, is emerging as a global public health problem since the syndrome was first described in 1981. The World Health Organization estimates that the total number of cases may be as high as 50,000 in Africa and 100,000 worldwide. As of August 1986, the largest numbers officially reported have been in the United States (21,517), Western Europe (2,568), Brazil (739), Central Africa (378), and Haiti (377) (Population Information Program, 1986b).

AIDS is caused by the human immunodeficiency virus (HIV, also known as HTLV-3 or LAV). The predominant mode of transmission is sexual activity—homosexual and heterosexual. In Central Africa and Haiti, cases have tended to be evenly divided between men and women. In the U.S., Europe and Brazil, cases have been predominantly among male homosexuals, although the number of cases due to heterosexual transmission is growing. For either homosexual or heterosexual transmission, risk increases with the number of sexual partners. Antibodies to HIV indicate exposure to the virus. Although it is not known if everybody infected with the virus will develop AIDS, those who are positive for antibodies are certainly at high risk. Antibodies to HIV are very common in some groups. For example, in 1985, 49 percent of male homosexual clients of an STD clinic in San Francisco were found to be antibody-positive. Prevalence of infection is particularly high among prostitutes. Prevalence among female prostitutes in Nairobi rose from 4 percent in 1981 to 59 percent in 1985. However, evidence of infection is not restricted to prostitutes. In 1984, 6 percent of the Mama Yemo Hospital staff in Kinshasa had antibodies (Population Information Program, 1986b, Table 1). Another important mode of transmission is exposure to contaminated blood. In the United States and other developed countries this route has been associated with intravenous drug users, hemophiliacs (recipients of concentrated blood products), and recipients of blood transfusion. In 1984, U.S. studies of intravenous drug users and hemophiliacs showed that the prevalence of antibody was 58 percent and 46 percent respectively (Population Information Program, 1986b, Table 1). Exposure through the blood supply may now be substantially reduced by excluding high-risk blood donors, screening donated blood for antibodies to HIV and inactivating HIV in concentrated blood products. In many developing countries, these procedures are difficult to institute because of their expense and because of the difficulty in identifying high-risk individuals. The common reuse of syringes in health care facilities in developing countries may also add to the risk but the effect of this practice is difficult to measure.

AIDS is predominantly reported in ages 20-49 in all countries. Deaths among this age group have a disproportionately disruptive effect on society. The impact of AIDS is multiplied because some people leave areas where many are dying of AIDS (Hooper, 1986). AIDS is also becoming more common in children as infants acquire the infection from their mothers. This is a greater problem in Africa where more women have the infection, but it is a growing problem elsewhere. The danger of AIDS extends beyond the very serious consequences of the infection itself to its potential impact on delivery of health care services to all children. One fear is that reuse of needles will facilitate the transmission of AIDS in routine immunization programs. Some groups are promoting the single-use disposable syringe, but this is costly (WHO, 1986a). Another fear is that children infected with HIV may be harmed by vaccines against some other diseases. The U.S. Advisory Committe on Immunization Practices recommends that infected children not be given live virus and live bacterial vaccines (e.g., measles, oral polio, BCG). Also, children residing in the same household with a person infected with HIV should not be given oral polio virus vaccine, because the live virus can be transmitted (CDC, 1986c). It should be noted that these recommendations are intended for children residing in the United States. In many developing countries, the cost of identifying infected children may be prohibitive. Major signs of pediatric AIDS are weight loss, chronic diarrhea or prolonged fever, but these symptoms are common in developing countries and are not specific for AIDS (WHO, 1986b). AIDS may change the overall cost-benefit balance in immunization programs. Mortality rates in children may rise due to AIDS itself or the indirect effect on reduced levels of immunization.

The relationship between infection and disease needs to be better understood. AIDS is clearly a new disease, even in central Africa. In Kinshasa, Zaire, cases of cryptococcal meningitis (an opportunistic infection) increased sharply in 1981 (Piot et al., 1984). In Kigali, Rwanda, cases of oesophageal candidiasis (another opportunistic infection) increased sharply in 1983 (Van de Perre et al., 1984). In Lusaka, Zambia, cases of an aggressive form of Kaposi's sarcoma increaded in 1983 (Bayley, 1984). All three diseases are found in association with AIDS in these countries. On the other hand, the fact that antibodies in Africa are widespread suggests that HIV has been around for some time. It may be that some antibodies represent exposure to closely-related viruses. Distinct variants of HIV have been documented.

The impact of AIDS is only just beginning to be felt. Since it is spread primarily as a venereal disease, interruption of transmission will require major behavioral modification among highly sexually active people. It is known from the theory of venereal disease that the groups with the largest number of sexual partners are primarily responsible for transmitting venereal disease (Hethcote and Yorke, 1984). Further, as the virus becomes more prevalent, the potential for exposure through contaminated blood becomes greater. The research to produce new drugs and vaccines is proceeding at a great pace. The race is on between the transmission of AIDS and development of new methods of control.

## III.  MODEL BUILDING

Mathematical models of the population dynamics of disease may aid in the analysis of disease control. The construction of models requires explicit formulation of assumptions concerning the relationships among transmission, morbidity and mortality. A better understanding of these relationships may improve the accuracy of predictions and the evaluation of control strategies. The structure of models also emphasizes the common features of disease control in populations so that each special case does not have to be approached in isolation. This section mentions some special considerations in using models of selective disease control.

Models of selective disease control require at a minimum specific identification of the disease of interest. The trend for a group of diseases does not necessarily reflect the trend for any particular disease in the group. For example, in the late nineteenth century in England, smallpox deaths were declining as measles deaths increased (Mercer, 1986, p. 138). Even a common name for a particular disease may actually refer to different diseases with different etiologies.

Models of specific diseases also have to distinguish between the process of infection and its effect on morbidity and mortality. The effect of a disease may be influenced by the availability of rapid diagnosis and the effectiveness of treatment. Age, genetic background, nutritional status and other diseases of the patient also influence the outcome. The time of illness and death does not necessarily coincide with time of infection. As in AIDS, it is possible for infection to occur years before overt signs and symptoms. As in measles, death attributable to the infection may occur more than a month past clinical illness. It is incomplete to summarize this effect as an age-specific case-fatality rate. Yet models attempting to include many biological, social and economic determinants of mortality are forced to compress effects into this form (Barnum et al., 1980).

It may be useful to model transmission explicitly. The ability of a person to transmit an infection does not necessarily correlate with morbidity and mortality. Asymptomatic malaria cases may be a reservoir of infection. Programs that focus on transmission may be quite different from programs that focus on morbidity and mortality. For example, treatment of malaria cases reduces morbidity without affecting transmission. Changes in transmission may result in both changes in age-specific patterns as well as overall incidence. In general, reduction of transmission tends to increase the age at first infection and the time interval between subsequent infections (if immunity is not acquired).

The concept of an underlying model of disease transmission and control can be illustrated with and expression R defined for malaria as follows:

$$R = \frac{ma^2bc \; \exp(-\mu\tau)}{r\mu}$$

where

m  is the ratio of the density of the biting mosquito population to the density of the human population;

a  is the rate of biting on humans by a single mosquito (number of bites per unit time);

b  is the proportion of bites by sporozoite-bearing mosquitoes that result in infection;

c  is the proportion of bites by uninfected mosquitoes on malarious people that result in infection;

r  is the rate of recovery of humans ($1/r$ is the average duration of infection);

$\mu$  is the rate of mortality for mosquitoes ($1/\mu$ is the average lifetime of a mosquito);

$\tau$  is the incubation period in the mosquito (time from infection until sporozoites are present in salivary glands).

The expression R is the basic reproduction rate of malaria which is the average number of secondary cases of infection generated by a single infected person in a population of susceptibles (Aron and May, 1982). During the period of infection, one person will infect, on average, $mac/r$ mosquitoes. Only a fraction of these mosquitoes, $\exp(-\mu\tau)$, will survive the incubation period to infect, on average, $ab/\mu$ people during its remaining lifetime. R is the product of these terms. Clearly, only if R exceeds unity will malaria spread.

The basic reproduction rate elucidates the dynamics underlying the observed incidence of malaria. The basic reproduction rate indicates the potential for transmission from a single individual and consequently the difficulty in controlling and eradicating malaria. Even where malaria transmission has been eliminated, the potential remains and may be realized as shown by recent evidence of transmission in California (CDC, 1986d).

The application of this concept does, however, have limitations. Estimates of the actual transfer of infection (parameters b and c) have been highly variable. The impact of infection on the human host is not addressed. Moreover, where malaria transmission is well established, acquired immunity is an important determinant of epidemiological patterns. These areas are now the subjects of active research investigation.

# IV.  SELECTIVE DISEASE CONTROL

Selective disease control may provide an important option for reducing mortality. Diseases to be selected should have high prevalence or high mortality. A contributing factor seen in all three case studies may be a degree of weakening induced by the disease that increases susceptibility to other diseases. Even as mortality levels decline, these diseases will continue to adversely affect the well-being of their host populations. Disease prevention programs, which can produce relatively quick results, may be an extremely effective way to target scarce health resources (Walsh and Warren, 1979).

The method of disease control is also important. One reason that control of specific diseases is often assumed to drain resources from primary health care is that the 1950s malaria eradication campaign of the World Health Organization relied on specialized teams to spray insecticides. This effort could not be sustained. If the program resulted in eradication, the campaign could be discontinued. On the other hand, continued spraying without eradication became a costly burden. In contrast, smallpox vaccine was relatively easy to administer and required less specialized personnel. Moreover, smallpox transmission had features favorable for eradication. The offspring of the successful eradication of smallpox is the Expanded Program on Immunization of the World Health Organization.

Selective disease control however is not a total substitute for other programs in public health. Improvements in nutrition, water sanitation and maternal/infant care help to reduce mortality. These changes may ultimately have greater impact but the impact slowly develops over many years (e.g., Preston and van de Walle, 1978). Nevertheless, activities targeted against specific diseases have made a noticeable demographic impact, as discussed for malaria control in Sri Lanka (Meegama, 1986) and smallpox vaccination in Europe (Mercer, 1985). Since multiple factors affect mortality, multiple pathways to low mortality exist. Historical examples of mortality decline should inform debate, but should not limit options, especially when technological advances such as vaccines are available.

# ACKNOWLEDGMENTS

Anouch Chahnazarian and Henry Mosley provided helpful comments on various drafts. This work was supported by the Andrew Mellon Foundation and the Johns Hopkins Biomedical Research Support Grant.

# REFERENCES

Aaby, P., Bukh, J., Lisse, I.M., and Smits, A.J. (1981). Measles vaccination and child mortality. *Lancet* ii:93.

Anderson, Roy M. (1982). Directly transmitted viral and bacterial infections of man. In *Population Dynamics of Infectious Diseases* ed., Roy M. Anderson, London and New York: Chapman and Hall, pp. 1-37.

Aron, J.L., and May, R.M. (1982). The population dynamics of malaria. In *Population Dynamics of Infectious Diseases* ed. Roy M. Anderson, London and New York: Chapman and Hall, pp. 139-179.

Barnum, H., Barlow, R., Fajardo, L. and Pradilla, A. (1980). *A Resource Allocation Model for Child Survival,* Cambridge, Mass: Oelgeschlager, Gunn & Hain.

Bayley, A.C. (1984) Aggressive Kaposi's sarcoma in Zambia, 1983. *Lancet* i:1318-1320.

Black, F.L. (1982). Measles. In *Viral Infections of Humans, 2nd ed.* (ed.) A.S. Evans, New York and London: Plenum Medical Book pp. 397-418.

Black, F.L., Berman, L.L., Borgono, J.M. et al. (1986). Geographic variation in infant loss of maternal measles antibody and in prevalence of rubella antibody. *Amer. J. Epidem. 124*:442-452.

Bruce-Chwatt, L.J. (1985). *Essential Malariology (2nd ed.)*, New York: John Wiley & Sons.

Cantrelle, P., Diop, I.L., Garenne, M., Gueye, M., and Sadio, A. (1986). The Profile of Mortality and its Determinants in Senegal, 1960-1980. In *Determinants of Mortality Change and Differentials in Developing Countries,* Population Studies No. 94, New York: United Nations, pp. 86-116.

Centers for Disease Control. (1986a). Measles—United States, First 26 Weeks, 1986, *Morbidity and Mortality Weekly Report 35*(33):525-533.

Centers for Disease Control. (1986b). Outbreak of malaria imported from Kenya. *MMWR 35*(36):567-573.

Centers for Disease Control. (1986c). Immunization of children infected with HTLV-III/LAV. *MMWR 35*(38):595-606.

Centers for Disease Control. (1986d). *Plasmodium vivax* malaria—San Diego County, California: 1986, *MMWR 35*(43):679-681.

Cox, D.R., and Lewis, P.A.W. (1966). *The Statistical Analysis of Series of Events,* London: Methuen, Chap. 9.

D'Souza, S. (1986). Mortaility Structure in Matlab (Bangladesh) and the Effect of Selected Health Interventions. In *Determinants of Mortality Change and Differentials in Developing Countries,* Population Studies No. 94, New York: United Nations, pp. 117-144.

Ewbank, D., Henin, R., and Kekovale, J. (1986). An Integration of Demographic and Epidemiologic Research on Mortality in Kenya. In *Determinants of Mortality Change and Differentials in Developing Countries,* Population Studies No. 94, New York: United Nations, pp. 33-85.

Fernando, D.F.S. (1985). Health Statistics in Sri Lanka, 1921-1980. In *Good Health at Low Cost* (eds.), S.B. Halstead, J.A. Walsh and K.S. Warren, New York: Rockefeller Foundation, pp. 79-92.

Halsey, N.A., Boulos, R., Mode, F., Andre, J., Bauman, L., Yaeger, R.G., Toureau, S., Rohde, J., and Boulos, C. (1985). Response to measles vaccine in Haitian infants 6 to 12 months old: influence of maternal antibodies, malnutrition and concurrent illnesses. *New England Journal of Medicine 313*(9):554-549 (August 29).

Henderson, R.H. (1984). An example of vaccine application: The Expanded Programme on Immunization. In *New Approaches to Vaccine Development* (ed.), R. Bell and G. Torrigiani, Schwabe & Co., Basal, pp. 506-515.

Hethcote, H.W. and Yorke, J.A. (1984). Gonorrhea Transmission Dynamics and Control. *Lecture Notes in Biomathematics, Vol. 56,* Berlin Heidelberg, New York, Tokyo: Springer-Verlag.

Hooper, E. (1986). An African Village Staggers Under the Assault of AIDS. *New York Times,* Sept. 30, 1986, pp. C-1, C-3.

Kasongo Project Team. (1981). Influences of measles vaccination on survival pattern of 7-35-month-old children in Kasongo, Zaire. *Lancet* i:764-767.

Meegama, S.A. (1986). The Mortality Transition in Sri Lanka. In *Determinants of Mortality Change and Differentials in Developing Countries,* Population Studies No. 94, New York: United Nations, pp. 5-32.

Mercer, A.J. (1985). Smallpox and epidemiological-demographic change in Europe: The role of vaccination, *Popualtion Studies, 39*(2):287-307.

Mercer, A.J. (1986). Relative trends in mortality from related respiratory and airborne infectious diseases, *Population Studies, 40*(1):129-145.

Piot, P., Quinn, T.C., and Taelman, H. (1984). Acquired immunodeficiency syndrome in a heterosexual population in Zaire. *Lancet* ii:65-69.

Population Information Program. (1986a). Immunizing the World's Children. *Population Reports,* L-5.

Population Information Program. (1986b). AIDS—A Public Health Crisis. *Population Reports,* L-6.

Preston, S.H., and Van De Walle, E. (1978). Urban French mortality in the nineteenth century, *Population Studies, 32*(2):275-297.

Schindler, L.W. (1985). The Development of a Malaria Vaccine. In *Status of Biomedical Research and Related Technology for Tropical Diseases, OTA-H-258,* Washington, D.C.: U.S. Government Printing Office, pp. 225-245.

United Nations. (1985). *World Population Prospects, Estimations and Projections as Assessed in 1982, Population Studies, No. 86,* New York: United Nations.

Van de Perre, P., Rouvroy, D., and LePage, P. et al. (1984). Acquired immunodeficiency syndrome in Rwanda. *Lancet* ii:62-65.

Van de Walle, E. (1985). Anatomie d'une epidemie de rougeole vue par la lorgnette d'une enquete a passages repetes, Seminar on Estimation de la mortalite du jeune enfant de (0-5 ans) pour guider les actions de sante dans les pays en developpement, Centre International de l'Enfance, Paris.

Walsh, J.A., and Warren, K.S. (1979). Selective primary health care. An interim strategy for disease control in developing countries, *New England Journal of Medicine, 301*(18):967-974.

World Health Organization. (1986a). Choice of syringes for the EPI. *Weekly Epidemiological Record 61*(6):41-43.

World Health Organization. (1986b). WHO/CDC case definition for AIDS. *Weekly Epidemiological Record 61*(10):69-73.

World Health Organization. (1986c). *Eighteenth Report of the WHO Expert Committee on Malaria,* WHO Technical Report Series, No. 735, Geneva: World Health Organization.

# HEALTH INFORMATION FOR PUBLIC HEALTH POLICIES AND SERVICES IN DEVELOPING COUNTRIES

Huda Zurayk

## I. INTRODUCTION

Most developing countries face a priority need to organize, as part of development planning, effective and efficient processes for delivery of public health services, in view of the poor levels of health experienced by population groups and the lack of qualified input resources that could be devoted to their improvement. A necessary, though certainly not sufficient, condition for organization of such processes is the availability of health information systems that can delineate the health needs, and monitor the progress towards preset goals. Such systems are practically nonexistent, however, in the countries where the need for improvements in the health sector is greatest, and are generally of low quality wherever they exist. Organizing information systems must thus be seen as a process that moves in parallels and is linked with the process of development of public health policies and services.

**Research in Human Capital Development, Vol. 5, pages 57-73.**
**Copyright © 1988 by JAI Press Inc.**
**All rights of reproduction in any form reserved.**
**ISBN: 0-89232-508-9**

The aim of this paper is to address the issue of health information in developing countries, concentrating on the content and the strategies for developing the necessary systems, while taking into account the realities of the context in which they are established. The illustrations are drawn mainly from experiences in Arab countries, but the issues of relevance to developing countries in general are given priority consideration.

It is important to note first that developing countries which have established some health information systems have generally modelled such systems on those in developed countries, despite differences in level and pattern of organization of the health care sector. Moreover, they have tended to consider the information systems mainly as "neutral data banks" that cumulate information and produce health indicators with little attention given to the potential for the dynamic interplay of statistics and health services at every level of the delivery system (Murnaghan, 1981: 309). Following the Alma-Ata declarations (WHO, 1978), a shift in health policy towards implementation of primary health care has occurred in most developing countries, and has made such information practices particularly inadequate (Murnaghan, 1981: 308). This chapter emphasizes the necessity for congruity in the development of health information systems in developing countries with the process of implementation of primary health care delivery systems.

The functions of an information system can be summarized into two main processes: the process of determination of relevant information needs and of expressing them in quantifiable indicators; and the process of organizing manpower, equipment and other resources for acquiring and analyzing the data needed (White, 1980, p. 298). Accordingly, this presentation shall be divided into two sections. The first section considers the minimum core of information items and indicators that can describe health problems in developing countries and evaluate interventions aimed at their solution. The second section focuses on the strategies of organization of resources for data acquisition and processing that can raise the quality of contribution of the health information system to development of public health policies and services. In addressing the issues of content and organization of resources, reference will be made to an overall National Health Information System (NHIS) made up of many component systems.

## II.   CONTENT OF A NATIONAL
## HEALTH INFORMATION SYSTEM

The possible scope of a NHIS is very wide, particularly with integration of some social and economic indicators (Murnaghan, 1981, p. 305). In the U.S. for example, 190 quantifiable objectives have been developed for disease prevention and health promotion; these are tracked over time and space by systematic monitoring and surveillance systems, and by periodic surveys (Green et al., 1983, p. 18). To maintain acceptable quality in the output from a NHIS, however, the system's scope must be delimited by the nation's capability for implementation. A limitation of scope is particularly relevant for developing countries where Ministries of Health have insufficient funds or expertise to manage an elaborate system (Murnaghan, 1981, p. 306). Nevertheless, flexibility must be built into these systems from the beginning to permit gradual expansion in scope, and responsiveness to changes in the organization of the health care system (Steinwachs, 1985, p. 607).

To maintain the comprehensive usefulness of the body of data produced by the NHIS, the limitation in scope must come less from coverage of concepts in the health care system and more in terms of depth of their representation. The concepts to be covered can be derived from a simplified model of the health care system (Figure 1). The model represents health care resources as being utilized by the community through a process which affects the health status of the population (White, 1980, p. 306). Each of the four components of the health care system, the community of concern, the level of resources, the process of utilization and health status are summarized by concepts that need to be translated into health indicators (Murnaghan, 1981, p. 314; White, 1983, p. 306-307). The depth of representation, in terms of number and complexity of indicators, must be determined by each nation according to the objectives of its public health policies and available resources.

Some developing countries have derived an extensive list of indicators of these concepts (General Health Secretariat of Gulf Countries, 1981) which is difficult to implement at the first stage of NHIS develpment. Indicators must be given priority based on their simplicity and their immediate usefulness to public health policy and services, with a sensitivity to the context of concern. As an illustration of such a process Murnaghan (1981) has suggested a list of indicators that could serve as a uniform minimum core of information for developing countries which emphasize primary health care. These suggested indicators are shown in Table 1, arranged according to the components of the model presented in Figure 1.

This core of indicators represents information needs that primarily serve planning and management purposes, at central or perepheral levels. It is important to recognize, however, that the information needs at the periphery also include items that are operational i.e., directed toward improvement of a particular task. Table 2 presents an illustration of information items of this nature, indicating for each the relevant task. The indicators of Table 1 and the information items of Table 2 illustrate a core that can guide developing countries in determining the content of a natural health information system at an early stage.

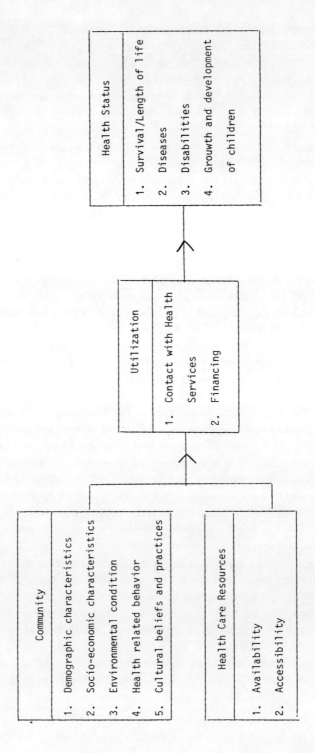

*Figure 1.* Uniform Minimum Information Concepts Derived from Simplified Model of the Health Care System

*Table 1.* Illustrative List of Indicators for
National Health Planning and Evaluation in a Developing Country

*Community*
1. Demographic characteristics
    population size
    age structure
    rural-urban distribution
    rate of growth
2. Socioeconomic characteristics
    literacy rates of adults by sex
    proprotion of persons below a specified income
3. Environmental conditions
    proportion of households with adequate supply of safe water and basic sanitation
4. Health-related behaviors
    proportion of persons with less than the minimum food intake

*Health care resources*
1. Availability
    number of primary care personnel per 10,000 population by type and geographic area.
    number of hospital beds per 10,000 population by type of hospital and geographical area.
2. Accessibility
    proportion of population within a specified travel time from a continuous source of primary
        health services, a community hospital or other continuous source of referral (secondary
        level) service.

*Utilization*
4. Contact with health services
    primary care visits and number of persons visiting or visited per 1,000 population by year.
    hospital discharges and number of people discharged per 1,000 population by year.
    proportion of births attended by trained health personnel.
    proportion of school-entry age children having completed basic immunization series.
2. Financing
    proportion of GNP spent on health
    ratio of expenditures for primary health care to expenditures for hospital inpatient care.

*Health Status*
1. Survival and length of life
    life expectancy at birth
    infant mortality
    three principle causes of death in age groups 0-4, 5-14, 15-44, and 45+
    maternal mortality rate
    deaths in children and young adults from pneumococcal pneumonia.
    deaths in children under 6 from diarrhea.
2. Diseases
    incidences and/or prevalence of selected communicable diseases of major health importance
        to the population.
    list in order of frequency of 10 to 15 most commonly reported health problems in the
        population
    incidence per 1,000 births of neonatal tetanus.
3. Disabilities
    persons with sick days per 1,000 and value of sick days per 1,000 during past 14 days.
    persons per 1,000 with disabling impairment and chronic diseases.
    proportion of population resident in long-term health care institutions.

*Source:* Rearranged from Murnaghan, 1981:314-15.

*Table 2.*  Illustrative List of Information Items
for Special Services at the Periphery

| Information item | Relevant Task |
|---|---|
| 1. Births | well-baby and post-natal care |
| 2. Deaths | counseling and support |
| 3. Infectious diseases | control and prevention |
| 4. Pregnancies | prenatal care |
| 5. Hospitalizations | follow-up care |
| 6. Special conditions, such as: | special care |
|     diabetes | |
|     disability | |
|     epilepsy | |
|     mental problem | |
|     repeated reproductive loss | |

# III. STRATEGIES FOR ORGANIZATION OF RESOURCES

The aim of strategies adopted by a NHIS for organization of human and material resources is the adequate and cost-effective provision of information needed by the health delivery system. In developing countries, the orientation toward primary health care puts specific demands on the decentralization of the loci for utilization of information and on its flow within the delivery system. Moreover, availability of resources is limited, which imposes the requirement for a dynamic organizational pattern that can make efficient and effective use of such resources.

## A.  Orientation towards Primary Health Care

The most important characteristic of a primary health care delivery system is the contact it maintains with individuals, families and communities through heavy emphasis on the grass-root level of care and participation (WHO, 1978). Implementation of a primary health care system thus usually involves a shift from centralized health care where secondary and tertiary level institutions receive the bulk of financing and attention, to a system where the expanse of activity is at the periphery. A second important characteristic of a primary health care system is its reliance on a network of linkages between the periphery and the more specialized institutions to ensure a continuum of care for the population.

To serve the needs of a primary health care delivery system, a NHIS must reflect these organizational characteristics of the delivery system. A decentralization in information handling activities must take place which parallels the decentralization of delivery of services. In addition, a flow of information along the network of the delivery system must occur to serve the purposes of referral and follow-up.

*Strategy 1:    "Decentralization in information handling."*

In many developing countries in which some components of the NHIS have been developed, the main purpose of the system is still considered to be the reporting of events and indicators to the central government for use in planning of services. Quite often the operation of the information system has become a routine activity which is inadequately monitored for accuracy, completeness and continuing utility. Collection occurs at health service institutions, while processing and analysis take place in a detached manner at the central level. The case of Egypt serves as an illustration of such a process.

In *Egypt,* statistics on births and deaths, infectious diseases, characteristics of health manpower and on activities of health institutions are collected at the smallest unit level in the periphery and forwarded periodically with no processing to the district level. District level totals are cumulated and the records are passed on to the governate level. At that level, totals are also cumulated, and the records are then passed on to the Center for Information and Documentation at the Ministry of Health in Cairo where processing and report generation are undertaken. The reports are circulated at the central level of the Ministry where they are supposed to be used for planning purposes. These reports do not feed back to the periphery which remains a passive contributor to the system. In fact, there is a clear delineation in information functions within the structures of the system whereby the periphery, is in charge of collection of information, the Center of Information and Documentation for the design and analysis activities, and the management of the Ministry of Health for using the information in developing public health policies and planning services. (Oral reporting during meeting with Dr. Zaher Iskandar, director of the Center of Information and Documentation at the Ministry of Health, Cairo November, 1985).

Such a centralized system of information handling is not suited to the needs of a primary health care system. If some initiative in planning of services is to be transferred to the periphery, then with it must come the ability to undertake some data processing at the periphery. The information can be utilized directly in planning and delivery of services at that level. However, achieving an effective process of decentralization in information handling is not a straightforward task. The experience of Bahrain presents an instructive illustration in this respect.

*Bahrain* is a Gulf country and as such it differs from developing countries in two important respects. First, it has a small population of less than half a million persons, and second, its financial resources are plentiful. Yet, it is precisely because of these two characteristics that Bahrain has been able to rapidly implement a primary health care system. Moreover, Bahrain is similar to most developing countries in the relatively low level of skills and the easy attitude to work of its manpower, and in that respect its experience can be useful to consider.

The population of Bahrain has been divided into captive groups mostly along geographical lines, and a process of remodeling of existing health centers and of building new ones has developed rapidly, so that each population group is served by a well-staffed and equipped health center. These health centers are linked to a large government hospital which has also undergone a process of improvement. The development of components of the NHIS has moved parallel to these activities. In particular, a health center component has been developed and implemented at the Hidd Health Center on an experimental basis. The system is based on an encounter form which is completed for every patient visiting the health center. The forms are analyzed periodically at the health center to show load of patients per attendant and per session during days of the week, as well as time spent with attendant and types of complaints by age and sex. The health center has acquired a micro-computer which is used to continuously enter the information from the encounter forms and to do the periodic processing in a timely fashion. Yet, despite these achievements, the aims of decentralization are not achieved, because the utilization of the information processed in planning the services of the health center is minimal. (Visit to Hidd Health Center, October, 1985).

What this illustrates is that the important bottleneck to a useful decentralization in information handling is not necessarily the lack of human and computer facilities at the periphery. Although it is extremely unlikely, for example, for periphery areas in most developing countries to acquire computer facilities, the task of analysis can be undertaken manually and can be simplified to suit any conditions. The difficulty lies in the lack of ability of personnel at the periphery to interpret and use the processed information, as discussed later in this chapter.

*Strategy 2:  "Interaction of the NHIS network with the delivery system network."*

The primary health care delivery system provides the individual with referrals to specialized institutions, and follow-up care at community level upon discharge. For optimum operation of such a system there must be a parallel information exchange between the components of the system on events of importance to the health care of the individual and his/her family. An illustration of the workings of such a process from Bahrain is presented.

*Bahrain* has one main government hospital, the Salmaniyah Medical Center, to which patients are referred either by health centers or by private physicians. A hospital discharge system summarizing the episodes of illness was implemented in 1978 in the Salmaniyah Medical Center, and has been operating smoothly since then. It produces periodic reports on the characteristics of discharges from the hospital. The system is generally underutilized within the hospital for operational purposes (such as selection of outlier cases for quality assurance investigations) and for research purposes. However, it has achieved successfully a process of feedback of information to health centers on discharged patients.

The identification number of the health center in which a patient is registered is entered on the admission section of the Admission and Discharge Summary Sheet of the Salmaniyah Medical Center. Upon discharge of the patient from the hospital, a copy of the Summary Sheet is automatically forwarded to the indicated health center. The Summary Sheet is filed in the patient's medical record at the health center, providing the physician at the health center with the necessary information about the hospital stay. The exchange of information in the other direction, from the health center to the hospital, is done briefly through information on the referral slip. Once the health center information system is implemented in all health centers, summary information from the encounter records can be listed in order of visit to the health center, and forwarded to the hospital or to the specialized clinic upon referral of the patient. The physician of the specialilzed institution can thus review a summary of the medical history of the patient, particularly as related to the care sought at the health center preceding referral to the hospital (Zurayk, 1980).

The interaction of the NHIS with the delivery system is important, even beyond the networks of patient flow. Information produced by some components of the NHIS, independent of health delivery institutions, can prove useful to these institutions. A web of information networks can be developed, some linking service institutions together and others linking components of the NHIS outside the delivery system to units within it. An illustration of the second type of linkage is presented, again from experience in Bahrain.

The birth registration system is located at the Ministry of Health in Manama, the capital city of *Bahrain*. The system has achieved acceptable levels of coverage and timeliness of registration. Information on births is transferred from the Ministry to the Central Statistical Office, where it is analyzed, using the central computer system, for statistical purposes. A recommendation was made to add the identification number of the health center in which the mother is registered to the birth certificate. This would make it possible for the computer to print on a weekly basis a list of births in each health center, indicating for each birth the expected immunization schedule according to the date of birth. The list would be sent to the nurse in charge of the well-baby clinic and would help her organize her work and achieve the desired immunization coverage for the children registered in the health center. Unfortunately, this information exchange between the birth registration system and the health center was difficult to implement, mainly because it involved the collaboration of agencies in more than one Ministry (Hamadeh, 1980).

## B.   Efficient and Effective Utilization of Resources

As indicated earlier, the scope of a NHIS must be delimited by the availability of resources, and can expand gradually with the growth of resources. At any stage of development and with any set level of resources, however, the scope can be expanded by efficient organization.

*Strategy 3:   "Building on existing systems."*

In many developing countries, some systems for collection and processing of vital and health statistics are already operational with different levels of validity, reliability and coverage. In initiating a systematic organization and development of a NHIS, therefore, it is useful to begin by taking stock of existing systems and evaluating their quality. Some systems may have to be replaced, but others can prove valuable, and may require none or a manageable degree of improvement to become serviceable. An illustration from Lebanon is used to demonstrate such a process.

In *Lebanon,* a task force on information was appointed by the Minister of Health in 1982 to plan for the gradual implementation of a NHIS. The task force considered its first responsibility to be the delineation of information needs of the Ministry and the evaluation of existing systems that can provide the information to meet some of these needs. Figure 2 presents a matrix developed by the task force that links information needs expressed as vital and health events and processes to systems that could provide indicators to represent them.

Two sources of information were located on physicians practicing in Lebanon. The Ministry of Health requires every eligible and qualified physician seeking to practice in Lebanon to register at the Ministry, showing all the necessary documents, in order to be given a license to practice. After examining the registry, however, it became clear to the task force that the registry could not be used as a source of information on the characteristics of physicians practicing in Lebanon because it has no mechanism to update the information related to changes in qualifications or movements of physicians within or outside the country.

The second source located on physician manpower was the Order of Physicians. This is a professional organization to which eligible and qualified physicians must belong in order to be allowed to practice in Lebanon. Since the order collects annual dues from members, it employs persons to contact the physicians periodically to seek information regarding any changes in their qualifications, area of practice, or residence. For privacy considerations the order would not allow access to its files, but it was ready to prepare summary reports that would give sufficient information on the distribution and characteristics of the physician manpower in Lebanon. In relying on this

| Information Needs | | Possible Sources of Data | Birth Registration | Death Registration | Infectious Diseases Reporting | Facility Registration | Order of Physician | Hospital Discharge System | Population Census | Health Module or Morbidity Survey | Special Surveys |
|---|---|---|---|---|---|---|---|---|---|---|---|
| Population | Population Characteristics | | | | | | | | X | X | X |
| | Births | X | | | | | | | X | X | X |
| | Deaths | | X | | | | | | | X | X |
| Resources | Facilities | | | | X | | | | | | X |
| | Manpower | | | | | X | | | | | X |
| | Financial | | | | | | | | | | X |
| Morbidity | Causes of Death | | X | | | | X | | | X | X |
| | Hospital Discharge Diagnosis | | | | | | X | | | | X |
| | Outpatient Causes of Visit | | | | | | | | | X | X |
| | Infectious Diseases | | | X | | | X | | | X | X |
| | Chronic Conditions | | | | | | X | | | X | X |
| | Disabilities | | | | | | | | | X | X |
| | Home Illnesses | | | | | | | | | X | X |
| Utilization | Hospital Utilization | | | | | | X | | | X | X |
| | Health Center Utilization | | | | | | | | | X | X |
| | Physician Utilization | | | | | | | | | X | X |
| Health Determinants | Environment | | | | | | | | | X | X |
| | Life Styles | | | | | | | | | X | X |
| | Cultural Habits | | | | | | | | | X | X |

*Figure 2.* Matrix Linking Information Needs to Possible Sources of Data

system, the Ministry was saved resource allocation to develop an update mechanism for its registry at a time when such resources could be valuably utilized towards meeting other of its priority information needs (Lebanese Ministry of Health; Task Force on Information, 1983).

*Strategy 4: "Training nonspecialized manpower."*

Decentralization of information handling adds to the responsibilities of health services personnel, tasks for which they are largely untrained. At the first level, community health workers and the paramedical staff of the health centers are responsible mainly for the collection process and for some simple data analysis and presentation. Such personnel need training in the scientific methods of data handling. Moreover, such training must emphasize the usefulness of the information generated in improving performance and planning of the health workers' daily activities. Training programs for community health workers usually cover knowledge and skills in many areas of public health, but rarely do they include an introduction to the concepts of biostatistics and epidemiology. Only through acquisition of awareness, knowledge and skills can the community health workers adequately perform the required data handling tasks (Shah, 1985).

At the second level of interaction with the NHIS come the physicians at the health centers whose role within the primary health care system extends to the care of the community, and the management of the services of the health center. It is essential for such physicians to acquire an understanding of the usefulness of statistics in community diagnosis and in evaluation of interventions aimed at improving the health of the individual and the group. To be effective, however, training of physicians in the sciences of information must not be limited to a classroom activity, but must also take place within the physicians' work environment and cover the information skills needed to assist the physicians in performing their jobs.

At the last level of interaction come the health managers and policy makers at intermediate and central levels. They are the utilizers of output from the NHIS, mainly for planning purposes. It is the responsibility of statisticians at various levels of the NHIS, through frequent workshops and continuous contact with these administrators and policy makers, to gradually foster their skill to express clearly their information needs, and to interpret the measured indicators in a manner that is useful for planning and policy making activities.

*Strategy 5: "Training and efficient organization of specialized manpower."*

The managers and operators of the NHIS are statisticians and statistical workers who occupy positions, in accordance with their level of education, at statistical offices and information centers at intermediate or central levels of administration of the health delivery system. Statistically at higher levels of education are usually of low availability in developing countries. In addition, in most countries qualified statistical workers are not being prepared in sufficient numbers. Colleges of health sciences have given most attention to the production of nurses, who are the most needed resource within a primary health care system, followed by other specialists such as sanitarians, laboratory technologists and medical records personnel. In contrast to these front-line workers, the activities of the statistical worker are of a "backstage" nature. Nevertheless, it is important to give full recognition to the role of the statistical worker as a member of the health team, and to support training programs that produce statisticians in sufficient diversity of levels and in sufficient number according to foreseen need.

Within the framework of a primary health care delivery system, the functions of the statistical resource of the NHIS must stretch beyond the confines of offices at intermediate and central levels to maintain contact with the collection processes at the periphery and within health institutions. As such, the responsibility of the statistical resource is not only the design of component systems of the NHIS, but also involves the monitoring of their implementation and operation. In fact, an important function of the statistical resource is to assist health personnel at the periphery, and within health institutions, to utilize the information generated in these loci in improving their planning and delivery of services.

The responsibilities of the statistical resource can be organinzed in a two-tiered format, whereby the involvement of the statistical workers at intermediate levels with the periphery is large, while the statisticians at the central level communicate less with the periphery and more with statisticians at the intermediate levels. In view of the probable shortage of well-trained statisticians at intermediate levels, the communication between the central and intermediate levels is essential to maintain a dynamic system of monitoring and feedback, and to ensure adequate analysis and utilization of the information at intermediate administrative levels.

*Strategy 6:* *"Utilization of a variety of methods for data acquisition."*

The process of data collection within components of a NHIS usually involve routine collection methods, but also include some reliance on sample surveys and specialized studies. In most developing countries, as the systematic development of a NHIS is organized, a process of building infrastructures of the routine systems must take place. Moreover, the scope of the system is limited by scarce resources. There arises a need, therefore, to rely more heavily than at later stages on sample surveys and alternate methods. This allows the health system to collect information on essential health concepts outside the scope of the NHIS, to evaluate the information yielded by the components of the NHIS, and to learn about particular situations quickly. Responsibility for design and implementation of such interventions rests with the statistical resource at intermediate and central levels, and may occupy a significant portion of their work effort in the first stages of organization of the NHIS. However, such activity gradually diminishes as the routine systems become well-established. As an illustration of the use of an alternate to routine methods, the activity of the Faculty of Health Sciences at the American University of Beirut, in a particularly acute phase of the war in Lebanon, is presented.

*Lebanon* has been in a continuous state of war since 1975, which has taken different forms throughout the duration at various places within the country. For Beirut city, the siege imposed in 1982 following the Israeli invasion of Lebanon resulted in the breakdown of most of the services in the city, including water, electricity and garbage collection, which endangered the health situation of the inhabitants of the city. The governmental and nongovernmental agencies wishing to participate in alleviating this situation needed to be informed quickly of the health problems that were emerging in the city. Under these conditions, and in the absence of functioning routine systems of information that could reach these agencies, the Faculty of Health Sciences organized an emergency surveillance operation which relied on two methods of data collection: a sample survey of the inhabitants, and active surveillance of a sample of health institutions in the city.

First, the population in the besieged city of Beirut was sampled, using area sampling methods, and families living in apartments and in displacement centers were interviewed regarding major health problems. Second, the relevant records of the major hospitals and of a sample of dispensaries and health centers were reviewed frequently to detect cases of infectious diseases and locate their place of occurrence. A team of students was trained and utilized to undertake the interviewing and surveillance. It was an intensive activity in a short period of time which assisted in directing the emergency health activities in a period of crisis (Faculty of Health Sciences, American University of Beirut, 1983).

*Strategy 7:* *"Involvement and support of schools of public health."*

Strategies 4 and 5 have emphasized the need for training of manpower that would be responsible for tasks within the NHIS, as well as training of personnel that would utilize the output of a NHIS at various levels of operation of the health care system. The Schools of Public Health in developing countries have an important role to play in these training programs by developing both degree programs in the information disciplines and short training courses for medical and health personnel. The quality of these training programs is enhanced by the participation of the schools in the systematic process of organization of the NHIS. Through such participation, schools of Public health also contribute to the process of design and implementation of routine systems, as well as of sample surveys and active surveillence processes, as discussed in Strategy 6.

Some further details of the experience of the Faculty of Health Sciences at the American University of Beirut are presented.

In 1983, the Faculty of Health Sciences participated in establishing the Directorate of Planning at the Ministry of Health in *Lebanon,* which consisted of three units: the unit of planning, the unit of epidemiologic surveillance, and the unit of health information systems. One faculty member was in charge of each unit and supervised a team of employees in establishing the unit, and developing and implementing its work program. Students from the faculty participated in the work of the units as part of their training, and many continued to serve as employees following graduation. The Directorate of Planning now continues to operate, with much reduced input from the faculty, despite difficult circumstances in the country (Kutran, 1984).

Following its experience with the Emergency Health Surveillance activities, the Faculty of Health Sciences also established, in 1983, a Population Laboratory with the objectives of: (1) providing faculty and students with the opportunity to be involved in continuous and collaborative community research, and (2) channeling the research effort toward the identification of health needs at the community level, and the development and testing of instruments for information gathering needed by Ministries of Health in Lebanon and the region. The Population Laboratory has succeeded in obtaining funding from different sources to conduct health surveys in locations representing important typologies of Lebanese life. Through such surveys, it aims to arrive at a diagnosis of the health situation and the needs for intervention in these and similar locations throughout the country. The real challenge of bridging of the gap between the processes of information gathering and analysis, and the processes of translation of the findings into action-oriented policies remains. Lebanon in its current situation presents a particularly difficult case in this respect (Zurayk and Armenian, 1985).

*Strategy 8: "Development of computer resources."*

Computer systems of various forms can contribute to the process of analysis, storage and retrieval of information within a NHIS. Their acquisition is restricted, however, by the availability of financial resources. In addition, their efficient operation requires a sufficient level of skill in computer data handling among the personnel and users of the system. It is necessary for the introduction of computerized systems in the organization of a NHIS in developing countries to be gradual and selective. Such a planned process of growth has the added advantage of avoiding an untimely expansion of scope of the NHIS, in response to over-investment in computer resources.

Implementation of computer systems needs to be most selective at periphery areas. In addition to cost consideration, it is a better learning process for periphery areas to emphasize first the simplicity of collection and processing of information through a limited manual system. Health and paramedical personnel can thus achieve in-depth interaction with information handling without the complexity of understanding a computer system.

The use of computers at intermediate and central levels, on the other hand, is critical. In planning computer facilities, it is a good strategy, particularly for intermediate levels, to achieve some independence from a central computer system through the use of micro-computers. This allows for interaction with the information processed, whereas relying on a central computer facility within the Ministry or some other agency imposes definite limits on flexibility of contact with the data. Of course, when financial resources allow, a system of micros can be linked to a central system for larger memory, scope and speed in data analysis.

## IV.  CONCLUSIONS

The development of computer technology and its capacities for data linkages and complex data analysis have created a large gap in information handling potential in developed and developing countries. To strive to copy sophisticated systems is, therefore, an inefficient, frustrating and unwise process for meeting the information needs of public health policies and services in developing countries. While attempting to develop computer potential, much can be achieved through simple systems as long as the characteristics of relevance, accuracy and timeliness of the information provided to the administrators and policy makers are secured. Priority consideration should be given to the need to develop the human element at every level of interaction with the health information system, in order to ensure that adequate information is generated and that it is utilized appropriately in the planning and delivery of health services.

## ACKNOWLEGMENT

I would like to acknowledge with thanks the contribution of Fadia Saadeh, instructor in the Faculty of Health Sciences, in the preparation of this paper.

## REFERENCES

Faculty of Health Sciences, American University of Beirut. (1983). Emergency Health Surveillance Project, July-November 1982. *Weekly Epidemiological Record, 58* (2):7-9.
General Health Secretariat of Gulf Countries. (1981). Mimeographed report: Study of information and unified indicators that are used in the process of comprehensive health planning in member countries.

Green, L., Wilson, R., and Braver, K. (1983). Data requirements to measure progress on the objectives for the nation in health promotion and disease prevention. *American Journal of Public Health, 73*:18-24.

Hamadeh, R. (1980). Mimeographed report: Child Immunization Information System. Bahrain Ministry of Health, Office of Professional Standards and Systems Analysis.

Kutran, K. (1984). Mimeographed report: Progress Report on the Work of the Unit for Health System Planning. Lebanese Ministry of Public Health, Unit for Health System Planning.

Lebanese Ministry of Health, Task Force on Information. (1983). Mimeographed report: A general framework for an information system at the Ministry of Public Health.

Murnaghan, T. (1981). Health indicators and information systems for the year 2000. *Annual Reviews in Public Health, 2*:299-361.

Shah, U. (1985). Epidemiology training: a necessity for primary health care. *Journal of Epidemiology and Community Health, 39*:194-196.

Steinwachs, D. (1985). Management information systems, new challenges to meet changing needs. *Medical Care, 23* (5):607-622.

White, K. (1980). Information for health care: An epidemiological perspective. *Inquiry, 17*:296-312.

WHO. (1978). The Alma-Ata conference on primary health care. *WHO Chronicles, 32*:409-30.

Zurayk, H., and Armenian, H. (eds.). (1985). In *Beirut 1984, a Population and Health Profile.* American University of Beirut.

Zurayk, H. (1980). Mimeographed report: Progress Report and Priorities for Action for the Bahrain Ministry of Health Information System. Bahrain Ministry of Health, Office of Professional Standards and System Analysis.

# PART II

# OVERVIEW AND COMMENTARY

# THE IMPACT OF WATER AND SANITATION ON HEALTH AND DEVELOPMENT

Alan L. Sorkin

This paper is fundamentally concerned with the interrelationship between water, sanitation, health and economic progress. One objective is to provide a synthesis of the literature regarding the relationship of water supply and modern sanitation to health status. Although the connection seems inherently plausible, it has not been rigorously demonstrated. A second focus of the paper concerns selected economic aspects of water supply and sanitation programs. The relationship between water supply and economic development as well as financing issues are discussed in some detail. The above interactions are considered exclusively in terms of the developing countries.

In 1980, some 1.1 billion people in developing countries lacked sewerage facilities and an almost equal number did not have access to safe water. Given this reality, and considering expected population growth to 1990, over two billion people will have to be provided with water and modern sanitation

**Research in Human Capital Development, Vol. 5, pages 77-98.**
**Copyright © 1988 by JAI Press Inc.**
**All rights of reproduction in any form reserved.**
**ISBN: 0-89232-508-9**

facilities during the 1980s to meet the goals of the United Nations Drinking Water and Sanitation Decade. (see below)

Safe water supplies and adequate sanitation facilities for the world population by 1990—the aims of goals of the International Drinking Water and Sanitation Decade (1981-1990) are unrealistic. The World Health Organization estimated that only 22 percent of the rural population in developing countries have "reasonably safe" drinking water and 15 percent have sanitary human waste disposal facilities. (Seventy percent of the population in developing countries reside in rural areas.)[1]

Even if the funds, manpower, and management capability were available, the objectives for the decade could not be fulfilled. The greatest constraint is the paucity of skilled (including not only professional and technical workers) and semiskilled health and sanitation workers.

Estimates regarding the percentage of population covered by water or sanitation must be used carefully and with full understanding of how they were obtained. For example, the degree of rural coverage is usually based on a comparison between the reported size of the rural population served and the size of the total rural population. However, nearly all of the dispersed people served by wells or rudimentary aqueducts are often excluded from the rural "population served" figure, while all the dispersed population is generally included in the "total reported population." This situation can cause major discrepancies between the level of coverage reported and the true figure.

One of the fundamental problems in meeting the goals of the International Drinking Water and Sanitation Decade is the high cost of conventional sanitation services. Very general estimates based on existing per capita costs indicate that up to $60 billion would be required to provide a universal water supply, and from $300 to $600 billion would be needed to provide sewerage facilities for everyone. Per capita investment costs for sewerage alone range from $150 to $650, which is far beyond the ability of many recipients to pay,[2] and is considerably greater than the financial capabilities of international lending agencies.

# THE INTERRELATIONSHIP BETWEEN WATER SUPPLY, SANITATION AND HEALTH

A convenient supply of safe water and the sanitary disposal of human wastes is fundamentally necessary for good health. Water that is contaminated with pathogens can spread disease, and water that is located far from home results in the loss of productive time and energy by the water carrier. Moreover, inadequate facilities for excreta disposal increase the risk of transmitting disease and illness pathogens from sick to healthy individuals. Over 50 infections can be transferred from a diseased person to a healthy one because of poor excreta disposal methods. Given the existing level of malnutrition in developing countries, these diseases have high mortality rates, especially among children.

It is the poor who suffer the most from a lack of water and sanitation. This occurs not only because they lack the income to provide for the necessary facilities, but also because they are unaware of how to minimize the ill effects of the unsanitary conditions in which they live. As a result, the debilitating effects of endemic disease reduce the productive capacity of those individuals who already have low incomes.

## Relationship of Lack of Water and Impure Water to Particular Disease Conditions

There is some evidence that the shorter the distance from a family's home to protected water, the lower is the incidence of diarrhea.[3] Moreover, those families with water inside the house tend to have the lowest diarrheal infection rates, persons with water nearby (but outside) the home have the next lowest, and those with the water source farthest away from the house have the highest rates of infection. The ease with which reasonably good water can be obtained by users seems to be a key factor in terms of the incidence of diarrhea.

Related factors contributing to the decline in mortality from diarrheal diseases are the availability of some form of sanitary excreta disposal facility, the quality and quantity of the water supply, and the degree of health education within the community (see Table 1).

While water supply and sanitation are certainly important in controlling diarrhea, the most important factor in terms of child morbidity and mortality is the nutritional state.[4] This assertion is based on the assumption that the usual route of transmission is by hand to mouth and not by some single controllable source such as the quality of domestic water. Thus, the nutritional state of the child host is frequently more important in the etiology of the disease than the method of transmission. However, there remains some uncertainty regarding the above argument since a thorough examination of possible trade-offs between water supply and nutrition has not been completed.

As one might expect, research pertaining to skin diseases indicates that prevalence is inversely related to the quantity of water available for use. The closer the family to a protected water source, the greater the probability that family members will use water in larger quantities and that they will have a reduced incidence of skin disease.[5]

Community water supplies and modern sanitation can bring about an important reduction in cholera mortality. Existing research indicates a decline in rates of from 0 to 70 percent.[6]

Cholera is a "waterborne" disease and, therefore, the quantity of water available has nothing to do with infection rates. Protected water supplies in a specific area are associated with significantly lower cholera infection rates

*Table 1.*   The Effect of Water Supply
and Sanitation Programs in 24 Nonintervention Studies

| Parameter Affected | Number of Studies | Percent Reduction in Diarrheal Diseases (Median) |
|---|---|---|
| Water Quality | 6 | 30 |
| Water Availability through Standpipes | 11 | 34 |
| Water Quality and Availability | 4 | 40 |
| Excreta Disposable | 8 | 40 |

*Source:*   Adapted from John Briscoe, "Water Supply and Health in Developing Countries: Selective Primary Health Care Revisited," *American Journal of Public Health,* September, 1984, vol. 74, no. 9, p. 10.

in that area. Although people can travel out of the protected area, contract cholera, and bring it back into the region, the spread of cholera will be limited if there is a protected supply of water. Improved and protected excreta disposal facilities have been shown to be another important factor in the control of cholera.

With regard to the general prevention of cholera, an interesting study on the costs of alternative ways to prevent this disease was undertaken in the Philippines. Since existing evidence indicates that available anti-cholera vaccines are of limited usefulness, the costs and effects of immunization were compared with the costs and effects of providing simple privies in rural Philippine communities. The conclusion was that "sanitation (excreta disposal) proves both to be more effective and less expensive than vaccination, especially in long-term programs for control and elimination of cholera from endemic areas."[7]

Typhoid fever is another "waterborne" disease. Existing studies show that a safe water supply and proper sanitation can reduce mortality from 60 to 80 percent.[8] A simulation exercise was completed comparing the costs and effects of improved sanitation with that of immunization. It was concluded that anti-typhoid vaccine that gives high and long-lasting immunity is actually less effective and more costly in the long run than is the construction of privies.[9]

Schistosomiasis or bilharziasis is a "waterbased" disease; that is, a disease where a necessary part of the life cycle of the infecting agent occurs in aquatic animals. The disease results from infection by several species of worm which, as larvae, develop inside certain types of snails. Approximately a month after entering the snail, the larvae are shed back into the water and at this point can penetrate a person's skin upon contact.

Safe water and good sanitation can reduce deaths from schistosomiasis by approximately 50 percent.[10] One study indicated that children living in houses that did not have indoor water taps had higher schistosomiasis infection rates than children who lived in homes with such facilities. It was also shown that water supply or sanitary facilities designed to make it unnecessary for people to go near snail-infected waters generally resulted in reduced human infection rates.[11] Research in St. Lucia indicated that it was possible to encourage people to stay away from snail-infested creek water. This was done by providing alternative water facilities such as piped water to each house, community laundry and shower facilities, and swimming and wading pools for children. Tentative results indicate that "recurrent costs of the household water supplies project in the Riche Fond Valley are lower than the annual cost of mollusciding operation in a nearby valley, and after a few more years overall costs of the water supplies will probably be no greater than those of mollusciding."[12]

## METHODOLOGICAL PROBLEMS IN WATER AND SANITATION RESEARCH

There are four major methodological problems with studies that purport to demonstrate the relationship between water, sanitation and health. These are (1) lack of adequate control, (2) the one-to-one comparison, (3) confounding variables, and (4) failure to record facility usage. Each of these will be discussed in turn.

Without an adequate control group, it is impossible to distinguish between health gains resulting from water supply or sanitation improvements and health benefits that would have occurred anyway because of social, economic or environmental change. Moreover, even if no health changes appear to have occurred, no conclusions can be made because in the absence of health or sanitation improvements, health status might have declined. Alternatively it is possible that without the water and sanitation facilities health might have improved but these facilities could have resulted in the spread of infection.

Even when control communities are specified and observed for comparison with the experimental communities, it is not unusual to select a particular control community and compare it with a single experimental community. A one-to-one community comparison is analogous to basing a conclusion on the effect of a medical treatment solely on the differential response between two persons, one treated and one untreated. The sample size in each category is only one and any conclusions would lack statistical validity.

Inadequate control of confounding variables is also a major problem regarding most research of this kind.[14] Completely controlling for the large number of confounding variables that might influence the various health indicators is probably an impossible task, except in the case of a randomized intervention with sufficient numbers of villages in both groups. It is generally necessary to select only those variables which will have an important confounding effect. Thus, for example, in the case of studies of excreta disposal facilities and diarrheal disease, the major confounding variables are water supply, socioeconomic status and level of education.

Confounding variables may be dealt with in several ways. Intervention and control group selection can be based on comparability with respect to confounding variables. Alternatively, these two groups can be selected on some other basis and confounding variables can be controlled at the data analysis stage by comparing matched subsamples. These two approaches may also be combined.

Water supplies or sanitation facilities themselves have no direct impact on health. Health gains depend on the level of use and by whom they are used. It is essential to record usage activity in detail especially for the age group which has the highest incidence of disease and thus serves as the main source of infection for others. For example, in the case of diarrheal disease, it is necessary to record the defecation behavior in young children which is the group least likely to use the sanitation facilities.[15]

Collaboration between engineers (who study interventions) epidemiologists (who study health impacts) and social scientists (who study intervening processes) has been limited. This lack of interdisciplinary collaboration must be overcome if new studies of the impact of water supply and sanitation on health are to provide really new information and insights.

## WATER AND ECONOMIC DEVELOPMENT

It is generally true that a potable water supply for village residents of any region of a developing country is a necessary condition for significant economic growth and development. However, by itself, a potable water supply is usually insufficient to stimulate economic development. Thus the lack of natural and human resource development in a region may preclude an increase in economic activity even after the introduction of a piped water supply.

Part of the problem is that water for human consumption will not directly cause a change in economic output. If a long-term increase in output is one of the goals of rural water supply investment, then the latter probably should be broadened to include additional facilities or programs that complement the water program. For example (in arid regions or areas with a dry season), if a village water supply system is designed to permit the watering of livestock and the irrigation of small gardens, the likelihood that the water system will have a significant impact on the local economy is substantially increased. Providing resources for complementary programs such as health education, sanitation, feeder lots, and marketing information should also increase the probability that the water supply program will have a positive impact in terms of development.

# ECONOMIC BENEFITS THROUGH IMPROVED HEALTH

A study of the association between health and water supply systems that accurately predicts their effects on economic development and health improvement has not yet been conducted. This is because social, economic, and physical conditions vary greatly among target populations precluding accurate generalizations. Moreover, when such a study is conducted in rural areas of developing countries, sampling problems and difficulties of uncontrollable exogenous factors greatly increase the probability of significant errors in the results.[16]

Even if health effects could be accurately predicted, a related problem is that there is a considerable degree of unemployment and under-employment in the rural areas of developing countries. Therefore, a rural water supply program that is designed primarily to improve the health of the labor force may have very little impact on economic output and earnings. Moreover, most studies have shown that water-related health improvements are greatest among children. These youthful beneficiaries are not members of the labor force.

Conventional wisdom maintains that by concentrating water supply investment in so-called rural "growth points," the impact of the investment on economic development will be enhanced. With regard to water supply investment, it is possible that the village water systems, together with complementary investment programs similar to those discussed above, could reduce rural-to-urban migration rates. However, there is little evidence that, in the short run, a rural water supply program by itself will have any effect on outmigration.[17] Moreover, in the long run, if the water supply program results in a healthier, more potentially productive, rural population, the lack of rural employment opportunities would probably result in an increase in outmigration.[18] However, while the short-run outmigration effects of a rural water supply program are doubtful, it is likely that potable water supply systems can be used to encourage the concentration of previously dispersed rural populations into more economically viable village units.

If a rural water supply or waste disposal program brings about reduced water-related disease rates, and thus a healthier population, it is conceivable that the rate of growth of some categories of expenditures currently made for health and medical services could be reduced. Specifically, fewer funds might be necessary for vaccination programs (typhoid, cholera), hospital and health center facilities and equipment, physicians and staff, drugs and medicines, and transportation for health purposes. Little empirical information is available regarding the impact of water supply investments on total health expenditures.

# INCREASED TIME FOR PRODUCTIVE WORK

A nearby water supply system reduces the time required for obtaining the water needed for drinking, washing and preparing food. Those who must obtain water for family use will have more time to devote to other activities. The provision of water for the family in the rural areas of most developing countries is the primary responsibility of women and children. Because of the distance from the water source to the home, family members may spend one to four hours per day carrying water.[19]

After the introduction of a potable water supply system, women would be able to spend time formerly used in carrying water in activities which increase economic output and earnings. Alternatively the water system could result in an increase in her leisure time. If there is an overall or seasonal shortage of labor, this may make it possible to increase overall village output and income.

The impact of the installation of a convenient village water supply system on the time spent by women and children in carrying water has been studied in a number of countries. In the Lowlands of Lesotho, 30 percent of families spend over 160 minutes per day collecting water.[20] As a result of the Zaina scheme in Kenya about 100 minutes per household per day are saved from the water collecting activity.[21] In East Africa rural families spend up to 164 minutes per day carrying water; in Eastern Nigeria families spend up to 300 minutes per day collecting water.[22]

However, in a study of nine Tanzanian villages where agricultural work occupied the largest share of time of a majority of married women, these individuals were asked what they would do if they had more time available. Less than half said they would spend it on agricultural work.[23]

In another study carried out in the small village of Kpomkpo in Southeast Ghana, women were asked how they would allocate their time if a new water system saved them about twelve hours per week.[24] There responses were distributed as follows:

| Activity | Hours | Percent |
|---|---|---|
| Directly Productive | 6.8 | 57 |
| Household Jobs | 4.2 | 35 |
| Leisure | 0.9 | 8 |
| Total | 11.9 | 100 |

In the above example, the women did, in fact, have the opportunity to engage in productive work, which involved cassava and charcoal production. As a result, an estimate of the value of the time which would not have to be used fetching water was made by multiplying the average returns to labor from cassava and charcoal production (by month) times 0.57, the time saved in obtaining water. In this case, it was assumed that the returns to labor were constant, that is marginal returns were equal to average returns.

However, even if there were no evidence that the time saved from no longer carrying water is directly used for productive activities, "saving time is development, for time saved from humdrum tasks is time to invest in human capital."[25] Thus priority should be given to technologies that reduce the time women and children spend obtaining wood and water and preparing food.

## COST EFFECTIVENESS OF HEALTH AND SANITATION PROGRAMS

The World Bank has estimated that the cost of providing water supplies and sanitation to all those in need by the year 2000 will range from $135 to $260 billion. Construction of a rural community standpipe costs $20-$26 per capita, and rural sanitation costs $4 to $5 per capita. In urban areas the costs are $31 and $23 respectively.[26]

The above cost figures are primarily for public standpipes, which are generally not highly effective in reducing morbidity and mortality from water related diseases. Water connections inside the house are typically necessary to encourage the hygienic use of water. For example, shigella-caused diarrheas decreased 5 percent with outside house connections but fell 50 percent when sanitation and washing facilities were available within the home.[27]

Walsh and Warren indicate that from a cost-effectiveness standpoint water supplies and sanitation are far less effective in comparison with other health interventions (see Table 2). They conclude that selective primary health care is far more cost-effective than any of the other health interventions.

These results have been severely criticized by Briscoe[28] who argues that in cost-effectiveness calculations it is the *net* rather than the *gross* cost which should be used. In the case of water supplies this can make a major difference since many poor people (particularly in the cities) presently pay substantial amounts of money for poor quality water supplies.

In terms of cost-effectiveness analysis, the net economic cost of water supply improvements may be far less than the total cost of the project. This is because a large percentage of total costs represent redirected expenditures that were previously incurred by the population for a poor quality water supply service.

Moreover, in the case of water supply and sanitation, infant death reduction is one result but not the only outcome. In the Walsh-Warren analysis (see Table 2), water supply and sanitation programs are compared with interventions aimed specifically at reducing infant mortality. Not surprisingly, they conclude that the programs which affect only infant mortality are more effective than

*Table 2.*   Estimated Annual Costs of
Different Systems of Health Intervention

| Intervention | Per Capita Cost | Cost Per Infant and/or Child Death Averted |
|---|---|---|
| Basic Primary Health | | |
| Range | $0.40-$7.50 | 144-20,000 (I) |
| Median | $2.00 | 700 |
| Mosquito Control for Malaria | $2.00 | 600 (I) |
| Onchocerciasis Control Program | $0.90 | Few infant and child deaths |
| Mullosk Control for Schistosomiasis | $3.70 | Few infant and child deaths |
| Community Water Supplies & Sanitation | $30-$54 | 3600-4300 (I,C) |
| Narangwal Nutrition Supplementation | $1.75 | 213 (I) |
| Selective Primary Health Care | $0.25 | 200-250 (I,C) |

*Notes:*   I denotes infant
C denotes child
1 delivered by village health workers
2 in this case, delivered by mobile units

*Source:*   Adapted from Julia Walsh and Kenneth Warren, "Selective Primary Health Care: An Interim Strategy for Disease Control in Developing Countries," *The New England Journal of Medicine,* vol. 301, no. 18, November 1, 1979, p. 973.

programs which have multiple impact. However, even with the above criticisms, it is unlikely that community water supplies and sanitation are as cost-effective as selective primary health care.

# RURAL WATER PROGRAMS

Rural sociologists have developed the term "rurban" by combining the words rural and urban. The term refers to those population centers (i.e., villages) that are located in areas where most of the people make their living from agriculture, hunting, fishing, or any combination of these occupations.[29]

In developing rural water programs the most common approach has been to first construct those water systems which have the lowest costs. This has resulted in most of the systems having gravity supplies or wells, with a relatively large (15 to 20 percent) community contribution toward the construction cost. The tendency has been to emphasize water and sanitation projects in the high income rural areas. The approach has been justified on the grounds that it permits the quickest flow of funds into the program. The money can

Table 3. Characteristics of the Rural Program

| Type of Program | Population Served | Source | Distribution Systems | Water Delivered | Local Organization | Financial Recovery |
|---|---|---|---|---|---|---|
| Well | Dispersed | Well or protected spring | None | At well only | None | None |
| Rudimentary | Semi-concentrated | Pumped well or protected spring | Simple | Public fountains plus a few patio connections | Little, mainly for operations and maintenance | Little or none |
| Rurban | Concentrated with 500 person core | Well, spring, or treatment plant | Serves rural plus nearly concentrated areas | Patio connections and a few public fountains | Strong for operations maintenance, administration, and rate collection | Recovery for operations, maintenance, local administration, and reserve |

Source: Adapted from David Donaldson, "Overview of Rural Water and Sanitation Programs for Latin America," *Journal of the American Water Association*, May, 1983, p. 227.

subsequently be used for supplying water to areas with higher costs, thereby providing the maximum possible coverage in the shortest time.

The rural water programs constructed since 1960 have consisted of three types:

1.   Protected springs or wells—These basic programs involve developing a single source of water such as a spring or a well that is equipped with a hand pump to serve a number of scattered families. The operation of such a system is not dependent on a community organization and is usually maintained and paid for by central government funds at no cost to the users.

2.   Rudimentary aqueducts—A rudimentary aqueduct uses a well or spring supplemented by a small storage tank to provide limited distribution of water to a semi-concentrated population through public fountains and a limited number of patio connections. The users pay a small sum but depend heavily on the government to maintain, operate, and expand such systems.

3.   Individual house connections—This type of program is usually designed to serve communities with a central core of at least 100 houses. These systems, often called "rurban" systems (see above), normally consist of a protected spring, a pumped well, or a treatment plant that delivers water to a storage tank. The system supplies water through house or patio connections and makes minimal use of public fountains. A local water board, assisted by the national program, operates, maintains, and administers the system and collects water fees.[30] The characteristics of the different rural programs are summarized in Table 3.

Experience has shown that each of the three types of programs discussed above should be considered steps in an evolutionary process. For example, in one country it was found that community wells attracted households, and the population increased around 10-12 percent near the community wells. When the density became sufficiently high, local demand became so great that rudimentary aqueducts, using the original wells as the water source, were developed in several locations. This change from wells to rudimentary aqueduct systems took an average of 12 to 15 years. In piped systems a similar change from public fountains to patio connections took an average of eight to ten years. It was found that progress from one stage to the next could be advanced if coordinated efforts replaced independent programs.

## CASE STUDY

In Bhutan the lack of a safe drinking water supply is the chief cause of disease. The mortality rate of children increases sharply after the first year, mainly because of unhygienic weaning practices and the lack of clean water. Thus,

64 percent of major diseases in Bhutan are water related.[31] The mountainous terrain imposes severe burdens on the family's time and energy in regard to obtaining water, especially for women. When available, the water is too cold for bathing during most of the year. There is no tradition of sanitary disposal of human and animal waste.

In Bhutan the water supply and sanitation programs must be developed together. Fecal-borne diseases accounted for 72 percent of all infections reported in 1979. Understanding of personal cleanliness is minimal and when "Western-style" flush toilets have been installed, these tend to become clogged up by dry materials such as leaves and twigs because of local cleansing habits.

Responding to this acute need for clean and reliable drinking water and for adequate sanitation, the Bhutan government has outlined an ambitious plan for 1981-87.[32] It proposes to eliminate water and sanitation-related health problems in the rural sector and expects that by the year 2000, some 4,500 villages will have clean water and the majority of families will have the appropriate types of sanitary latrines.

Bhutan has a large number of streams, rivers, and springs. It has been demonstrated that the most economical method of using them to bring water to villages is with the gravity flow system. Once properly installed, these systems require very little maintenance and they can be combined with a filtration system of gravel and sand to make the water drinkable. Because rural settlements in Bhutan are small and scattered, the cost of providing piped water is quite high. While plastic pipes are cheaper than iron ones, the total cost is approximately $7,500 per scheme and the 1981-87 plan will mean an investment of about $34 million for the fittings, pipes, and equipment.

## FINANCING COMMUNITY WATER SUPPLY

The financing schemes used for rural and urban projects are often quite different. In urban projects the most frequently used approach is to set the water rate at a level which recovers the total costs (i.e., the operational, loan, and administration costs, as well as a reserve for future expansion). Thus, each project is expected to be a self-sufficient entity. Because of their smaller size and the widespread poverty of the rural population, rural projects usually cannot be financed in a similar manner.[33]

In Latin America, the financing of a rural project is usually made up of three elements: local contribution of labor, construction materials and/or cash (15-20 percent of the project cost); an international loan for pipes, fittings, and pumps (50 percent); and an annual grant to cover program overhead and operational expenses (30-35 percent). The cost of operation and maintenance, as well as partial repayment of the loan, is borne by the community. The program covers the remaining loan expenses from its yearly appropriation (in one major country the rural aqueducts pay for all of the loan costs). In other parts of the world the grant portion is higher as the communities repay less of the loan costs.

At the present time, many governments are heavily subsidizing the construction and operation of rural water systems. Because of the uncertainty regarding continuation of funds, this type of subsidy requires a project by project approach. Rather than rely on government subsidies, experience has shown the benefits of using revolving funds to support these programs. (See below). In addition, the revolving funds—once they become self-sustaining—can be used to supplement community self-help for other undertakings designed to improve quality of life in rural locations.[34]

Rural construction is frequently subsidized, at least in part, with national and state funds. It is also common to borrow funds abroad for such projects, including funds to cover some local currency requirements. Some countries have a policy of providing major concessions to local communities for repayment of debt on water and sanitation facilities, or make no effort to collect the full costs from those who benefit from the facilities. In such situations, it should be asked whether borrowing foreign funds (on which substantial interest is charged) is sound policy.

For a given investment over a 15 to 20 year period, a country may build more rural systems with its own money than it would with borrowed money by an amount equivalent to the interest paid. Moreover, if it obtains, for example, a 5 percent 20-year loan, it will pay $1.6 million in interest for every $1 million of principal received.

However, an alternative view is that systems will get constructed earlier with borrowed money, and so the anticipated improvements in public health and living standards will be realized almost immediately.[35]

## Financing Operation and Maintenance

Regarding water systems, it is typically found that about one half of total costs reflects operation and maintenance activities. Thus, every community, regardless of size, must generate revenue covering at least the full cost of operation and maintenance from the sale of water and services. Without adequate and continually available funds for the operation and maintenance of a system, investment in that system will fail to generate satisfactory returns. This is true because the full benefits of a water supply or modern sanitation system are realized only when the facility is available for people to use all of the time.

Most water supply cost estimates have overlooked the investments that will be needed for major repairs and replacements. At the municipal level, efficient water organizations can usually provide financing for some major items that wear out through reserves that are generated via the provision of services.

Generally, overall annual depreciation of a water system is commonly estimated at 1.5 to 3.0 percent of the facility's cost. Most international agencies recommend that charges for water cover depreciation or debt service, whichever is larger, as well as the operation and maintenance costs.[36] When the organizations responsible for providing water and sanitation services are following sound financial policies, it will normally be possible to absorb occasional large expenditures from built-up reserves.

Subsidies for operation vary widely, ranging from the situation in which the water utility is owned and operated by the regional agency, to the opposite extreme in which the municipality assumes the entire operational responsibility. The majority of projects fall somewhere between the above cases, with federal or state agencies providing technical assistance and some financial subsidy.

## REVOLVING FUNDS

A formal definition of the term revolving fund is "a fund that is continually replenished as it is used, either through further appropriation or by income generated by the activity that it finances."[37]

It terms of a rural water program, a revolving fund implies the establishment of a monetary account, on a regional or national level, to finance the construction of the individual community projects. The funds that are lent out are recovered by having the assisted community make repayment to the revolving fund. As the repayments are made, thay are reloaned to finance additional projects. The method of obtaining the original financing for the fund, the terms of the loans, and the terms of the repayment, vary considerably. Various approaches have been evolved to adapt the revolving fund concept to the social and economic potential of the community and to the financial realities of the country as a whole. The adaptation to local conditions is one of the strengths of this method of financing.

In general, the establishment of revolving funds has followed these overall patterns:[38]

1. A grant is used to obtain the initial funds. These funds are maintained by relending the payments as they are collected.
2. The fund is created by means of a loan, and then maintained by using the surplus income produced by the difference between the payments and conditions for amortizing the loan and the payments made by the communities.
3. A third pattern is for the fund to be infused with the income generated by community reimbursement of a loan (national or international) which is serviced by the national government.

# MANPOWER PROBLEMS

Water and sanitation systems which should operate with good routine maintenance have frequently become inoperable after less than five years. The technologies may be appropriate and low in cost, but the manpower needed for maintenance and operation is usually allocated elsewhere or not trained at all. The shortage of manpower is obvious at the professional, technical, and semiskilled levels. International aid offers technical assistance in the form of advisors or consultants, but because too few local people qualify as effective counterparts, these advisors are quickly absorbed into the bureaucracy. Initially hired on a temporary basis, the expatriate too often comes a permanent or simipermanent employee. The system becomes self-perpetuating as expatriate contracts are renewed. This form of aid is welcomed by donors who want to keep funds "in-house" and highly visible, and by the expatriate who may find it increasingly difficult to find comparable employment at home.[39]

Because water and sanitation activities can be placed under a variety of governmental jurisdictions, the issue concerning training programs is complex. At the professional level, sanitary engineers are qualified through postgraduate engineering courses, which follow undergraduate studies in civil engineering. Since sanitary engineering curriculums often emphasize theoretical knowledge, water ministries have sometimes been required to establish their own training programs in order to provide practical information to recent graduates.

Training courses have generally developed individually, corresponding to divisions in institutional responsibilities with each group responding to its own confined market. For sanitation-oriented personnel, this has led to dead-end careers and frustration. However, water supply and sanitation are interdependent. The fact that responsibility for their implementation is often the duty of separate ministries does not eliminate the need for training curriculums to include material concerning both water and sanitation. Lack of knowledge in both sectors results in mistakes by field workers. This lack of coordination can result in, for example, the water supply authority installing shallow wells topographically below latrines that have been located with the advice of the health ministry. Moreover, water supplies are frequently installed without related education on how water can be used to improved health. Without any improvement in hygiene, water can hardly be expected to have any significant impact on health.

# TRAINING PARAPROFESSIONAL RURAL WATER TECHNICIANS

One of the most critical problems facing rural development of water supplies and sanitation programs is the severe shortage of intermediate level technicians.

At the apex of the skill spectrum are the civil engineers involved in this field. Unfortunately, most civil engineers working in developing countries come from relatively affluent, urban backgrounds. This often has the result of separating them culturally from their poor, often illiterate, rural clients. Thus, many of these engineers are unwilling to spend days and weeks in the field and are often unable to communicate effectively with the villagers. Moreover, civil engineers are scarce and expensive to train and employ in developing countries.

At the opposite end of the skills distribution there are masons, plumbers, and other tradesmen who may actually be more qualified than engineers to deal effectively with rural people. However, they are unable to perform many of the technical tasks associated with design and construction.[40]

Agua del Pueblo (see below) has developed a training course to deal with the shortage of intermediate-level technicians. A comprehensive modular curriculum is based on the actual tasks to be performed by program personnel. Paraprofessional technicians who are trained in the course graduate with a practical knowledge of project planning and administration, community promotion and organization, surveying, hydraulic design, construction techniques, health education, latrine construction, operation and maintenance procedures, soil and water conservation, and other essential activities. After graduation, these technicians are able to plan, design, and construct village water projects with a minimum of supervision.

The first rural water technicians learned their skills on the job while working in Agua del Pueblo's construction programs. Because of the need for such human resources in other organizations, Agua del Pueblo later developed a structured six-month training program.

## CASE STUDIES OF FINANCING AND MANPOWER DEVELOPMENT FOR RURAL WATER PROGRAMS

The government of Brazil has established a water and sewer revolving fund that makes loans to the states in order to establish loan funds that, in turn, are used to pay for the construction of small community water systems. Once the system is in operation, the consumer pays the state water agency on the basis of metered use or, in some cases, a flat rate. The rates charged vary among the states, with the poorer ones obtaining a lower rate of interest on loans from the federal government, than those with higher per capita incomes. This permits the former to charge lower water rates. In all cases, however, the states must repay the loans to the federal government. The loans are indexed to the cost of living and, therefore, maintain their real value, an essential requirement in a country where inflation can be as high as 90 to 100 percent per year. Any subsidy to the local community in terms of reduced water rates is a matter of state policy.

Federal funds for water supply are administered by the Brazilian National Housing Bank (BNH), the custodian of social security funds. This federal agency has a cautious lending policy, and delinquency in amortization has not been a serious problem. In the states, however, there has been considerable difficulty in maintaining water rates at a level that will repay the cost of the system as well as covering operation and maintenance. Many of the states in the poorer parts of Brazil have had to subsidize the water systems of smaller communities.[39]

The major difference between the Brazilian approach and what is normally understood as a water/sanitation revolving fund is that the funds, after being repaid to BNH, do not necessarily find their way back out to other water and sanitation projects—because they may be used in a number of other sectors where BNH has interests.

Since 1977, Agua del Pueblo, in cooperation with the Behrhorst Clinic Foundation and the Guatemelan Ministry of Public Health, has adminsitered a program of "soft" project loans to communities from a revolving fund. An analysis of the costs for three communities that participated in this program in 1981 showed that community contributions of materials, contracted labor, and the value of voluntary labor, were on average 81 percent of total costs. Amortization payments are recycled through the revolving loan fund and are used to make subsequent loans to other communities for water projects.

At the same time, the program develops invaluable local skills and experience in the management of credit. Most of these communities have had no previous experience with credit. In several villages the experience acquired in managing project loans has subsequently been applied to obtaining loans from other institutions for additional self-initiated community improvements. For example, the village of Pacul negotiated another loan from the government's agricultural development bank shortly after the water project was completed. This second loan allowed the construction of a small-scale irrigation system that resulted in significant improvements in crop yields.[40]

A successful project loan program involves administrative and financial training for members of local water committees. These individuals must manage the loan, maintain financial records, collect monthly payments from each family, and deliver payments to the water program offices. None of the water committees that participated in the training program are behind in their payments to the revolving fund.

Training village personnel in practical skills required for operation and maintenance of the program is essential for program success. During construction of Agua del Pueblo projects, selected villagers were trained to identify system breakdowns, to repair pipes, to clean valves and tanks periodically, and to repair or replace faulty faucets. A maintenance fee of 35 cents per family per month was collected and the proceeds were retained in the community for this purpose. A small supply of replacement pipes, accessories, and a few simple tools for use in the village were included in the original project budget. Local water committee members were taught how and where to acquire other supplies when needed, and were encouraged to call on Agua del Pueblo officials if problems arose that could not be solved locally. To date all completed systems are fully operational. Some Agua del Pueblo assistance was required after the disastrous 1976 earthquake to repair major damage promptly, but all routine operation and maintenance functions have been competently managed since that time by trained villagers using locally collected funds.

Another example of a national program serving small villages is the one developed in Panama with the assistance of the Agency for International Developement. In 1972 and 1976, loans totaling $13.3 million were approved by AID for improving rural health in Panama. Approximately $6 million was allocated for public health, primarily through construction of piped water systems for villages with 250-500 residents.[41]

Many of the systems were originally operated by diesel or gasoline pumps. Because of rising fuel costs, about half had been converted to gravity systems by 1980. A random evaluation at that time of 26 of the systems showed that 16 of them were functioning well with effective management, adequate maintenance, and regular collection of user fees. The other 10 were having some problems, but it appeared that they would be resolved in the near future.

This relatively successful piped water program has several important characteristics: (1) the existence of trained community personnel, (2) monthly charges for water ranging from $0.25 to $3.00 per household (the higher fees were for the fuel-operated systems), (3) community participation in the installation of the systems, (4) use of the system for most household needs, and (5) good quality water. In addition, the project was reported to be useful because the implementation process encouraged self-reliance and the emergence of effective local leadership.

In the communities judged to be too small for piped systems, AID loans partially financed the installation of 1600 hand pumps. It was estimated that after some time, about half were not operative. An evaluation suggested that hand pumps could be made more reliable if communities assumed some responsibility for pump maintenance and repair, and if pumps that were more easily repaired were used.

The following conclusions are based on the evaluation report:[42]

1.  The organization of a national effort to construct piped water systems is likely to be successful only if it is preceded by small-scale programs that permit development of managerial expertise and use appropriate system designs.

2.  Rural piped water systems are more likely to remain in operation when there is demand for household water, when community residents participate

in obtaining and maintaining the system, and all persons have equal access to the water.

3.  Small rural water systems require periodic monitoring and technical support to remain operational and safe. Regular inspection visits by a back-up team provide opportunities to resolve difficulties before they threaten the operation of the water system.

4.  Some mechanism must be available to enable communities to finance the cost of expansion, major repairs, or conversions to alternative energy sources, i.e., program funding or revolving funds.

5.  Chemical treatment of filtration may be avoided if groundwater is clear and potable, even in piped water systems larger than those contemplated under current AID loans.

6.  Training for rural sanitarians should be updated and the division of labor between engineers and village personnel reviewed.

## NOTES AND REFERENCES

1.  McGarry, M., and E. Schiller, "Manpower Development for Water and Sanitation Programs in Africa," *Journal of the American Water Works Association,* June, 1981, p. 282.

2.  The World Bank, "Appropriate Technology for Water Supply and Sanitation: A Summary of Technical and Economic Options" (mimeographed), December, 1980, p. 1.

3.  Saunders, R., and J. Warford, *Village Water Supply: Economics and Policy in the Developing World* (Baltimore, Maryland: The Johns Hopkins University Press for the World Bank, 1976), p. 39.

4.  Scrimshaw, N.S., "Synergism of Malnutrition and Infection: Evidence from Field Studies in Guatemala," *Journal of the American Medical Association,* Vol. 212, June, 1970, pp. 1685-1692.

5.  Saunders, R., and J. Warford, op. cit., p. 40.

6.  Azurin, J.C., and M. Alvero, "Field Evaluation of Environmental Sanitation Measures Against Cholera," *Bulletin of the World Health Organization,* Vol. 2, 1972, pp. 985-987; R. J. Levine, M. R. Khan, and S. D'Souza et al., "Failure of Sanitary Wells to Protect Against Cholera and Other Diarrheas in Bangladesh," *Lancet,* Vol. 2, 1976, pp. 86-89.

7.  Cyjetanovic, B., "Sanitation versus Vaccination in Cholera Control: Cost Effectivenss and Cost-Benefit Aspects," in *Strategy of Cholera Control* (Geneva: World Health Organization, 1971), pp. 17-24

8.  Zahere, M., B. G. Prasad and K. K. Govil et al., "A Note on Urban Water Supply in Uttar Prodesh," *Journal of the Indian Medical Association,* Vol. 38, 1962, pp. 17-82.

9.  Cjetanovic, B., B. Grab, and K. Uemura, "Epidemiological Model of Typhoid Fever and Its Use in Planning and Evaluation of Antityphoid Immunization and Sanitation Programs," *Bulletin of the World Health Organization,* Vol. 45, No. 1, pp. 53-75.

10.  Jordan, P., "Schistosomiasis-Research to Control," *American Journal of Tropical Medicine and Hygiene,* Vol. 26, 1972, pp. 877-887; M. Khalil, "The Relation Between Sanitation and Parasitic Infections in the Tropics," *Journal of the Royal Sanitary Institute,* vol. 27, 1926, pp. 210-215.

11.  Saunders, R., and J. Warford, op. cit., p. 41.

12. Jordan, P. et al., Control of Schistosoma Mansoni Transmission by *Provision of Domestic Water Supplies in St. Lucia: A Preliminary Report* (New York: The Rockefeller Foundation, 1974), p. 36.

13. Deborah Blum and Richard Feachem, "Measuring the Impact of Water Supply and Sanitation Investments on Diarrheal Diseases: Problems of Methodology," *International Journal of Epidemiology,* Vol. 12, No. 3, p. 360.

14. Blum and Feachem, op. cit., p. 361.

15. Briscoe, John, "The Role of Water Supply in Improving Health in Poor Countries (with special reference to Bangladesh)," *American Journal of Clinical Nutrition,* November, 1978, Vol. 31, pp. 2100-2113.

16. Saunders, R., "Economic Benefits of Potable Water Supplies in Rural Areas of Developing Countries," *Journal of the American Water Works Association,* June, 1975, p. 315.

17. Levy, M., and W. Wadyki, "Lifetime Versus One-Year Migration in Venezuela," *Journal of Regional Science,* Vol. 12, No. 3, 1972, p. 407.

18. Riddell, B., and M.E. Harvey, "The Urban System in the Migration Process: An Evaluation of Step-Wise Migration in Sierra Leone," *Economic Geography,* Vol. 48, July, 1972, p. 270.

19. White, G., D. Bradley, and A. White, *Drawers of Water: Domestic Water Use in East Africa* (Chicago: University of Chicago Press, 1972, p. 107).

20. R. Feachem, E. Burns, S. Cairncross, A. Cronin, P. Eross, D. Curtis, M. K. Kah, D. Lamb, H. Southall, *Water, Health and Development: An Interdisciplinary Education* (London, Tri-Med, 1978).

21. Carruthers, I.D., *Impact and Economics of Community Water Supply: A Study of Rural Water Investment in Kenya* (London, Agrarian Development Unit, Wye College, 1973).

22. White, Bradley and White, op. cit., p. 93.

23. Warner, D., *Rural Water Supply and Development: A Comparison of Nine Villages in Tanzania,* Economic Research Bureau Paper No. 69.17 (Dar es Salam: University College, 1969), p. 14.

24. Dalton, G. E. and R. N. Parker, *Agriculture in South East Ghana,* Vol. 2 (Reading, United Kingdom, University of Reading, 1973).

25. Birdsall, N. and W. P. Greevey, "The Second Sex in the Third World: Is Female Poverty and Development Issue?" Workshop on Women in Poverty. Washington, D.C., International Center for Research on Women, 1978, pp. 1-36.

26. Walsh, Julia and Kenneth Warren, "Selective Primary Health Care: An Interim Strategy for Disease Control in Developing Countries," *New England Journal of Medicine,* Vol. 301, No. 18, November 1, 1979, p. 971.

27. Hollister, A. C., M. D. Beck, A. M. Gittlesohn et al., "Influence of Water Availability on Shigella Prevalence in Children of Farm Labor Families," *American Journal of Public Health,* Vol. 45, 1955, pp. 354-362.

28. Briscoe, John, "Water Supply and Health and Development Countries: Selective Primary Health Care Revisited," *American Journal of Public Health,* Vol. 74, No. 9, September, 1984, pp. 1009-1013.

29. Davee, R., "Rural Water Supply Services: Community Financing," Special Meeting of Ministers of Health Interm REMSA/INF112.

30. Donaldson, D., "Overview of Rural Water and Sanitation Programs for Latin America," *Journal of the American Water Works Association,* May, 1983, pp. 226-227.

31. Nath, U. R., "The Cost of Water," *World Health Magazine,* April-May, 1983, p. 7.

32. Nath, U. R., op. cit., p. 9

33. Donaldson, D., "Rural Water Supplies in Developing Countries," *Water Resources Bulletin,* Vol. 8, No. 2, April, 1972, p. 394.

34. Ibid.

35. Shipman, H., "Strategies for Financing Water and Sanitation Projects," *PAHO Bulletin,* Vol. 15, No. 3, 1983, p. 211.

36.   Shipman, H., op. cit., p. 212.
37.   Donaldson, D., "Rural Water Supplies...," op. cit., p. 396.
38.   Shipman, H., op. cit., p. 213.
39.   Karp, A., and S. Cox, "Building Water and Sanitation Projects in Rural Guatemala," *Journal of the American Water Works Association,* April, 1982, pp. 166-167.
40.   Wagner, E. G., "The Latin American Approach to Improving Water Supplies," *Journal of the American Water Works Association,* April, 1983, p. 170.
41.   Mechan, R., and A. Viveros-Lang, "Panama: Rural Water-Project Import Evaluation" (draft), Washington, D.C.: Agency for International Development, November, 1981.
42.   Donaldson, D., "Overview of Rural Water...," op. cit., p. 229.

# DETERMINANTS OF DRUG IMPORTS
# TO POOR COUNTRIES:
## PRELIMINARY FINDINGS AND IMPLICATIONS
## FOR FINANCING PRIMARY HEALTH CARE

David W. Dunlop and A. Mead Over

## ABSTRACT

Financing Primary Health Care in poor countries has become an important implementation problem which must be resolved in order for the successful achievement of the international objective of Health for All by the Year 2000. In the last several years increasing attention has been devoted to the resolution of this financing problem by countries of the third world and also by donors. Willingness to pay for health care services as well as social insurance schemes have been considered and analyzed in various settings. However, such domestic resource mobilization efforts fail to take into consideration that a large share of the resources necessary to operate a health care delivery system in poor countries comes from nondomestic sources and, thus, requires foreign exchange.

**Research in Human Capital Development, Vol. 5, pages 99-125.**
**Copyright © 1988 by JAI Press Inc.**
**All rights of reproduction in any form reserved.**
**ISBN: 0-89232-508-9**

A foreign exchange shortage affects a population's health status as a result of four linked effects. These four effects are (a) the *allocation* of scarce foreign exchange towards or away from health care inputs, (2) the altered *production* process resulting from changed availability of foreign-exchange-using resources, (3) the altered *consumption* of health services resulting from changes in the relative prices of different health care services, and (4) the *health-status* effect of a changed mix of health care services.

The empirical part of this paper first presents data showing that foreign exchange typically comprises about 40 percent of the total cost of operating a health care system in a poor country. Most of this foreign exchange pays for imported drugs and the logistics of distributing them. The role of foreign imports is examined in the context of Tanzania's attempts to implement a primary health care strategy.

Then the empirical analysis focuses on the first link in the relationship between a foreign exchange shortage and a possible reduction in health status—the allocation effect. Using multiple regression analysis on time series data from seven countries, the paper explores hypotheses regarding the determinants of per capita drug imports. The results support the hypotheses that a country's macroeconomic health and its microeconomic supply of health care facilities influence per capita drug imports in expected ways in some countries but suggest that other factors— including some for which measures are not yet available—may be crucial to understanding and predicting the pattern of drug imports.

Under the assumption that the results of the ungoverned operation of the allocation, production, consumption and health status effects are quite negative, the paper concludes with a discussion of policies that could protect a nation's health status in periods of foreign exchange scarcity through interventions at each of these four stages. Opportunities for effective policy initiatives are available to both the affected countries and to donors.

# I. INTRODUCTION

In a recent *New York Times* article, the author, Sheila Rule, captures the essence of the health care delivery problems facing a poor country, Kenya, and the role of foreign exchange using resources in the provision of health care to those afflicted. She writes:

At a small health clinic here [in Kisumu, Kenya]...five nurses and a clinic officer are confronted with as many as 300 new patients a day...under Jomo Kenyatta, Kenya's first President after the nation gained independence more than 20 years ago, the Government developed a set of social programs that were virtually unrivaled in the region...The leader for the past six years, President Daniel arap Moi, has moved to strengthen the basic services. But the goal of adequate care for all increasingly appears unattainable [due to high population growth] combined with an unsteady economy [which place] growing pressures on the budget, erode living standards and overwhelm social services. The health workers (at the clinic) report shortages of everything from drugs to medical journals and books. At one center, four of five vans were out of commission recently because there was no money for repairs. At other times, there is not enough money to buy gasoline.[1]

In the above story, all of the items mentioned which are in short supply require foreign exchange to procure. Similar shortage problems exist in the health programs of a number of other poor countries, particularly in Africa.

At the same time, in another recent *Wall Street Journal* article (April 11, 1985), Art Pine reports on an increasingly serious possibility facing the IMF:

> the possibility that African countries may be unable to repay billions of dollars in IMF loans over the next two years...Both IMF and U.S. officials view economic prospects for the region as grim for the foreseeable future...[however] the industrial countries want to avoid widespread defaults to the IMF even if they have to subsidize repayment on the ground that defaults could undermine the effectiveness of the 146 country organization. A country that is too far in arrears isn't allowed to borrow more from the IMF until it resumes repayment. The IMF itself hasn't proferred any solution to the African problem, although it has been discussing the situation at length. For the IMF managing director, Jacques de Larosiere, is said to be taking a tough approach in demanding prompt repayment, in line with general fund policies toward borrowing countries. But U.S. officials say they doubt the organization can continue that posture indefinitely.[2]

The realities facing the IMF and the rural health workers in Kenya are in conflict. Most countries in Africa and many others in Latin America and Asia are facing, and will continue to face, severe balance of payment crises for at least the next five years. In 1984, the World Bank projected both continued slow GDP growth and eroding balance of payments for African and non-African countries throughout the 1980s.[3] Thus, the amount of foreign exchange available in most poor countries will be limited for the foreseeable future.

Concern for developing primary health care systems which are low cost has been expressed since the initiation of the primary health care strategy to achieve "Health Care for All by the Year 2000" in 1978.[4] In addition, many countries and donors have made significant progress toward financing, part of the recurrent cost of primary health care activities through local efforts—from fees for service to cooperative insurance schemes.[5] To note the importance of the financing problem, the World Health Assembly will address this matter in its next annual meeting in 1986. However, none of the above efforts have focused on the foreign exchange aspect of the problem which is the subject of this paper.

## II. AN ANALYTICAL FRAMEWORK

As was highlighted in the first story presented, a shortage of foreign exchange, which is a macroeconomic problem, is having substantial effects on the microeconomies of health care delivery in rural health clinics. The two issues which this paper wishes to raise regarding this link are (a) what are the effects of a foreign exchange shortage on the health care and the health status of poor countries? and (b) can "low cost" policies be devised to enable poor countries to manage a period of foreign exchange scarcity with minimal negative consequences for the health care delivery system?

A foreign exchange shortage in a poor country affects the health care provided and possibly the health status of its population via several intermediate causal links, none of which is well understood.[6] These links can be labeled as follows: (a) the allocation effect; (b) the production effect; (c) the consumption effect; and (d) the health status effect.

## A.  The Allocation Effect

Public and private decision makers, when faced with a reduction in foreign exchange availability, must decide how to allocate this reduction. These decisions reveal the preferences of these decision makers and of their constituencies as well as their perceptions of the political sensitivity of budget categories and of the likelihood that budget cuts in some sectors will be compensated by increased international assistance. This paper presents the results of an empirical investigation of the effects on expenditures on drug imports of these allocation decisions.

## B.  The Production Effect

As a consequence of the budgetary allocation decisions defined above, specific budget reductions often change the relative availability of inputs used in the production of health care services within each clinic and hospital. When certain resources such as drugs and other medical supplies are only sporadically available, the ability of health care providers to accomplish their work is eroded.[7]

Typically the ratios of imported drugs and gasoline to domestic labor input are greatly reduced when trade imbalances persist. Without adequate supplies of drugs and other medical supplies, and without the resources required to store, move, and secure them, and to supervise their use, the quantity and quality of basis curative medical care is eroded. When such deficiencies become apparent to the general public in any country around the world today, the perceived quality of care is eroded.

Finally, if the health care production process is inflexible, such that there is little substitutability between the foreign and domestically supplied inputs, a reduction in the availability of a fully utilized resource like drugs would inexorably lead to a reduction in total output by the system as a whole. Such inflexibility in the production process could be the result of specific service delivery protocols not easily amenable to change in the short run.

## C. The Consumption Effect

From the point of view of the consumer, the reduced productivity of the health care system operated by the government would imply either more trips and greater effort and/or higher side-payments to obtain any given level of health care from that system. These adjustments are equivalent to an upward shift in the supply of government provided health care services, such as that from $S_1$ to $S_2$ in panel (a) of Figure 1.

The consumer would react to this upward shift in supply by decreasing his consumption of government provided health care services (from $Q_1$ to $Q_2$) and either substituting private sector (from $q_1$ to $q_2$) health care or reducing health care consumption, or both. The increased demand for privately supplied care and/or drugs will increase their prices (from $p_1$ to $p_2$) and produce monopoly rents for their suppliers, at lease in the medium run. What has been observed in many countries around the world are long queues for a few days after the drugs and medicines have been delivered, with a significant decline in utilization after the initial flurry of activity. During the last half of the usual resupply period, few if any people attend the clinic, unless under great duress. Such fluctuating utilization patterns are most noticeable in the more remote areas of a country. Thus, without ensuring continuously available supplies of drugs and related inputs, governments will not be able to effectively alter the above-described utilization patterns, since service quality is not ensured.

## D. The Health Status Effect

The change in health status or family planning resulting from a change in either the amount or mix of health care consumption is not well understood.[8] The common presumption is that an adverse health status effect results when government production drops. Certainly preventive health service consumption falls since no other system provides such services. To the extent that the consumption of such preventive services improves the health of individuals and society, it is reasonable to conclude that a shift away from government provided health care may have an adverse effect on the health status of the population.

It is clear, however, that without significant and steady utilization of the rural services, the health care system cannot provide the continuity of curative medical care required to sustain high quality. Neither is there adequate utilization of the health care system so that the preventive services defined above can be widely diffused throughout a population such that herd immunity can be obtained, in the case of immunization, or that positive trends in mortality or fertility rates can be maintained. Thus, in order for the primary health care system to successfully operate and yield the positive social externalities which potentially exist, a continuous and regular supply of drugs must be available.

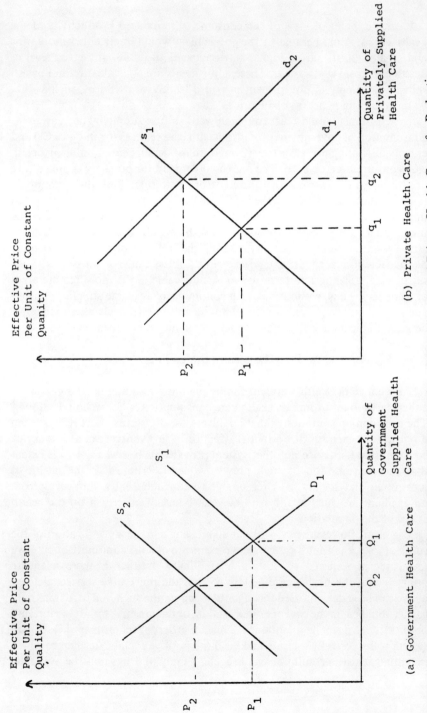

Figure 1.   Effects on Prices and Quantities of Government and Private Health Care of a Reduction

E.  Policy Intervention

The negative effects of a binding foreign exchange constraint, health care utilization, and, possibly health status could possibly be mitigated through policy interventions aimed at any of the above four links. First, governments could allocate a larger share of a shrinking foreign exchange budget to the health sector. Second, personnel of government health care entities and international health service researchers could be stimulated to discover and adopt techniques, contracting procedures, and other mechanisms that could conserve foreign exchange-using resources within the government sector of the health care system.

Third, attempts can be made to prevent the consumer from reducing consumption from the government operated subset of providers by improving its quality via maintenance of all complementary resources and thereby compensate for its increased cost. Fourth, the negative health status effects of any reduction in the consumption of services provided by government operated facilities may partially be alleviated by reallocating foreign exchange to the set of activities which have the most impact on reducing mortality and morbidity. This set may be within the traditionally defined health sector, or may be external to it, e.g., food consumption, housing, water and sanitation facilities, or education.

The design of policies to manage a period of foreign exchange scarcity without negative consequences for health care provision or health status, requires some understanding or reasonable presumptions about all four of the above defined linkages. However, this paper specifically focuses on the first linkage—the allocation effect.

## III.  IMPORTANCE OF FOREIGN EXCHANGE

A.  Foreign Exchange Share of Total Cost

The foreign exchange financing problem was identified by studies of the recovery costs of operating health care programs and facilities in poor countries.[9] While the proportions vary from country to country, and in part depending on the valuation methods used in cost analyses, the few studies presently available estimate that foreign exchange-using resources comprise about 40 percent of the total recurrent cost of a rural based health program (see Table 1.)[10] Imported drugs typically use most of the foreign exchange, and, in the case of Tanzania, represented over 90 percent of foreign exchange cost components. Such a figure of 40 percent by itself may or may not be relevant or impressive, depending upon the larger economic context of the country or the dynamics found within the health sector itself. In order to

*Table 1.*   Foreign Exchange Share of Total Operating
Costs of Government Health Facilities in Poor Countries

| | | Year of Estimate | | | |
|---|---|---|---|---|---|
| Facility Type | Country | 1969 | 1978/79 | 1981 | 1983 |
| Hospital | Tanzania | | 0.41 | | |
| | Uganda | 0.22 | | | |
| Health Center | Tanzania | | 0.53 | | |
| | Uganda | 0.39 | | | |
| | Indonesia | | | 0.37-0.46 | |
| Other Rural Units | Tanzania | | 0.38 | | |
| | Sudan | | | | 0.47 |
| | Indonesia | | | 0.22-0.51 | |

*Sources:*  1.  United Republic of Tanzania, *Evaluation of the Health Sector,* 1979, 2 vols. (Dar es Salaam: Ministry of Health, Sept. 1981).
2.  David W. Dunlop, "Underfinancing of Social Services in Tanzania: The Case of Primary Health Care," paper prepared for Office of Evaluation, AID, Washington, D.C., Feb. 1984.
3.  David W. Dunlop, The Economics of Implementing Primary Health Care Delivery in Sudan," paper prepared for USAID/Sudan, Sept. 1983.
4.  David W. Dunlop, *The Economics of Uganda's Health Service System: Implications for Health and Economic Planning,* unpublished Ph.D. dissertation, Michigan State University, East Lansing, Michigan, 1973.
5.  Peter Berman, *Equity and Cost in the Organization of PHC in Java, Indonesia,* unpublished Ph.D. dissertation, Cornell University, Ithaca, N.Y., 1984

ascertain its relevance, it is useful to present a case study of Tanzania which took a strong policy stand in 1971 to expand its health care system, particularly in rural areas.

### B.  The Case of Primary Health Care Development in Tanzania

Tanzania is fully engaged in the global movement to implement the primary health care strategy for achieving "Health for All by the Year 2000." In 1971 it changed its priorities and began to rapidly expand its rural based facilities. Although it never reallocated any operating funds away from urban based (hospital) services, additions to available government operating funds were disproportionately allocated to rural based health care services.[11] The data presented in Tables 2, 3, and 4 show the extent to which the health care system expanded over the two decade period from independence in 1961 to 1981, when the system significantly reduced its expansionary trends. Table 2 shows the rapid development of rural based facilities, with a doubling of the number of dispensaries, and a four-fold increase in health centers between 1971-1981. The number of hospitals also increased significantly during the same period but not to the same degree.

*Table 2.*  Trends in the Composition of Health Facilities
in Tanzania, 1961-1980

| Year | Number of Hospitals | | | Number of Health Centers | | | Number Dispensaries | | |
|------|------|-------|-------|------|-------|-------|------|-------|-------|
| | Govt | Total | Index | Govt | Total | Index | Govt | Total | Index |
| 1961 | 52 | 98 | 100.0 | 22 | 22 | 100.0 | 736 | 975 | 100.0 |
| 1970 | 60 | 119 | 121.4 | 69 | 69 | 313.6 | 1126 | 1395 | 143.1 |
| 1972 | NA | NA | NA | 105 | 105 | 477.3 | NA | 1491 | 152.9 |
| 1974 | 80 | 139 | 141.8 | 129 | 129 | 586.4 | NA | 1670 | 171.3 |
| 1976 | 82 | 141 | 143.9 | 161 | 161 | 731.8 | NA | 2078 | 213.1 |
| 1978 | 92 | 151 | 154.1 | 194 | 194 | 881.8 | 1972 | 2547 | 261.2 |
| 1980[1] | 98 | 157 | 160.2 | 235 | 235 | 1068.2 | 2134 | 2709 | 277.8 |

Notes and Sources to Table 2.

*Notes:*

1.  Estimated from Table 02B,MOH, *Inventory of Health Facilities,* 1978, which in 1978 included facilities under construction, and assumed completed on 1980.

*Sources:*

1.  Table 4, pg. 32, Oscar Gish, *Planning the Health Sector* (London: Holmes and Meier, 1975).

2.  Tables X, XI, XII, pgs. 28-30 in Albert Henn, *Tanzania Health Sector Strategy* (Dar es Salaam: USAID/Tanzania, February 1980).

3.  Tables 01, 02A, 02B, pgs. 572-574, Ministry of Health, *Inventory of Health Facilities 1978, Main Report* (Dar es Salaam: Ministry of Health, August 1979).

*Table 3.*  Trends in Selected Skilled Health Personnel in Tanzania, 1972-1980

| Personnel Category | Year | | | | | % Increase 1972-1980 |
|------|------|------|------|------|------|------|
| | 1972 | 1974 | 1976 | 1978 | 1980 (est) | |
| Medical Officers | 494 | 603 | 683[1] | 772 | 830 | 68 |
| (% Tanzanians) | 39.5 | 53.7 | 52.1 | 55.0 | 84.0 | |
| Assistant Medical Officers | 140 | 160 | 193 | 250 | 300 | 114 |
| Medical Assistants | 335 | 485 | 770 | 1176 | 1200 | 258 |
| Rural Medical Aides | 578 | 506 | 1049 | 1736 | 2800 | 384 |
| Nurse/Midwives "A" | 877 | 1000 | 1100 | 1300 | 1540 | 75 |
| Nurse/Midwives "B" | 2382 | 3000 | 3720 | 4900 | 5025 | 111 |
| Health Auxiliaries | 290 | 370 | 455 | 545 | 800 | 176 |
| MCH Aides/Village Midwives | 700 | 850 | 960 | 1900 | 2700 | 286 |

Notes and Sources to Table 3

*Note:*

1.  25 Cuban and 60 Chinese doctors are excluded from each year's figures.

*Source:*

2.  Table XV, pg. 34 in Albert Henn, *Tanzania Health Sector Strategy,* (Dar es Salaam: USAID/Tanzania, February 1980).

*Table 4.*   Drug and Medicinal Product Imports, Tanzania, 1960-1982

| Fiscal Year | Total Imports Mill. T. Shs. Current | Total Medicinal & Pharmaceutical Products(Mill.T.Shs.) | Percentage Medicinal & Pharmaceutical is of Total Imports | Per Capita Medicinal & Pharmaceutical Products in Constant 1975 T.Shs[1] |
|---|---|---|---|---|
| 1960 | 518.0 | 13.4 | 2.60 | 3.55 |
| 1962 | 945.5 | 14.6 | 1.55 | 3.48 |
| 1964 | 879.5 | 18.3 | 2.08 | 4.13 |
| 1966 | 1285.0 | 22.4 | 1.74 | 4.37 |
| 1968 | 1531.7 | 28.4 | 1.85 | 4.89 |
| 1970 | 1939.2 | 45.1 | 2.33 | 6.85 |
| 1972 | 2597.6 | 55.5 | 2.14 | 7.05 |
| 1974 | 5429.6 | 107.2 | 1.97 | 9.05 |
| 1976 | 5354.7 | 122.0 | 2.28 | 7.12 |
| 1978 | 8815.6 | 201.0 | 2.28 | 8.86 |
| 1980 | 9238.4 | 259.2 | 2.81 | 7.23 |
| 1981 | 9120.0 | 228.0 | 2.50 | 4.87 |
| 1982 | 8392.0 | 193.0 | 2.30 | 3.18 |

Notes and Sources to Table 4
*Note:*
The deflator used is the Tanzanian National Consumer Price Index based on prices in 18 towns as reported in IMF, *International Financial Statistics Yearbook,* 1981 and updated per information obtained at USAID/ Dar es Salaam. A preferred deflator would be a midical and pharmaceutical specific import price index; however, data for such an index are unavailable. Data on world consumer prices indicate a similar upward trend in prices and would show a similar pattern to the one indicated. Population data were obtained from the IMF, *International Financial Statistics Yearbook,* 1981 and updated based on the annual population growth rate obtained from the 1978 census.
*Sources:*
1.  East African Community, East African Customes and Excise Department, *Annual Trade Report of Tanzania, Kenya, and Uganda,* for various years ending December 31, 1974.
2.  Ministry of Finance, Tanzanian Customs Department, *Annual Trade Report of Tanzania for Year Ended December 31, 1980,* Dar es Salaam.
3.  Ministry of Finance, Tanzanian Customs Department, Transmittal Letter, May 11, 1982 to USAID/Dar es Salaam.

Table 3 also shows the expansion of manpower cadres during the 1970s which complement the rural focus depicted in the facility date presented in Table 2. Medical Assistants, Rural Medical Aids, and MCH Aids were cadres which expanded more rapidly than others in order to staff the growing number of rural based facilities.

Finally, the data in Table 4 show the gradual buildup in real drug availability (a complementary resource to the other two in providing health care services) during the 1960s, and the expansion which occurred after the 1971 rural focused policy shift. The significant decline which started in 1979, after the last coffee boom year of 1978, has not ended, with the only source of imported drugs coming from the support provided by the Danish Government. Since 1974, after the first oil price increase, the government of Tanzania has had increased difficulty in financing imports due to its increasingly adverse trade balance.[12]

## C. Trends in Real Pharmaceutical Imports

The importance of the above analysis for Tanzania is that the dates clearly show a change in the mix of resources used to provide health care for a large share of the country's population living in rural areas. In Tanzania this change in resource mix appears to be related to the above mentioned macroeconomic changes which occurred in the late 1970s. One may conclude that when such a trend in the availability of one important input manifests itself, it is likely that significant dislocations will occur throughout the health care system as described in the framework section of this paper.

Real per capita pharmaceutical import trend data are analyzed in Section IV for each of the seven case study countries incorporated into this paper— Ivory Coast, Jamaica, Peru, Sri Lanka, Sudan, Tanzania, and Thailand. While the absolute amount of imported drugs per capita may vary from country to country, as is indicated by different units along each Y axis, the trends for all countries show a similar downward pattern since the late 1970s, with some patterns, e.g., Ivory Coast, Jamaica, Sudan, Tanzania and Thailand being very striking. The other two countries, Sri Lanka and Peru, started their downward trends earlier in the early 1960s when both countries encountered their first balance of payments difficulties.

In the section that follows, an empirical analysis seeks an improved understanding of the factors which affect the pattern of real per capita pharmaceutical imports in these seven countries. Both macroeconomic and other control variables are incorporated into the analysis. The empirical findings and policy implications conclude the paper.

# IV.  A MODEL OF THE FACTORS WHICH CONSTRAIN PHARMACEUTICAL IMPORTS

The empirical analysis seeks to determine the factors which define the foreign exchange resource constraint facing health care systems (both public and private) in poor countries, as measured by per capita medicinal and pharmaceutical imports. The foreign exchange constraint variable on which the empirical analysis focuses is real per capita pharmaceutical product imports (SITC Code #541), over 90 percent of which is comprised of drugs and similar items (SITC Code #541.7). It is hypothesized that pharmaceutical product imports are influenced by a number of independent variables which can be grouped into distinct sets. The first set includes several macroeconomic forces, such as (a) the size and growth of total economic activity, as measured by GDP, (b) the balance of payments situation as measured by the trade balance and the size of that balance relative to the size of GDP, and (c) government expenditure patterns as defined by the government consumption share of GDP and the magnitude of the goverment deficit as defined as a share of total government expenditures. The assumed relationship between these measures and the dependent variable is defined more precisely below.

Besides such macroeconomic forces, there are three other sets of variables which could influence the pattern of pharmaceutical imports. These are: (a) the health status of country's population, as measured by life expectancy at birth and the infant mortality rate; (b) the nature and growth of the country's health care system, as indicated by yearly population-to-physician and population-to-hospital bed ratios; and (c) macroeconomic and health sector specific policy variables. This last category of variables includes the existence and market share of a domestic pharmaceutical industry, and the extent to which external donors (both public and private) are providing financial assistance for the procurement of pharmaceutical products.

Of particular concern to the authors is the extend to which macroeconomic forces, i.e., trends in GDP, the balance of trade, and government fiscal policy as defined by its share of GDP and the extent of deficit financing, are associated with the availability of pharmaceutical imports. The other independent variables control for differences among countries with respect to health status, the health care system, resource availability, and the policy environment.

## A.  The Model and Data

The principal econometric specification of the model in this exploratory analysis can be stated as follows:

RRXIMP/C  =  f(GDP, TB, GSHR, HS, POPDOC, POPBED, DONSHR), where

RRXIMP/C  =  real per capita pharmaceutical imports, 1980 = 100, over the 1950-1982 period, or as close to that period as the data will allow;

GDP  =  gross domestic product as measured in real terms RGDP, 1980 = 100, or its growth rate, RGDPDOT;

TB  =  balance of trade as measured by merchandise exports minus merchandise imports, F.O.B., TBAL, or a lagged version of TBA, TBALLAG;

GSHR  =  Government consumption share of GDP;

HS  =  health status, as measured by either LEXP, life expectancy at birth, or INMORT, infant mortaility;

POPDOC  =  the population-doctor ratio;

POPBED  =  the population-hospital bed ratio;

DONSHR  =  the share of total pharmaceutical product imports financed by international biliateral and multilateral agencies.

DIMFSB    =  whether the country had an IMF standby agreement,
             1=standby agreement; and
DPHC      =  whether the country had a primary health care policy,
             1=such a policy

In this study, country specific data from seven countries have been analyzed. The results are presented in the following section of the paper. The seven countries include Ivory Coast, Jamaica, Peru, Sri Lanka, Sudan, Tanzania, and Thailand. The criteria used to pick these seven include; (a) diversity by geographical region, (b) variance in economic performance over the 1950-1985 period, (c) diversity in per capita income, and (d) diversity in the macroeconomic and health sector policy context. In a subsequent section, comparative country specific data are presented in Table 6 to show the diversity as defined above.

The analysis presented in this paper has assumed that the ordinary least squares linear regression model applies, such that (a) the functional form of the relationships between the dependent and independent variables are assumed to be linear, (b) there is no omitted variable bias, and (c) there is no significant serial correlation. Given the nature of the statistical findings as presented in Table 7, these assumptions are generally supported. This analysis, however, represents a "progress report" on further empirical analysis being conducted, and which will be reported in a subsequent paper.

## B.  Hypothetical Statistical Relationships

Table 5 presents the hypothesized statistical relationships between the dependent variable drug imports and the independent variables. With respect to the macroeconomic variables, per capita pharmaceutical imports are hypothesized to be positively related to the size and growth rate of total economic activity as defined by GDP. It seems reasonable to expect that as income rises, the demand for pharmaceuticals would also increase as is the case for most other goods and especially for health care.[13]

Since the late 1970s and particularly during the recent global economic recession, the balance of trade, i.e., exports minus imports, has generally been negative in many poor countries. It is assumed that the balance of trade represents a long-run measure of a country's capacity to import. Since the economic structure of many countries has changed considerably over the 1970s in part due to the two oil price increases, it is hypothesized that the balance of trade would be positively related to changes in real per capita pharmaceutical imports.[14] A lagged effect of the balance of trade is also investigated, with the assumption being that there may be a time lapse between a change in foreign exchange availability and import changes.

*Table 5.*  Hypothetical Empirical Relationship Between Dependent Variable,
Real Per Capita Pharmaceutical Imports, and Independent Variable

| | |
|---|---|
| *I.  Macroeconomic Variables* | *Assumed Partial Sign* |
| 1.  GDP | + |
| 2.  GDP growth rate | + |
| 3.  Balance of Trade | + |
| 4.  Government Consumption share of GDP | + |
| *II.  Health Status* | |
| 1.  Life Expectancy at Birth in Years | + |
| 2.  Infant Mortality | − |
| *III.  Health Care System: Supply Variables* | |
| 1.  Population per Doctor Ratio | − |
| 2.  Population per Hospital Bed Ratio | − |
| *IV.  Policy Environment* | |
| 1.  Donor Financed Share of Imported Drugs | ? |
| 2.  Existence of IMF Standby | − |
| 3.  Existence of PHC Policy | − or 0 |

Most recent macroeconomic analyses conducted by international
organizations express concern regarding the chronic nature and increasing size
of government budget deficits. Often, government deficits are incurred to finance
the recurrent cost of government programs, including health programs. As
governments are increasingly encouraged to live within their means, government
programs must curtail all expenditures, including those on imported items, such
as drugs. Since a sizable share of pharmaceutical imports were for use in publicly
supported facilities, as government consumption expenditures rose, or declined,
as a proportion of GDP, the recurrent expenditures for health and other
government programs including expenditures for drugs are hypothesized to vary
accordingly. It is assumed that a positive relationship would tend to hold
between the government consumption share of GDP and pharmaceutical
imports, even though the health sector recurrent expenditure share of total
government spending varies as well.[15]

Other factors besides the above mentioned macroeconomic variables affect
pharmaceutical imports. Thus, it is considered important to control for health
status as well as the possibility that the supply of health care providers might
also affect pharmaceutical imports. With respect to health status, it would have
been the authors' preference to include a variable that measured change in
disease patterns in the population, since disease specific therapeutic
requirements vary significantly. Certainly chronic diseases such as heart
disease, or diseases that require a significant recuperation period, e.g., TB,
require more costly therapeutic regimens than the normal bout of diarrhea,

or other common infectious or parasitic diseases found in poor countries. Unfortunately such information is not readily available for most countries. Thus, as a distinct second best, two aggregate health status measures are employed, life expectancy at birth and infant mortality.[16] In countries and locales where careful study has been conducted,[17] it has been demonstrated that increased life expectancy in poor countries is primarily accomplished by reducing prevalent childhood diseases such as measles, malaria, and diarrhea. These and other similar diseases are relatively easy to treat. Thus, the drug requirements to provide adequate medical care to a population whose life expectancy is increasing will rise concomitantly. Thus, it is reasonable to assume a positive relationship between life expectancy and per capita drug imports. The same reasoning would lead one to expect a negative relationship exists between infant mortality and drug imports.

To the extent that utilization of health care services in any country is associated with the supply of health care providers, and that the demand for drugs is a derived demand from increased utilization,[18] it was considered important to control for changes in the supply of health services as measured by various population-to-resource ratios. The two ratios employed in this analysis include (a) population per physician, and (b) population per hospital bed. It would be useful to analyze how changes in the mix of health service resource availability, for example toward more paraprofessional health care workers and primary care clinics, might affect the demand for and use of pharmaceuticals. Since long-term trend data on such variables are not readily available, the hypothesis investigated in this study is that the demand for drugs increases as the number of physicians and/or hospital beds increase relative to growth of the population. Thus a negative relationship is posited in Table 5.

Increasingly, international donor agencies have provided drugs and other medical supplies to countries as part of a health project. In addition, some donors have included drugs on the list of approved items available for import financing via a donor specific commodity import program (CIP). Whether such donor financing substitutes for or complements drug imports financed by the country itself is unclear. Nevertheless, to the extent that information is available on donor drug financing for two sample countries, it is incorporated in the empirical analysis, with no prior assumption regarding the direction of impact.

## C. Omitted Variables

There are several important omitted variables which require incorporation in future analysis. They include (a) the time when in-country (domestic) pharmaceutical manufacturing capability occurred, (b) the market share of domestic manufacturers, (c) the changing preferences of consumers for imported drugs relative to traditional medicines, and (d) the raw material import share of domestically manufactured drugs. Data on these important factors which undoubtedly affect pharmaceutical imports are not readily available to the authors as yet. It is anticipated that it may be possible to incorporate these factors in subsequent analyses.

In addition, it is important to ascertain how certain macroeconomic and health sector policy changes may affect drug imports. Certainly, aggregate import flows are reviewed given the IMF's policy change requirement prior to and during annual standby agreements (SBA's), Extended Fund Facilities (EFF's), and the Paris Club policy change requirements pursuant to entering into negotiations about public and private debt rescheduling. Other bilateral and multilateral donors are also increasingly concerned about policy changes regarding chronic trade imbalances and government recurrent cost commitments, particularly where the government plays an important role in the economy and has maintained policies that have led to chronically high budget deficits. Thus, it is important to include variables that incorporate the impact of these macroeconomic policy factors.

The country's implementation of a primary health care policy and an essential drugs program, as well as the way it allocates available foreign exchange to finance drug imports by private pharmacies, can have important outcomes with respect to (a) what is imported and (b) which groups in the population are the principal beneficiaries. It is unclear, however, how a primary health care policy may affect aggregate drug imports, particularly without complementary changes in the size and the way in which the entire health care system is managed. However, one can assume that an essential drugs program would either reduce or leave unchanged the value of pharmaceutical imports, depending on the extent to which (a) the prior drug list was affected by the new policy, and (b) procurement efficiency was affected.

The omission of these variables, though unavoidable at this stage of the research, biases the estimated coefficients of all included variables and thus limits the strength and policy implications of any conclusions which might be drawn from the empirical results. With this caveat, the next section represents the results of these preliminary empirical explorations.

## V.  EMPIRICAL RESULTS

### A.  A Comparison of Case Study Countries

Seven countries were selected according to the four criteria specified earlier: geographic diversity, diversity in per capita income, differences in economic growth performance, and varying health and economic policy contexts. Some descriptive data on the selected countries, Ivory Coast, Jamaica, Peru, Sri Lanka, Sudan, Tanzania and Thailand, are presented in Table 6.

Table 6: Comparative Economic and Health Indicators on the Seven Countries

| Country | (1) Pop.1982 Mil. | (2) GNP/ Cap. 1982 | (3) Growth Rate in GNP/ Cap. 1961-1982 | (4) Life Exp. at Birth 1982 | (5) Pop. Growth Rate 1972-1982 | (6) Pop. per Phys.1981 | (7) Current Account Balance, Mill. $ | | (8) Govt. Consumption Share of GDP | | | (9) PHC Policy Year Adopted | (10) Essential Drugs Policy Year Adopted | (11) IMF Standby # Years |
|---|---|---|---|---|---|---|---|---|---|---|---|---|---|---|
| | | | | | | | 1970 | 1979 | 1961 | 1975 | 1982 | | | |
| Ivory Coast | 8.9 | 950 | 2.1 | 47 | 4.9[1] | 21,140 | −26 | −560 | 11.7 | 16.9 | NA | Not Adopted | Not Adopted | 1 |
| Jamaica | 2.2 | 1330 | 1.7 | 73 | 1.5 | 2,830 | −145 | −47 | 9.5 | 18.3 | 22.9 | since 1978 | since 1984 | 6 |
| Peru | 17.4 | 1310 | 1.0 | 58 | 2.8 | 1,390 | 284 | 1,055 | 9.2 | 13.6 | 13.5 | since 1979 | since 1981 | 23 |
| Sri Lanka | 15.2 | 320 | 2.6 | 69 | 1.7 | 7,170 | −47 | −203 | 14.6 | 9.3 | 8.3 | since 1979 | since 1975 | 14 |
| Sudan | 21.2 | 440 | −1.4 | 47 | 3.2 | 8,390 | −29 | −151 | 7.9 | 13.8 | 13.3 | since 1977 | since 1984 | 11 |
| Tanzania | 19.8 | 280 | 1.9 | 52 | 3.4 | 17,560 | −29 | −457 | 11.2 | 17.1 | 13.4 | since 1971 | since 1983 | 5 |
| Thailand | 48.5 | 790 | 4.5 | 63 | 2.4 | 7,110 | −234 | −1,945 | 9.6 | 10.4 | 13.1 | since 1978 | since 1981 | 5 |

Source: World Bank, *World Development Report*, 1984, (Washington D.C.: World Bank, 1984)

Notes: (1) The rate of natural increase of the domestic population in Ivory Coast is about 3.0% per year. The additional population growth rate is due to net immigration from surrounding countries.

(2) Jamaica is presently under a multi-year Extended Fund Facility. Ivory Coast was under an EFF from 1980 ato 1984

(3) Y = Yes, N = No.

The seven countries provide geographic diversity with two countries being from Asia, two from Latin America, and three from Africa—both East and West. In this group, economic performance over the two decade period has varied from negative per capita growth in Sudan to the strong performance registered by Thailand (nearly 5.0 percent p.a.). Per capita income levels also vary from the low figure of $280 for Tanzania to over $1,300 for both Jamaica and Peru. Latin American countries register the highest average, with Asian and African averages being lower though similar.

Most all countries have seen their current account balance go from a marginally negative position in 1970 to a more adverse position by the end of the decade of the 1970s. More recent data from most countries would suggest that current account balances become even more negative by the mid-1980s. According to the data presented in Table 6, only two of the seven countries, Jamaica and Peru, had improved their current account position during the 1970s.

There is diversity in the share of GDP represented by government consumption expenditures among the seven countries, with nearly a three-fold difference indicated between the highest (Jamaica) and lowest (Sri Lanka) figures in 1982. In addition, there has been considerable changes recorded among the seven countries in the size of the government expenditure share over the 1970-1982 period. With the exception of Sri Lanka, the changes recorded suggest that government expenditures have risen more rapidly than the growth in GDP.

Second, differences exist between the countries with respect to (a) health status as measured by life expectancy, (b) population growth, and (c) the supply of physicians, There is a twenty-six year difference between life expectancy in Ivory Coast and Sudan, and Jamaica. Clearly, Africa has the lowest life expectancy and the population to physician ratio also indicated that there are relatively fewer highly trained persons available on that continent to provide health care. Population growth is also highest among the three countries in Africa, averaging over 3.0 percent p.a. The two Latin American countries have the largest physician supply relative to population, but there is little regional pattern with respect to life expectancy.

Third, health policy changes have progressed at different speeds in the seven countries. As of 1984, one country, Ivory Coast, had not adopted either a Primary Health Care or Essential Drugs policy. On the other hand, Tanzania had de facto adopted a PHC policy in 1971,[19] and Sri Lanka had introduced an essential drugs program in 1975. Most countries adopted an essential drugs program after adopting a PHC policy.

Finally, there is variable experience with IMF assistance. Peru, and to a lesser extent Sri Lanka and Sudan, have had a long-standing relationship with IMF policies and programs designed to improve their economic performance. The IMF intervened early in Peru and Sri Lanka due to their long-standing balance of payment difficulties. Even though both Thailand and Tanzania are encountering trade imbalances in the mid-1980s, in 1984 they did not have IMF Standby agreements.

## B. The Empirical Findings

Table 7 presents a preliminary set of the empirical results of the analysis conducted on time series data from seven countries, Ivory Coast, Jamaica, Peru, Sri Lanka, Sudan, Tanzania, and Thailand. The estimated equations for five of the seven countries explain over 75 percent of the variation in the dependent variable, adjusted for the number of observations, as measured by $\bar{R}^2$. For the other two countries, Sri Lanka and Thailand, $\bar{R}^2$ is about 0.50, and the equations for each of these countries contain several statistically significant coefficients. The F statistics indicate that each equation as a whole is statistically significant at the 0.01 level. Since the hypothesis of zero autocorrelation cannot be rejected at the 5 percent significance level for any of the equations, serial correlation is not a problem.

### 1. Macroeconomic Variables

The present findings are mixed with respect to the specific hyotheses summarized in Table 5. On the one hand, the positive relationship between RGDP, or its growth rate, RGDPOT, is statistically confirmed in three of the seven equations. In the case of the other four countries, however, the results suggest a negative sign, although in each case the relationship is not statistically insignificant.

In five of the seven equations, trade balance or the lagged (by one year)value of the trade balance is statistically significant. In three of the five significant cases, however, the sign is unexpectedly negative. In the two cases where a relationship is significantly positive, the trade balance is lagged by a year. While it is encouraging to obtain significant results in a majority of the cases, the mixed signs imply a need for further theoretical and empirical thought.

In five of the seven cases the government share variable, GSHR, has the expected positive coefficient, even though the relationship is statistically insignificant in four of the five cases. However, the coefficient for Thailand is significantly negative, perhaps because of the strong private pharmaceutical sector there.

To summarize the findings with respect to the macroeconomic variables, in all seven country equations, at least one macroeconomic variable is statistically significant with respect to the dependent variable, per capita pharmaceutical imports. In addition, in three countries, Ivory Coast, Jamaica and Thailand, two macroeconomic variables are statistically significant, and in four countries, Ivory Coast, Jamaica, Peru and Sudan, the statistically significant variable

*Table 7.* Selected Preliminary Empirical Results of OLS Linear Regression Analysis of the Factors Affecting Real per Capita Pharmaceutical Imports into Seven Poor Countries, 1950-1982

| Variable | Ivory Coast | Jamaica | Peru | Sri Lanka | Sudan | Tanzania | Thailand |
|---|---|---|---|---|---|---|---|
| Constant | 0.2399 (0.002) | −100.957 −(0.931) | 97.2559 (10.344)*** | 101.182 (1.672)* | 49.6915 (1.973)* | 108.496 (1.144) | 39.9677 (6.331)*** |
| RGDP | −0.0026 −(0.115) | 0.0111 (2.105)** | | | 0.0095 (3.009)** | −0.00002 −(0.039) | −0.0059 −(1.307) |
| RGDPDOT | | | 0.5428 (1.826)* | | | | |
| RGDPDOTL | | | | −0.1619 −(0.870) | | | |
| TBAL | | | −0.00014 −(0.063) | −0.0080 (1.666)* | −0.0045 −(0.874) | −0.0020 −(3.440)*** | −0.0017 −(1.775)* |
| TBALLAG | 0.0455 (2.937)** | 0.0845 (2.502)** | | | | | |
| GSHR | 2.9659 (1.765)* | 0.8060 (1.047) | −0.1694 −(0.300) | 0.4473 (0.909) | 0.1676 (0.422) | 0.1305 (0.219) | −0.8406 −(1.843)* |
| LEXP | −0.2326 | 1.5972 (0.849) | | −0.4476 −(0.686) | | | |

| | | | | | | | |
|---|---|---|---|---|---|---|---|
| INMORT | | | | | | 0.4420 (2.341)** | 0.3406 (0.861) |
| POPDOC | 4.7008 (2.159)** | | | 1.6779 (0.603) | -0.0789 -(0.259) | -2.5614 -(2.350)** | |
| POPBED | -24.7869 -(0.103) | -135.944 -(6.540)*** | -221.553 -(1.800)* | -66.5151 -(3.875) | -12.1527 -(2.638) | -12.0608 -(4.371)** | |
| DIMFSB | -4.5291 -(1.469) | | | | | | |
| DPHC | -24.6607 -(2.839)** | | | | | | |
| DONSHR | | | | -0.1731 -(1.828)* | | 0.1241 (1.840)* | |
| N | 22 | 27 | 30 | 32 | 21 | 30 | 28 |
| $R^2$ | 0.76 | 0.85 | 0.76 | 0.49 | 0.91 | 0.86 | 0.55 |
| F | 12.97 | 18.49 | 22.54 | 5.48 | 25.00 | 20.10 | 6.32 |
| DW | 1.82 | 1.55 | 2.37 | 1.46 | 1.29 | 2.18 | 1.34 |

Notes:
1. * = stastically significant at 0.10 level
2. ** = statistically significant at 0.05 level
3. *** = statistically significant at 0.01 level
4. t statistic is in parentheses

carries the hypothesized sign. While these findings do not overwhelmingly support the assumed relationships, they do suggest that macroeconomic forces play an important role in determining the availability of imported drugs in poor countries.

## C.  Other Findings

It is important to point out several other findings presented in Table 7. First, the "second best" measures of health status appear to be just that. A statistically significant finding is observed in only one out of four countries where such data were available and, in that one case, the expected negative relationship between infant mortaility and drug imports was not confirmed. The life expectancy variable is not significant at all and its sign is inconsistent.

Second, the population to doctor ratio appears statistically significant in only two of the five countries' equations where such data were available. The signs were also inconsisitent both for the statistically significant coefficients as well as for the other equations.

Third, while the assumed relationship between drug imports and the population to doctor ratio was not empirically supported, the findings with respect to the population to hospital bed ratio, appear highly significant. The correct sign appears in all countries for which data were available, and the coefficient is statistically significant in every case except one. These findings lend credence to the idea that as the health care system expands, particularly in the form of hospitals, thereby reducing the population to hospital bed ratio, the derived demand for a complementary drug supply increases. Additional study is required to determine whether such a finding would hold for a similar change in rural based primary health care facilities.

Fourth, the findings on the donor share for the two countries (Tanzania and Sudan) for which data were available indicate their statistical significance. However,since the sign of the relationship is positive in one case (Tanzania) and negative in the other (Sudan), it is unclear whether donor financing is viewed as a complement as would be the case for Tanzania, or as a substitute, as in Sudan. Further study of this factor is warranted on a case by case basis. In part, the relationship would depend on country decision makers' perceptions of how reliable and long-term the donor financial assistance may be, in conjunction with the extent to which (a) donors impose certain conditions on this form of assistance, and (b) the country views the potential for improved economic performance which can lead to increased procurement on its own.

Finally, for one country, Jamaica, the equation presented includes two policy dummy variables: (a) the existence of an IMF Standby Agreement, and (b) the existence of a primary health care policy. Both policy variables have negative signs which indicate a reduced level of per capita pharmaceutical imports during the years in which either item was in effect. At present, it is too early to fully interpret this particular finding and particularly whether either can be considered as an efficiency shift parameter in the use of pharmaceutical imports. Certainly the results are tantalizing and warrant further investigation.

## VI.   CONCLUSIONS AND POLICY ALTERNATIVES

There are several important policy conclusions and resulting policy implications that emerge from the present study. With regard to conclusions, it is important to first note that the data presented in this paper clearly show that since the late 1970s there has been a significant reduction in the supply of pharmaceutical and related products for use by health care providers in many poor countries. Second, the empirical analysis conducted on seven countries provides supporting evidence for the basic premise in this paper that a principal reason for the reduced supply of pharmaceutical items is poor economic performance since the late 1970s. This poor performance has led to a situation where foreign exchange earnings have been insufficient to finance drug and other medical supply procurements.

Third, the paper reviewed the impact a health care delivery system drug shortage has on the successful implementation of many important preventive health service programs which are based on a well functioning basic health service delivery system for wide dissemination. The case of Tanzania is representative of many poor countries where donors helped to expand the supply of rural health workers and facilities, and where drugs are now in short supply (with the exception of the assistance provided by DANIDA). Donor assistance is now vital in financing the necessary complementary foreign exchange using recurrent cost of health activities during the readjustment period of that country and in others as well. Tanzania and other countries have been hard pressed to sustain service levels and maintain preventive programs, especially immunization programs, due to foreign exchange shortages.

### A.   Responsibilities of Countries

In order to weather the present foreign exchange crisis in the health sector, it is important for poor country governments to work together with local private health providers. Ministries of Health must develop the capacity to fully anticipate the implications of a changing macroeconomic environment on the functioning of health care institutions. They must develop the internal capacity to analyze the cost structure of each health care providing entity in order to ascertain the extent to which it relies on foreign exchange using inputs to operate. Where possible, alternative, local sources of supply that do not rely on foreign exchange should be encouraged. Such analyses must become a central component of the dialogue between the Ministry of Health and the

Ministry of Planning, Treasury and Central Bank, which often has jurisdiction over the allocation of foreign exchange.

In addition, people with responsibility for health and other social programs in poor countries must have the analytical capacity to determine how various government policies affect exports, which remains the largest single source of foreign exchange earnings for any country. It is particularly important to monitor agricultural price policies which often adversely affect agricultural exports as well as exacerbate local food production. Careful monitoring of donor recommendations with respect to policy change is also required in order to develop an independent assessment of what may result as a consequence of donor recommendation.

Certainly if countries can implement ways to reduce the supply of nonessential drug imports and purchase and manage their procurements more wisely, the available supply of foreign exchange using resources can have a greater impact on service provision, and, hopefully, on the health status of the people. The efforts of the essential drug programs of both WHO and UNICEF are noteworthy in this regard. However, it is important to carefully monitor all procurements by both the public as well as the private sectors, in order to ascertain the implemented effectiveness of these programs. Further, each country must determine the most cost-effective alternative in terms of foreign exchange use for transporting and storing pharmaceuticals and other items. It becomes increasingly apparent in other sectors of the economy that private sector transporters and warehousing services work better.

Finally, it is increasingly important for countries to analyze the impact on service delivery of the possible substitution of local currency using resources for foreign exchange using ones. In some countries there are times when considerable substitution may be feasible, whereas in others it may not be possible. However, it is important to ascertain how the local currency raised by cost recovery (financing) efforts is used. If countries use these additional resources to train and employ more health workers per unit of available drugs, it is possible to worsen the provision of health care as well as frustrate efforts to reduce the government wage bill.

## B.   Responsibilities of Donors

First it is important for donors to understand how their individual "marginal" project or activity contributes to the overall macroeconomic performance of countries, particularly as such activities expand to country-wide programs. Such activities, while noble in intent, may not only contribute to a general recurrent cost problem, but also to a foreign exchange financing problem, particularly if the IMF becomes involved. It is vital to improve the analysis of how the project articulates not only with envisioned development plans, but also with realistic trends in foreign exchange availability. This is particularly true for health programs which typically have a 40 percent foreign exchange element. (In contrast, foreign exchange comprises only about 10 percent of the cost of a typical primary education program.)

Second, it is important for donors to use their resources to help countries find ways to reduce the foreign exchange requirements of health systems, not only in the pharmaceutical area, but also in many other program components. The recurrent cost of solar-powered communication systems, which can also improve supervision is but one possible example. Other possibilities exist in refrigeration and sterilization technologies.

Third, it is important for donors to finance studies of the cost structure and resource mix between local currency and foreign exchange components in the private health care sector. Such studies may provide useful insights into how public sector health care systems can utilize foreign exchange resources more wisely.

Finally, donors can become more facile in considering how certain recurrent costs can be capitalized, and, thus, financed in the "traditional" way. Just as spare parts for vehicles and other equipment are included in projects in the irrigation, power, and industrial sectors, why not include not only the initial drug component for a health project, but also the foreign exchange to continually replenish the stock? Such a foreign exchange fund can be placed in an externally held account in the country's name and can be used to procure items required to sustain the project.[20] By developing the project in such a manner, fluctuations in foreign exchange earnings of a country will not adversely affect the success of social projects which have long-term developmental impacts.

## ACKNOWLEDGMENTS

An earlier version of this paper was prepared for the Joint U.K. and Nordic Health Economics Study Group Meeting in Vadstena, Sweden, July 3-5, 1985. Also various aspects of this research by the authors have benefited from Seminar discussions at Boston University and The Johns Hopkins University. Computer assistance was ably provided by Ms. Karen Secular and the manuscript was professionally typed by Mr. Ferd Wulkan.

## NOTES

1. *The New York Times,* Sunday, February 3, 1985, p. 41.

2. *Wall Street Journal,* Wednesday, April 11, 1985, p. 32.

3. World Bank, *World Development Report,* 1984, (Washington, D.C.: World Bank, 1984), pp. 36-38.

4. WHO, *Global Strategy for Health for All by the Year 2000,* (Geneva: WHO, 1981).

5.   Wayne Stinson; *Community Financing of Primary Health Care,* Series 1, No. 4, (Washington, D.C.: American Public Health Association, 1982). The PRICOR Project of AID has monitored a number of innovative health financing activities since 1983. In addition, the World Bank has encouraged "cost recovery" efforts in conjunction with investments in the health sector.

6.   The few studies of health status production or labor productivity in poor countries have not specifically focused on the importance of foreign exchange in that production process. See for example, Walter Galenson and Graham Pyatt, *The Quality of Labor and Economic Development in Certain Countries,* Special Study 68; Geneva: ILO, 1964; David Wheeler and John Harris, "Recurrent Costs and Basic Needs Strategies" Boston University, Boston, Mass: Sept. 22, 1979. While John Fiedler did not analyze the foreign exchange component, his study is based on household specific data. See John Fiedler, *Health and Development in El Peten, Guatemala,* Unpublished Ph.D. Dissertation, Vanderbilt University, 1985.

7.   This erosion is particularly acute when a primary task of the provider is to engage in preventive health care activities which can contribute positive externalities to society as a whole in the form of: (a) maintenance of high immunization rates, particularly after an initial mass campaign; (b) healthier babies and mothers as a consequence of increased use of ante-natal care; and (c) increased use of family planning services.

8.   An evaluation of a selected set of donor financed health projects has been conducted by D.C. Gwatkin, J.R. Wilcox and J.D. Wray, *Can Health and Nutrition Intervention Make a Difference?* Monograph #13, (Washington, D.C.: Overseas Development Council, 1980). The tentative findings from this evaluation, however, reveal how little we know about these linkages despite the many PHC programs which are now in operation.

9.   See for example, A. Mead Over, "Five Primary Care Projects in the Sahel and the Issue of Recurrent Costs." Paper prepared for the Harvard Institute for International Development, Cambridge, MA, 1981; David W. Dunlop, "Cost Implications of Selected Health Care Components and Programs." Paper prepared for the World Bank, (Washington, D.C., June 1984); and David W. Dunlop, "Primary Health Care: An Economic Analysis of the Problems Facing Implementation." Background paper prepared for WHO Informed Consultation on Economic Aspects of PHC, March 1-5, 1982.

10.   Table 3, p. 15, David W. Dunlop, "Cost Implications of Selected Health Care Components and Programs," ibid, 1984, and derived from Peter Berman, *Equity and Cost in the Organization of PHC in Java, Indonesia,* unpublished Ph.D. Dissertation, Cornell University, 1984.

11.   Holly Caldwell and David W. Dunlop, "An Empirical Study of Health Planning in Latin America and Africa," *Social Science and Medicine,* 13, (1979) and Oscar Gish, *Planning the Health Sector,* (London: Holmes & Meier, 1975).

12.   The details of the macroeconomic situation facing Tanzania is presented in David W. Dunlop, "Underfinancing for Social Services in Tanzania: The Case of Primary Health Care." Paper prepared for the Office of Evaluation, Policy and Program Coordination Bureau, AID, Washington, D.C., February 1984.

13.   Pp. 176-179, David W. Dunlop, *The Economics of Uganda's Health Care System: Implications for Health and Economic Planning,* Unpublished Ph.D. Dissertation, Michigan State University, 1973.

14.   However, Dunlop, ibid, was unable to find support for this hypothesis in time-series data for Uganda.

15.   At some future point, it would be useful to incorporate the health sector recurrent expenditure share variation into the analysis. At present it is not feasible given available data sources.

16.   The authors are fully aware of the measurement difficulties involved in both health status measures. Nevertheless since they are the most readily available, they were employed despite such difficulties.

17.   Ruth Puffer and Carlos Serrano, *Patterns of Mortality in Childhood,* Scientific Publication #262, (Washington, D.C.: PAHO, 1973).

18.   This relationship was investigated by Dunlop using data from Uganda. See David W. Dunlop, *The Economics of Uganda's Health Care System:...* op. cit., 1973.

19.   Oscar Gish, *Planning the Health Sector,* op. cit., 1975.

20.   For example, it may be negotiated that the government of the recipient country would undertake to replenish the fund out of foreign exchange earnings at an agreed upon rate, with the proportion contributed by the government increasing over the course of the project.

# THE HIDDEN COSTS OF ILLNESS
# IN DEVELOPING COUNTRIES

Jose deCodes, Timothy D. Baker,

and Debra Schumann

## ABSTRACT

It is fitting that in 1986, the year of a return of Halley's comet that this year's volume of Research in Human Captial and Development should have a paper with antecedents in the seventeenth century work of Edmund Halley. As may be seen in the background of this article, the money value of man and the cost of disease have a long history of development. This paper, following the volume's theme of Public Health and Development, attempts to show the value of applying old techniques, repeatedly revised over centuries to modern problems of setting public health policies to support development.

Research in Human Capital Development, Vol. 5, pages 127-145.
Copyright © 1988 by JAI Press Inc.
ISBN: 0-89232-508-9

# I.  INTRODUCTION

The full burden of illness in developing countries is frequently underestimated. Although health planners and decision-makers are usually aware of *direct* costs for prevention and treatment of illness, they often overlook the *indirect* costs, the losses in productivity due to short-term morbidity, long-term disability, and premature death. Failure to recognize the magnitude of indirect costs of illness may distort health program priorities and policies and lead to resource allocation which does not reflect the true burden of disease on society.

This study assesses the indirect costs of various categories of illness in relation to the direct costs for a poor, semirural area of northeast Brazil. Indirect costs are assessed by calculating the present, discounted value for future earnings lost through permanent disability or death, plus current losses from morbidity. This technique has been utilized to assess the economic cost of a variety of illnesses (Fein, 1958; Klarman, 1965; Rice, 1969; Conly, 1975; Araujo, 1973; Feldstein et al., 1973). In contrast to the U.S., where Cooper and Rice found the ratio of indirect costs to direct costs to be 1.5 in 1972 (Cooper and Rice, 1976), the indirect costs of illness are nearly seven times greater than direct costs in this Brazilian region. Our finding that the major cost of illness is the *hidden* loss of production from morbidity and mortality is probably typical of most developing countries. This information should assist decision-makers in setting more realistic priorities and policies for the health sector.

# II.  BACKGROUND

The calculation of indirect costs of illnesses is based on an assessment of the economic value of human life. Such assessments were made as early as 1693 by Halley (1942) and by Petty (1699), and subseqently refined by Dublin and Lotka in their book *The Money Value of Man.* (1946). Hu and Sandifer (1981) have synthesized the cost of illness methodology noting that over 230 separate cost-benefit analyses of illness have been undertaken. A number of these analyses utilize the human capital approach. (An alternative to the human capital approach is the "willingness to pay" to avoid death or disability approach; a method that estimates how much individuals say they would pay to avoid illness or injury.)

Although little has been published from low and middle income countries on the cost of illness, there is a large body of literature from developed countries. Recent articles on the cost of illness in developing countries include articles from Scandanavia dealing with the cost of diabetes and mental illness in Sweden (Johnson, 1983; Hertzman, 1983) and general illness in Finland (Vinni, 1983).

There have been a number of articles on cost of illness in the United States, both before the landmark study by Cooper and Rice (1976), and more recently. Of particular interest is the 1982 Milbank Fund Publication on the Cost of Illness Methodology, (Hodgeson and Meiners, 1982).

Several books dealing with the principles of measuring the cost of illness have appeared in recent years: *Health: What is it Worth? Measures of Health Benefits,* by Mushkin and Dunlop (1974) and *Principles of Economic Appraisal in Health Care,* by Drummond (1980). A recent textbook on *The Economics of Health in Developing Countries* (Lee and Mills, 1983) has two chapters that deal, in part, with the concept of the cost of illness. ("Economic Appraisal in the Health Sector" by Prescott and Warford and "The Economic Evaluation of Immunization Programs" by Creese.)

The cost of illness that could be prevented by immunization has received considerable attention in both developing and developed countries, as the information is of current importance in determining health policy. Recent studies by the National Academy of Sciences, Institute of Medicine have prioritized vaccine development on the basis of cost of illness. For developing countries, the smallpox cost studies are summarized in Russell's monograph, "Is Prevention Better Than Cure?" (1985).

The costs of measles, primarily in developed countries, have been analyzed in reports ranging from carefully detailed estimates of the cost of measles (Witte and Axnick, 1975) to such nihilistic dismissals of the entire cost of illness approach as: "calculation of savings resulting from a fall in mortality requires and estimate of the value of human life. This can only be arbitrary" (Cutting, 1980). Unfortunately, many health professional reject the concept of placing a value on human life and thus shirk their responsibilities in setting logical health program priorities.

The WHO Cost Benefit Analysis of Tuberculosis Control Programs, including BCG immunization, in Korea present a theoretical analysis, but lack detailed data. The strength of the of the cost of illness approach is shown by the substitution of estimates and approximations for detailed data still leading to reasonable conclusions (Feldstein et al., 1973).

Another key study in developing countires is the study of Years of Life Lost in the Countries of S.E. Asia by Meade (Meade, 1978). This study does not include the morbidity costs of illness and is based on WHO statistical reports of uneven quality on deaths by cause and age. It presents the very important concept of setting health priorities based on years of life lost rather than merely using the number of deaths.

In the United States, the Centers for Disease Control's influential publication, *Morbidity and Mortality Weekly Report* has recently started using potential years of life lost (PYLL) as a better measure of the cost of a disease than simplistically reporting total deaths.

In addition to the actual years of productivity lost from death and days of productivity lost from morbidity, there are two additional factors by which illness decreases productivity: (1) decreased output of sick individuals still on the job, and (2) decreased innovation and entrepreneurship of sick individuals. Malenbaum presents evidence supporting these factors in his chapter in an earlier volume of this Human Capital and Development series (Salkever et al., 1983). Sorkin gives a balanced discussion of the pros and cons of including these factors in the cost of illness estimates in his monograph on Health Economics in Developing Countries (Sorkin, 1976). Based on earlier discussions with Dr. Sorkin, our Brazilian study did not attmept to measure the costs of illness from the above two factors.

In summary, there is a large body of literature on the cost of illness in developed countries and well developed methods for calculating the cost of illness. There is still considerable disagreement on the details and variations of the methods of calculation, and even the appropriateness of using methods that place a value on human life. However, there is very little information on the cost of illness in developing countries. It is our purpose to present both a tested method and results that may be of value for replication in other countries desiring health economic information to help set health resources allocation policy.

## III.   THE STUDY AREA

This study was undertaken in the municipio of Itabuna, in the cacao region of the State of Bahia, Brazil. The study area was chosen because of the presence of a diversity of diseases and health and research agencies whose resources were available.

The municipio is located on a strip of land 50 km wide along the Atlantic Coast. The climate has heavy rainfall and high temperatures, with lower rainfall inland from the coast. The primary product is cacao (chocolate). Cattle raising, light industry and mining are the other main economic activities. In 1977 the population of the municipio was estimated to be 169,138 with 150,252 living in the county seat of Itabuna. Much of the marginal areas of the city would be considered semirural in most countries. Thirty percent of the municipio population was less than 10 years old in 1970; 32 percent of the population was economically active (deCodes, 1979).

Within the cacao region, investment in the urban economic sector has been low until recent governmental efforts to accelerate regional development. Sixty-six percent of the economically active population work in agriculture, 9 percent in industry, and 25 percent in the tertiary or service sector. Recent development efforts include the construction of a coastal road cross-cutting several municipios, including Itabuna, and the establishment of The Executive

Commission for the Cacao Development Plan (CEPLAC) in the region to provide financial credit, support the economy of the cacao industry, and carry out research.

## A. Health

The State of Bahia Secretariat of Health has a rgional office in Itabuna with the responsibility for epidemiological surveillance, reporting of transmissible diseases, death certification, and provision of health services to the 32 municipios of the cacao region. This program was started in Itabuna just before our survey.

Although communicable disease is underreported, available data showed a high level of preventable disease. For example, in 1975, the Foundation for Special Health Services (FSESP), reported 295 *new* cases of tuberculosis without previous treatment. In 1970, 35 cases of schistosomiasis, 44 cases of typhoid, 112 cases of diphtheria, 10 cases of tetanus neonatorum, 1,890 cases of dysentery and 1,050 cases of hookworm were reported in the municipio of Itabuna. These statistics do not completely reflect the low level of health in the municipio, because they are based only on the number of people seeking health care. However, with allowance for underreporting, they give an indication of the communicable diseases of the region. Although injuries are not reported, they are generally recognized to have a high incidence in the region.

The mortality rate reported for the city of Itabuna was 10/1000 population, infant mortaility was reported as 83/1000 live births, and proportional mortality (deaths over 50 years—total deaths) was 35 percent (deCodes, 1979).

# IV. METHODS

## A. Sources of Data for Morbidity and Earnings

Informants in 400 households in the city of Itabuna and 472 households in the rural area of the municipio were interviewed over the course of seven months, between July 1977 and February 1978.

The interviews were conducted by 10 CEPLAC interviewers trained and supervised by the senior author. Interviewers were rotated halfway through the study to check for interviewer bias. Three questionnaires were administered to the urban and rural samples. The initial questionnaire, applied on the first visit to every household, contained information on place of residence (rural district or city area), housing conditions, and demand and utilization of health services. The second questionnaire was administered in every monthly visit to all households. It detected changes in household composition during the period between visits, births and deaths, the occurrence of disease and injury morbidity in the family, and the number of persons affected during the previous month. The third questionnaire was administered during the last round of interviews and elicited background information of percentage reduction of productivity due to diseases or disability, children's participation in the labor force, monthly family income, and family consumption expenditures. Additional information was obtained on nutrition, children attending school, absenteeism from work, food patterns, water utilization and sewage disposal for the households.

## B.   Tuberculosis Morbidity Data Sources

Tuberculosis was selected as an example of a prevalent chronic disease. Special morbidity data was collected from the files of FSESP which has a well-organized TB clinic. Cases of tuberculosis for the year 1977 among permanent residents of the municipio were noted, with specific information about age, sex, source of diagnosis, date of beginning or end of treatment, and reported results.

## C.   Mortaility Data Source

Information on mortality was collected from the Secretaria da Saude Publica do Estado da Bahia (State of Bahia Secretariat of Health). This Department processes the death certificates for the whole state. Death information collected from this source included deaths to Itabuna residents occurring outside the survey area.

## D.   Direct Costs Data Sources

Direct costs of medical care were obtained from agencies providing care to the population of Itabuna in 1977. These include: The State of Bahia Secretariat of Health, FSESP, The National Institute of Medical Assistance and Social Welfare (INAMPS), The Agency from the Ministry of Social Security which provided health care to rural workers and their families (FUNRURAL), the agency responsible for distribution of basic drugs (CME), and the Prefeitura of Itabuna. Information on out-of-pocket expenditures (direct personal payments for physician services, hospital expenses, drugs or other services) was obtained from the community survey.

## E.   Analytical Framework

The basic technique for estimation of the cost of illness utilized in this study is similar to methods used by Weisbrod (1961) and Rice (1969), and Cooper and Rice (1976). Modifications were made to the technique as considered necessary for existing economic conditions and availability of data in the research area. The economic cost of illness was ascertained by examining *direct* and *indirect* costs.

## F.   Direct and Indirect Costs

*Direct costs* are defined as health expenditures by agencies providing direct or indirect health services to the population, plus out-of-pocket expenditures for health care. Direct costs include not only the subsidized price charged to the consumer, but also the costs to maintain the health system infrastructure: administration, supervision, training of personnel, amortized construction, and maintenance of physical facilities and equipment. Hospitalization, drugs, and professional services were the major components of direct costs.

*Indirect Costs of Mortality, Morbidity and Disability* are assessed by calculating the present discounted value of labor earnings lost through permanent disability and death plus current losses through morbidity.

*The Cost of Mortality* was ascertained in this study utilizing the Dublin and Lotka (1946) formula:

$$V_a = \sum_{n=a+\frac{1}{2}}^{\infty} \left[ y_n P_{a+\frac{1}{2}}^n \frac{1}{(1+i)^{n-a}} \right]$$

where a is the person's age group at his last birthday, i is the discount rate, $P_{a+\frac{1}{2}}^n$ is the probability of survival of a person in that age group, up to the end of the period, and $Y_n$, average earnings of a person in that age group. The *cost of morbidity* was measured by days lost from work, as ascertained from a survey of the rural and urban Itabuna population (total days are divided by 222 working days) to convert to years lost. The morbidity detected in the community survey was extrapolated to the total population and the five monthly interviews were extrapolated for the whole study year. For the case of tuberculosis, the cost of morbidity was estimated as the average period of treatment for known cases. The years' cost was multiplied by the appropriate age, sex, and location earnings factors. *Disability* was defined as sequella of disease or injury, preventing return to work after the acute phase. Total disability was uncommon and its future duration uncertain. Partial disability was hard to measure accurately. Therefore, disability was treated as long-term morbidity, thus possibly producing a small underestimate of total direct losses, due to this factor.

To estimate *losses of productivity* from mortality, morbidity or disability, seven factors were considered: (1) life tables constructed for the population; (2) earnings levels by age and sex; (3) consumption; (4) the value of housewives; (5) conversion of current earnings to "maximum monthly salary" value; (6) changes in productivity; and (7) the rate of discount. For the application of Dublin and Lotka's formula, two of these factors had to be determined from the study population, the expected length of work life of the individual and the probability of survival up to the end of the period. *Life tables* for the male and female populations of the municipio were constructed using the Reed-Merrill methods, and are available on request to the author. *Average earning values* for the population were estimated from the survey instrument, based on monthly income. Earning levels were grouped by age and sex to account for variation in income for males and females at specific ages in the Itabuna population. Calculation of average earnings were based on the total population, rather than solely on the economically active population, to correct for unemployment and underemployment.

No consensus has been reached on the importance of correcting for *consumption* to obtain the net earnings. Most economists, including Cooper and Rice (1976), do not deduct consumption from individual earnings, on the grounds that losses to *society,* and not the individual family, are being measured. Some authorities, including Weisbrod (1961) and Mushkin (1959), feel that in developing countries consumption *should* be deducted as essential consumption approximates earnings. As this study measures the burden of ill health to "society," consumption is not deducted.

*The value of housewives* in the municipio of Itabuna is calculated based on information obtained in the survey instrument. Women performing exclusively housework activities (not living alone) were attributed an average value based on male and female earnings by age group for seven different socioeconomic segments of the population.

## G.   Conversion of Cruzerios to Minimum Monthly Salary

A concern of this study is to show the cost of illness in real money value, not permitting high inflation rates for subsequent years to mislead future readers by the costs calculated in the study year. This was done by using a comparative value which would follow the fluctuation of inflation in subsequent years. In this study, the estimated cost of illness for the study year is presented in units of the minimum regional salary stipulated by the Brazilian Federal Government for the State of Bahia from May 1, 1977. A unit was equivalent to Cr $868.50 at the time of the study. By displaying costs in this way, it will be easier for readers in subsequent years to appreciate the present value of the cost of disease in the study year.

*Changes in Productivity* of the average worker over time is of consequence in calculating future earnings. However, there are so many unknown factors determining future worker productivity, ranging from the price of oil to development of new technologies and industries, that we did not attempt to predict the effects of future changes in productivity.

In order to calculate the present value of expected lifetime earnings, it is necessary to apply an appropriate *rate of discount* to convert the future earnings stream to its present worth. Although economists agree that a rate of discount must be used to convert future earnings streams to present value, they differ on the discount rate to be used. The higher the discount rate assigned, the lower will be the present value for a given money stream. Conversely, the lower the discount rate, the higher will be the value of the earnings in the future. The discount rate therefore will have an important influence on setting disease priorities. Klarman (1965) and Heath and Oulton (1973) suggest presenting two or more discount rates. In this study, three different rates of discount (4, 7, and 10 percent) were applied to make sensitivity tests possible for the different rates, showing how variation affects the results of the study. The 10 percent rate reflects the current value of money, being higher in developing than in developed countries. The 4 percent rate of discount probably would result in an overestimation of the cost of death considering possible future increases in productivity. The 7 percent rate of discount is our best estimate for the rate of discount appropriate for Brazil.

# V.  RESULTS

## A.  Mortality

Note:   The tables in the results section have been condensed from detailed working tables.

Mortality data for this study were compiled from death certificates supplied for residents of Itabuna who died anywhere in the State of Bahia in 1977. Population figures were estimated by expansion of the sample data obtained from the survey (deCodes, 1979).

Table 1 shows the number of deaths by sex and age. An estimate of the infant mortality rate for the municipio, 116.2 infant deaths per 1,000 live births, was obtained by dividing the total number of infant deaths (corrected for stillbirth misreporting) by the estimated live births (estimated midyear population in the 0-1 age group plus infant deaths). Fifty-seven percent of infant deaths occurred in the first 30 days of life. The estimated general mortality rate for the municipio was 8.68 per 1000 population.

Table 2 presents deaths by age and cause of death. Fifty percent of the total deaths for both sexes were classified as *ill-defined conditions*. The lack of

*Table 1.* Deaths by Age and Sex

| Age Group | Male | Female | Total |
|---|---|---|---|
| 0-1 | 373 | 303 | 676 |
| 1-4 | 57 | 62 | 119 |
| 5-14 | 34 | 22 | 56 |
| 15-34 | 57 | 47 | 104 |
| 35-54 | 73 | 69 | 142 |
| 55-74 | 135 | 104 | 239 |
| 75+ | 74 | 58 | 132 |
| Total | 803 | 665 | 1,468 |

*Table 2.* Deaths by Cause and Age

| Age | Gastro-enteritis | Tuber-culosis | Respiratory | Peri-natal | Injuries | Ill-Defined | Other | Total |
|---|---|---|---|---|---|---|---|---|
| 0-1 | 59 | — | 35 | 197 | 4 | 360 | 21 | 676 |
| 1-4 | 11 | 1 | 12 | 1* | 5 | 77 | 12 | 119 |
| 5-14 | 3 | — | 2 | 1* | 14 | 25 | 11 | 56 |
| 15-34 | 1 | 3 | 1 | 1* | 40 | 36 | 22 | 104 |
| 35-54 | 3 | 1 | 2 | — | 17 | 46 | 73 | 142 |
| 55-74 | 1 | 3 | 5 | — | 10 | 118 | 102 | 249 |
| 75+ | — | — | 5 | — | 3 | 76 | 48 | 132 |
| Total | 78 | 8 | 62 | 200 | 93 | 738 | 289 | 1,468 |

*3 miscoded by age

*Table 3.* Itabuna, Brazil, 1977: Estimated Annual Number of Episodes of Disease by Group, Total Population

| Age | Gastro-enteritis | Tuber-culosis | Respiratory | Injuries | Ill-Defined | Other | Total |
|---|---|---|---|---|---|---|---|
| 0-1 | 2,937 | 3 | 4,383 | 542 | 1,244 | 1,097 | 10,206 |
| 1-4 | 7,939 | 30 | 14,515 | 3,449 | 2,027 | 5,613 | 33,573 |
| 5-14 | 2,867 | 39 | 13,492 | 6,856 | 2,257 | 7,853 | 33,364 |
| 15-34 | 2,212 | 177 | 14,991 | 9,649 | 4,075 | 9,972 | 41,076 |
| 35-54 | 2,895 | 89 | 9,786 | 5,872 | 3,374 | 12,047 | 34,063 |
| 55-74 | 983 | 28 | 6,811 | 2,935 | 3,002 | 8,717 | 22,476 |
| 75+ | 194 | 3 | 451 | 609 | 190 | 1,119 | 2,566 |
| Total | 20,027 | 369 | 64,429 | 29,912 | 16,169 | 46,418 | 177,324 |

diagnosis indicated the deficiency of health services coverage in this region. In order of decreasing importance in *numbers* of deaths are: perinatal causes, injuries, gastroenteritis, respiratory disease and tuberculosis (a few tuberculosis deaths may be included among respiratory and ill-defined conditions). The proportions of deaths by case groups are similar for both sexes with the exception that deaths by injury is three times higher for males than for females. The distribution of deaths for urban and rural areas are similar with the exception of higher rates from ill-defined causes in the rural population, as expected in areas of poor medical coverage.

The estimated incidence of disease by age groups is shown in Table 3. Incidence of tuberculosis is based on all cases or residents treated by FSESP. Comparisons of rural-urban rates (from detailed working tables not presented) show that the incidence of gastroenteritis and tuberculosis is higher in the rural area while injury and respiratory diseases incidence is higher in the urban area. (The most frequent condition in the group of respiratory diseases was the common cold, followed by bronchitis.) Morbidity from ill-defined conditions, as expected, had a higher incidence in the rural areas.

# VI.   INDIRECT COST OF ILLNESS

## A.   Morbidity—Estimating Loss of Current Productivity

Table 4 shows the *total estimate* of years of work lost from acute morbidity in the municipio of Itabuna. This table illustrates the impact caused by different groups of disease on the active labor force. Injuries and other specific diseases were essentially of equal importance and were responsible for over 80 percent of all work time losses. Of total male work time losses, injuries were responsible for almost 50 percent. The group of "other specific diseases" was responsible for the greatest work time loss among females (63 percent

*Table 4.*   Estimated Number of Years of Work
Lost by Groups of Diseases, Total Population

| Age | Gastro-enteritis | Tuber-culosis | Respiratory | Injuries | Ill-Defined | Other | Total |
|---|---|---|---|---|---|---|---|
| 10-14 | — | 1 | 3 | 20 | 1 | 7 | 32 |
| 15-34 | 82 | 85 | 105 | 910 | 117 | 513 | 1,812 |
| 35-54 | 62 | 56 | 73 | 713 | 166 | 934 | 2,004 |
| 55-74 | 4 | 21 | 46 | 663 | 94 | 699 | 1,527 |
| 75+ | — | 3 | 2 | 3 | — | 153 | 161 |
| Total | 148 | 166 | 229 | 2,309 | 378 | 2,306 | 5,536 |

of urban female and 43 percent of rural female time loss). Injuries were second in importance, followed by respiratory disease, among urban females. In rural areas, ill-defined conditions was second in importance among females, followed by tuberculosis.

## Mortality: Present Value of Future Productivity

Table 5 shows the cost estimates of premature mortality in the total population by disease groups. Percentages of total costs for each disease group are given for the three rates of discount (4 and 7, 10 percent discussed in the previous section), illustrating how the magnitude of indirect costs are affected by different discount rates.

Analysis of mortality losses for the total population shows the large group of ill-defined conditions as the leading group under any rate of discount, probably because the lack of diagnosis is high in the very young. As expected, the magnitude and percentage of total losses from the ill-defined group decreases with higher discount rates. Gastroenteritis and respiratory diseases also show lower indirect costs from mortality at higher interest rates, as they occur more frequently in younger age groups. Tuberculosis and injury deaths show a relatively smaller decrease in indirect costs at higher discount rates due to the paucity of deaths in the youngest age groups. As expected, the cost for

*Table 5.* Premature Mortality Losses by Group of Diseases, at Different Rates of Discount (Values in Annual Minimum Salary Units), Total Population

| Group of Diseases | 4% Disc Rate | % | 7% Disc Rate | % | 10% Disc Rate | % |
|---|---|---|---|---|---|---|
| Gastro-enteritis | 2511.78 | 5.9 | 1019.53 | 4.6 | 500.51 | 3.5 |
| Tuberculosis | 294.55 | .69 | 194.93 | .88 | 195.69 | 1.4 |
| Injuries | 4870.84 | 11.5 | 3035.12 | 13.7 | 2142.12 | 15.0 |
| Respiratory | 1712.79 | 4.0 | 724.39 | 3.3 | 379.3 | 2.6 |
| Perinatal | 5908.13 | 13.9 | 2160.91 | 9.7 | 918.85 | 6.4 |
| Ill-defined | 19114.11 | 45.1 | 9452.37 | 42.6 | 5782.73 | 40.3 |
| All other | 7953.95 | 18.8 | 5611.34 | 25.3 | 4423.72 | 30.8 |
| All Diseases | 42366.15 | 100% | 22198.59 | 100% | 14342.92 | 100% |

Annual Minimum Salary Unit = Cr$ 10422.00

perinatal deaths are the most sharply decreased by higher rates of discount. Estimates for the rural population show a similar pattern except for higher losses from ill-defined causes.

## B. Total Indirect Cost

The total indirect cost from illness was obtained by adding the present value of future earnings losses, estimated at the 7 percent rate of discount, to the estimated current earnings losses from morbidity. This was caculated for the total population of the municipio and separately for the urban and rural population. The per capita values were converted to monthly minimum salary units to make international comparisons easier and provide a more stable measure in a country with triple digit inflation. Table 6 shows the total indirect cost for the total population. The cost of injuries is more than five times greater than any specific disease, greater than the whole group of ill-defined conditions, and only slightly smaller than the category "all other diseases combined." Gastroenteritis and respiratory diseases cause losses of approximately the same magnitude, about twice as high as tuberculosis.

Comparison of losses between rural and urban populations should not be made in absolute values, because of the difference in population sizes. However, the total indirect loss from each population segment was divided by the population, resulting in per capita indirect costs. The rural-urban differences were not remarkable on a percentage basis, probably reflecting the semi-rural character of the so-called urban population. The groups of injuries, "all other diseases," and tuberculosis have higher costs for morbidity than for mortality. Tuberculosis is a chronic and disabling condition, which may explain the higher cost for morbidity. Also, part of the tuberculosis mortality cost may be hidden

*Table 6.* Estimate of Indirect Cost from Illness for
Total Population (Values in Annual Minimum Salary Units)

| Group of Diseases | Mortality 7% Disc | Morbidity | Total Cost |
|---|---|---|---|
| Gastroenteritis | 1019.53 | 486.69 | 1506.22 |
| Tuberculosis | 194.93 | 657.44 | 852.37 |
| Respiratory | 724.39 | 640.46 | 1364.85 |
| Perinatal | 2160.91 | - | 2160.91 |
| Injuries | 3035.12 | 8239.61 | 11274.73 |
| Ill-defined | 9452.37 | 1293.88 | 10746.25 |
| All other | 5611.34 | 7470.82 | 13082.16 |
| All Diseases | 22198.59 | 18788.90 | 40987.49 |

in the costs of respiratory and "ill-defined conditions" mortality. The cost of mortality for gastroenteritis is higher than the cost of morbidity. This is explained by the prevalence of high infant mortality from gastroenteritis. These losses are derived from prospective earnings of young populations rather than from work losses from the productive population.

## C.  Comparison of Direct and Indirect Costs

Table 7 shows direct and indirect costs of disease for the total population by disease category. The total direct cost is high, but the indirect cost is almost seven times greater. The group of "other specific diseases" is responsible for more losses than any other group. The obvious reason is that there are many diseases in this category. The indirect cost of injuries is 16 times greater than the direct cost.

The relationship between direct and indirect cost for respiratory diseases does not follow the pattern of other disease groups as direct costs for respiratory diseases are higher than total indirect costs. This can be explained by the common cold, the most frequent respiratory condition observed, customarily causes little loss of productive time, but the symptoms lead to a high demand for medications purchased by out-of-pocket expenditure. Actually out-of-pocket expenses for respiratory diseases were greater than indirect costs. "Ill-defined disease" has high indirect costs and relatively low direct costs, perhaps showing the lack of physician care, as there are small out-of-pocket expenditures for the "ill-defined conditions" group.

Health expenditures for perinatal causes of death were estimated based on percentages from prenatal and perinatal care for all institutions, on specific expenditures from the nutrition program, and on the estimated number of

*Table 7.*   Itabuna, Brazil, 1977: Direct and Indirect Costs
of Diseases Value in Annual Minimum Salary Units

| Group of Diseases | Total Institution | Out of Pocket | Total Direct | Total Indirect | Total |
|---|---|---|---|---|---|
| Gastroenteritis | 286 | 350 | 636 | 1506 | 2142 |
| Tuberculosis | 130 | — | 130 | 852 | 982 |
| Respiratory | 210 | 1419 | 1629 | 1365 | 2994 |
| Perinatal | 57 | - | 57 | 2161 | 2218 |
| Injuries | 182 | 526 | 708 | 11275 | 11983 |
| Ill-defined | 26 | 425 | 451 | 10746 | 11197 |
| All other | 1147 | 1262 | 2410 | 13082 | 15492 |
| All Diseases | 2038 | 3983 | 6020 | 40988 | 47008 |

Annual Minimum Salary Unit = Cr$ 10422.00

births in the population year. No out-of-pocket expenses were reported from the sample. The total indirect cost for this group (exclusively mortality) is high compared to the cost of other groups because of the large number of future productive years lost.

Total indirect cost for gastroenteritis is more than twice the total direct health expenditures for the disease. Out-of-pocket expenditures for respiratory diseases exceeded the institutional cost. This is important, considering that the segment of the population most vulnerable to this illness is the lowest economic level. Per capita cost of illness is more than one quarter of the annual minimum salary, or 3.3 monthly minimum salaries per person!

In summary, the analysis shows an infant mortality of 116 and a general mortality of almost 9/1000 population. The deaths by cause show a high number of perinatal deaths, injuries, gastroenteritis, and respiratory disease. Unfortunately, a large number of deaths, almost 50 percent, were not well diagnosed. In terms of morbidity: gastroenteritis and tuberculosis are high in the rural areas, while injuries and respiratory diseases are high in the urban areas. The information presented on the indirect costs for mortality, at different interest rates, is presented to show the relative robustness of the estimates. The total costs of illness, both direct and indirect, were calculated and will be discussed in the following section of conclusions.

## CONCLUSIONS

This study compares direct and indirect costs of illness in a poor, rural and semi-rural Brazilian county with a small urban capital. It clearly shows that the indirect cost of lost productivity from illness is much greater than the direct health expenditure. Figure 1 shows the relative contributions of both components. This information is of major importance to public health planners.

Figure 2 shows the relationship of direct and indirect costs for our five disease groupings. Only upper respiratory disease caused more direct than indirect costs. This is to be expected as the "common cold" has very high prevalence and often entails purchase and use of medicine, but causes little morbidity and no mortality.

Figure 2 also indicates that injuries deserve high priority for public health program investment allocation. Occupational and road accidents are responsible for the majority of lost production from injuries.

The large size of the group of "ill-defined conditions" shows that physicians are rarely available to provide definitive diagnoses of cause of death. Thus, the highest rates of ill-defined deaths are in rural areas. The 0-4 deaths were responsible for most of the indirect costs, and consequently, most of the total cost for the "ill-defined" group. Undiagnosed, infectious diseases and malnutrition may play an important role in this "ill-defined" group.

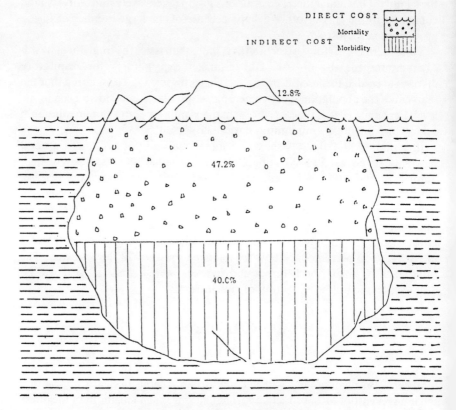

*Figure 1.*   Itabuna—Brazil, 1977
Proportion of Total Direct and Indirect Cost of Illness

The cost of gastroenteritis was less than expected. Perhaps some of the 0-4 ill-defined conditions are undiagnosed gastroenteritis.

The large size of the "other defined conditions" category points up a major problem. Simple primary health care programs now being planned to control a few major diseases will have no effect on over one-third of the cost of all illnesses.

In summary: This study has assessed the direct and indirect costs of various categories of disease for a rural area of Brazil. The study shows that the indirect cost of illness is much greater than the outlay for health expenditures in this rural municipio. Comparison of direct and indirect costs for each disease category should help health planners set health priorities and facilitate allocation of resources in a cost-effective manner.

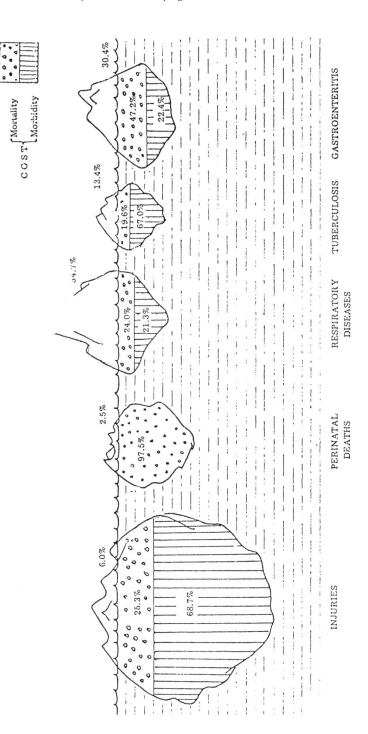

*Figure 2.* Itabuna—Brazil, 1977
Proportion of Direct and Indirect Cost of Illness by Disease Groups

As this methodology is applied in other developing countries it should be of great value to health planners in making the difficult decisions they face in the allocation of scarce resources within the health sector.

# REFERENCES

Araujo, J. (1973). *Aspectos Economicos de Saude.* (Thesis presented to the Faculty of Medicine of the Federal University of Bahia, Salvador, Brazil).

Conly, G. (1975). *The Impact of Malaria on Economic Development: A Case Study,* Scientific Publication No. 297, (Pan American Health Organization).

Cooper, B., and Rice, D. (1976). "The Economic Cost of Illness Revisited," *Social Security Bulletin* (February:21-36).

Cutting, W.A.M. (1980). Cost Benefit Evaluations of Vaccination Programs. *The Lancet,* September 20, p. 634.

deCodes, J. (1979). *Measuring the Economic Impact of Illness in the Municipio of Itabuna, Bahia, Brazil.* (Doctoral thesis, Department of International Health, The Johns Hopkins University School of Public Health).

Drummond, M.F. (1980). *Principles of Economic Appraisal in Health Care.* England: Oxford University Press.

Dublin, L., and Lotka, A. (1946). *The Money Value of Man* (New York: The Ronald Press).

Economic Aspects of Communicable Diseases. (1981). Report of a WHO Working Group. EURO Reports and Studies 1968. Regional Office for Europe, WHO, Copenhagen.

Feldstein, M., Piot, A., and Sundaresan, T.K. (1973). "Resource Allocation Model for Public Health Planning: A Case Study of Tuberculosis Control," *Bulletin of the World Health Organization,* Vol. 48, Supplement.

Fein, R. (1958). *Economics of Mental Illness* (New York: Basic Books).

Governo Federal de Brasil. Lei no 6 20S de Abril de 1975.

Halley, E. (1693/1942). An Estimate of the Degrees of the Mortality of Mankind, drawn from curious Tables of the Births and Funerals at the City of Breslow, with an Attempt to ascertain the price of Annuities upon Lives. Philosophical Transactions Vol. XVII, 1693, London. Reprinted Baltimore, MD; Johns Hopkins Press.

Heath, J., and Oulton, W. (1973). "A Cost-Benefit Study of Alternative Runway Investments at Edinburgh (Turnhouse) Airport," *Cost-Benefit and Cost-Effectiveness Studies and Analysis,* J. Wolfe (ed.) (London: George Allen Unwin Ltd.).

Hertzman, P. (1983). The Economic Cost of Mental Illness in Sweden. *ACTA-Psychiatr-Scand.* Nov., Vol. 68, No. 5, pp. 359-367.

Hodgson, T.A., and Meiners, M.R. (1982). Cost of Illness Methodology: A Guide to Current Practices and Procedures. *Milbank Memorial Fund Quarterly,* Summer, 60 (3), pp. 429-462.

Hu, T., and Sandifer, F. (1981). *Synthesis of Cost of Illness Methodology.* (Washington, D.C.: Public Services Laboratory, Georgetown University).

Johnson, B. (1983). Diabetes: The Cost of Illness and the Cost of Control: An estimate for Sweden. *ACTA-Med-Scand* (suppl.) 671, pp. 19-27.

Klarman, H. (1965). "Syphilis Control Programs," *Measuring the Benefits of Government Investments,* R. Dorfman (ed.), (Washington, D.C.: Brookings Institution).

Lee, K., and Mills, A. (eds.). (1983). *The Economics of Health in Developing Countries,* England; Oxford University Press.

Meade, M.S. (1978). Potential Years of Life Lost in Countries of S.E. Asia. *Soc-Sci-Med,* Vol. 14D, pp. 277-281.

Mushkin, S., and Collings, F. (1959). "Economic Costs of Disease and Injury," *Public Health Reports* 74, September.

Mushkin, S., and Dunlop, D.W. (eds.). (1979). *Health: What is it Worth? Measures of Health Benefits,* Elmsford, N.Y. Pergamon Press.

Petty, Sir William. (1699). Political Arithmetick, or a Discourse Concerning the Extent and Value of Lands People Buildings, Etc. London; Robert Clavel.

Rice, D. (1969). "Measurement and Application of Illness Costs," *Public Health Reports* 84:95-101.

Russell, L.B. (1985). *Is Prevention Better than Cure?* The Brookings Institution, Washington, D.C.

Salkever, D., Siragledin, I., and Sorkin, A. (1983). Research in Human Capital and Development, *Vol. 3, Health and Development,* Greenwich, Conn.: JAI Press.

Sorkin, A. (1976). *Health Economics in Developing Countries,* Lexington, MA: Lexington, Books.

Vinni, K. (1983). Productivity Losses Due to Illness, Disability and Premature Death in Different Occupational Groups in Finland. *Soc-Sci-Med,* 17 (3) pp. 163-167.

Weisbrod, B. (1961). *Economics of Public Health* (Philadelphia: University of Pennsylvania Press).

Witte, J.J., and Axnick, N. W. (1975). The Benefits from 10 years of Measles Immunization in the U.S. *Public Health Reports,* May/June.

# CHANGES IN HEALTH CARE DEMAND AND SUPPLY ACCOMPANYING ECONOMIC DEVELOPMENT

Peter Berman and Barbara A. Ormond

In the popular imagination, health is an important component of economic development—perhaps even one of its main goals. Economic development is expected to bring a combination of improved economic conditions and improved health care that will result in people's attaining longer lives, less disrupted by disease and disability. This implies that the major infectious diseases which account for the bulk of mortality and morbidity in poor countries will eventually be controlled or even eliminated, much as thay have been in the more developed countries today.

Experience proves these expectations to be well-founded. Low income countries that have experienced significant economic growth have seen rapid increases in the availability of health care and in the total volume of services provided, accompanied by measurable health improvements as shown by

Research in Human Capital Development, Vol. 5, pages 147-172.

increased life expectancy. In some countries, such improvements have also been reflected in changes in disease patterns. Infectious and parasitic diseases have decreased in frequency while chronic and degenerative diseases have become more prevalent. These changes in the level and pattern of demand for health services warrant closer attention because of the important implications for health planning and financing.

The aggregate statistics show a growing total demand for health services but they give little insight into changes in the composition of demand, such as shifts in the disease profile and changes in demand for particular types of providers or types of care. Higher income and urban populations may experience a disease profile similar to that of higher income countries, while lower income and rural populations still contend mainly with the diseases of underdevelopment. Differences in the level of household income may also be associated with changes in health care preferences, with demand for services of a higher perceived quality (physicians or hospitals versus paramedics or health centers, for example) rising with income. Furthermore, there are often significant differences in the need for, and access to, care within countries.

In addition to the effect of economic growth on demand and supply of health services, the development and dissemination of new health care technology has been an important factor in recent years in the changing structure of the health sector. Preventive care programs such as the expanded program on immunization (EPI) coordinated by the World Health Organization and diarrheal disease control programs emphasizing oral rehydration therapy are being promoted as affordable and fast-acting remedies to high levels of infant and child mortality. In contrast to such relatively inexpensive (on a per capita basis) and broad-scale programs, more and more expensive machinery and pharmaceuticals are available for the treatment of the chronic and degenerative diseases which are characteristic of the disease profile of high income groups.

This paper will discuss the experience of developing countries with regard to changes in the demand for and supply of health care. First, aggregate changes over time in health care supply, use, and expenditures and the relationship between these changes and increases in national income are examined. Then, differences in the pattern of use among different income groups are considered including differences in the relative importance of curative and preventive services, in the mix of private and public services, and between urban and rural areas. Recent household studies of the demand for health care in rural areas will also be reviewed to explore the micro-level implications of these aggregate changes. The concluding section of the paper will address the directions and levels of the changes that occur as countries move from low to middle income levels, how they can be better anticipated by planners, and their financial implications.

# I.   TRENDS IN ECONOMIC DEVELOPMENT AND THE DEMAND FOR HEALTH CARE: GUIDELINES FROM THEORY

## A.   Economic Growth and Aggregate Demand for Health Care

Historically, health services have been universally regarded as a "normal good," that is, the consumption of health services increases with rising income. In other words, health care is something that people seem to want more of as their ability to purchase goods increases. A recent international comparison of expenditures (using a sample of 20 countries) showed that as real GDP per capita rises, so does the percentage of GDP devoted to health. The lowest income countries spent an average of 2.9 percent of GDP on health while the highest income countries spent an average of 9.1 percent (Kravis, 1982). Growth in aggregate expenditures for health care has outstripped growth in aggregate income to a significant degree, a relationship that holds even among the wealthy (and healthy) countries of Europe and North America.

This trend, however, contains a paradox. Health care is not a typical consumption good like ice cream or furniture. Rather, it is used in large part to counteract the negative effects of illness. As incomes increase, people also tend to get healthier—mortality and morbidity rates decline. This rise in health status would suggest that, with rising income, people would consume less health services not more, at least after they had reached an initial satisfactory level of care. Yet the recent rapid expansion of health expenditures in the developed economies has not been accompanied by significant improvements in health status. The benefits of health care seem to have reached a plateau, while consumption continues to rise. What factors could explain these trends?

First, while it is true that populations become healthier as incomes rise, it is also true that their health needs change. Wealthier populations tend to be older populations. Chronic and degenerative diseases increase in frequency and infectious and parasitic diseases decline. The former may require lengthier and, thus, more costly treatment. They may also require more sophisticated technology further contributing to increased cost. The result could be rising health care expenditures paralleling improved population health.

A second line of argument involves the value of human capital. Economic development is generally accompanied by increases in the value of human labor from rising productivity. Health becomes a more valuable commodity as the opportunity cost of income foregone due to illness increases. Health services can be seen as an investment or maintenance expense to assure continued returns from the increasingly valuable asset found in human work time. Logically, then, increased income and returns to human work justify increased expenditures on maintaining human productivity (see Mushkin, 1965).

A third view related to the previous argument is that health care is a means, and only one of several means, of procuring the commodity truly desired by people—good health (Grossman, 1972). Health itself is at least a normal if not a luxury good, something for which there is a seemingly insatiable demand. Thus, as incomes rise more is spent on health. The proportion of income spent on health may even increase, implying an income elasticity of demand greater than one (for health, if not for health care). This trend may not show up in improvements in health status measures, which only crudely measure "health." Improvements in "health" at high income levels may be more subjective "quality of life" benefits that contribute to a greater sense of physical well-being and fitness without affecting morbidity or mortality indices.

A fourth hypothesis ascribes the trend of increasing health expenditures to institutional structures in the provision of health care: specifically the increased emphasis on specialized, high technology medicine; the lack of control of health care consumers over the amount of care they receive; and widespread use of third-party payment schemes. As mentioned earlier, changes in disease patterns may lead to increased use of more expensive therapies. Consumers also may have little control over the quantity of service they receive or their costs once they have initiated treatment. In addition, with health insurance the actual total cost of care may matter little to the individual, since the level of out-of-pocket payments they have to bear in the form of copayments and deductibles may be only a small proportion of the total cost.

All of these are plausible explanations for observed trends relating rising aggregate health care demand to increased income. Developing countries can probably expect similar trends—a general increase in health expenditures as national income rises; health care expenditures increasing as a proportion of household expenditures; and rapid expansion of the demand for health care even after the rate of gains in health status have declined.

## B.  Curative and Preventive Health Care

In considering the relative share of curative and preventive health care in overall demand, it is important to note that the distiction between cure and prevention is difficult to make precisely and is frequently hopelessly muddled in the data.

Some health services can clearly be classified as preventive and clearly identified as such in national data—especially when governments are the main providers of such services, as they are in many developing countries. These services include immunizations, prenatal and well-child care, and water supply and sanitation programs. One important difficulty occurs as preventive services are provided in the context of individual patient care, such as an outpatient visit to a physician. The majority of such contacts are probably curative in nature. A significant quantity of preventive services are certainly provided in this way as well. Thus, data presented below on "curative" care contacts probably overstate the amount of such services and underestimate the quantity of preventive care.

One would expect increases in demand for both curative and preventive care within the overall trend of increasing health care expenditures accompanying rising incomes. For preventive care, a number of factors would support this tendency. First, increases in education lead to more attention to health-maintaining behavior, including individual behavior and use of preventive services. This argument primarily posits a shift in preferences. Related to this and to the human capital views presented above, preventive services will be favored as a more efficient way of maintaining health as compared with curative care. Rational consumers seeking to assure health would invest marginal resources in prevention to avoid larger expenditures later on for treatment. This argument holds as well for governments and other provider institutions. For example, the efficiency gains of health maintenance organizations are attributed, in part, to increased emphasis on prevention.

While preventive care demand should increase with income, its growth may lag behind that of curative care in terms of aggregate expenditures. Preventive care is generally simpler and cheaper than curative, hence its efficiency. Thus, one would expect a trend of increasing expenditures for both types of care, but with an increasing proportion of total expenditure going to curative service. Preventive care may also substitute for curative to some degree, by preventing illness and hence future treatment. The rate at which this happens, however, will probably not exceed the rate of growth for new curative care. Overall, curative care will account for a larger and increasing proportion of overall health care consumption.

Public and private institutions such as national health insurance or third-party payment mechanisms may distort the balance between curative and preventive care, however. For example, some schemes cover curative care expenses, but not preventive. This approach has the perverse effect of pushing rational individual behavior away from increased use of preventive care. In recent years, the movement towards cost containment in the industrialized countries may have countered this trend. Insurance companies, health maintenance organizations, and others increasingly emphasize or require health promoting behavior or services in order to reduce the growth in costs.

## II. DEVELOPMENT AND THE SUPPLY OF CURATIVE AND PREVENTIVE SERVICES

Almost all developing countries, even the very poor, have seen dramatic expansion in the quantity of health services in the past several decades. In most cases the existing services are still inadequate, or inadequately distributed, to

Table 1.  Supply of Health Care in Twenty Developing Countries, 1965-1983

| | Physicians/10,000 population | | | Nursing pers/10,000 population | | | Hospital beds/10,000 population | | | GNP |
|---|---|---|---|---|---|---|---|---|---|---|
| | 1965 | MRE[a] | % change | 1965 | MRE[a] | % change | 1965 | MRE[a] | % change | growth rate[b] |
| Argentina | 15.87 | 24.81 | 56.33 | 13.33 | 14.71 | 10.29 | 62.50 | 54.05 | -13.51 | 0.50 |
| Bolivia | 2.67 | 5.10 | 91.23 | 4.15 | 6.20 | 49.41 | 24.39 | 17.99 | -26.26 | 0.60 |
| Brazil | 4.18 | 8.60 | 105.50 | 5.08 | 26.18 | 415.72 | 27.03 | 43.10 | 59.48 | 5.00 |
| Chile | 4.81 | 5.18 | 7.77 | 16.39 | 24.69 | 50.62 | 41.67 | 28.99 | -30.43 | -0.10 |
| Costa Rica | 4.93 | 10.00 | 103.00 | 17.54 | 29.67 | 69.14 | 41.67 | 33.67 | -19.19 | 2.10 |
| Dominican Republic | 6.13 | 4.15 | -32.37 | 3.70 | 11.20 | 202.35 | 29.41 | 28.49 | -3.13 | 3.90 |
| Egypt | 4.42 | 12.27 | 177.30 | 5.18 | 6.67 | 28.67 | 21.74 | 20.00 | -8.00 | 4.20 |
| Honduras | 1.83 | 3.21 | 74.68 | 5.95 | 14.29 | 140.00 | 15.87 | 12.80 | -19.33 | 0.60 |
| India | 2.06 | 3.93 | 90.96 | 0.91 | 1.86 | 104.09 | 5.99 | 7.91 | 32.02 | 1.50 |
| Indonesia | 0.31 | 0.87 | 175.98 | 2.22 | 4.35 | 96.09 | 6.90 | 5.60 | -18.86 | 5.00 |
| Ivory Coast | 0.48 | N.A. | N.A. | 3.30 | N.A. | N.A. | 18.52 | 16.98 | -8.32 | 1.00 |
| Jordan | 2.14 | 5.84 | 172.94 | 5.52 | 7.63 | 38.17 | 17.54 | 8.13 | -53.66 | 6.90 |
| Kenya | 0.94 | 0.95 | 1.81 | 5.05 | 18.18 | 260.00 | 12.66 | 16.64 | 31.45 | 2.30 |
| Malawi | 0.21 | 0.24 | 13.92 | 0.79 | 2.61 | 230.81 | 13.70 | 13.51 | -1.35 | 2.20 |
| Malaysia | 1.62 | 1.26 | -21.74 | 5.00 | 10.64 | 112.77 | 34.48 | 27.03 | -21.62 | 4.50 |
| Morocco | 0.83 | 0.89 | 7.23 | 4.41 | 5.46 | 24.04 | 15.38 | 11.79 | -23.35 | 2.90 |
| Senegal | 0.47 | 0.77 | 62.80 | 3.86 | 7.14 | 85.00 | 12.35 | 11.11 | -10.00 | -0.50 |
| Sri Lanka | 1.74 | 1.31 | -24.65 | 2.96 | 7.46 | 152.24 | 31.25 | 25.41 | -5.88 | 2.90 |
| Tanzania | 0.46 | 0.57 | 23.86 | 4.35 | 3.36 | -22.82 | 17.86 | 20.00 | 12.00 | 0.90 |
| Thailand | 1.38 | 1.46 | 5.53 | 1.98 | 4.13 | 108.26 | 8.55 | 15.20 | 77.81 | 4.30 |

[a]MRE = most recent estimate (1977-1983)
[b]Average annual rate of growth of GNP 1965, 1983

Source:  supply date:
World Bank, World Tables (3rd edition), (Baltimore: JHU Press, 1983)
PAHO, Program Budget, 1986-1987, PAHO Document No. 187, March 1985
UN, Statistical Yearbook, various years

Source:  GNP growth rate:
World Bank, World Development Report 1985, (New York: Oxford University Press, 1985)

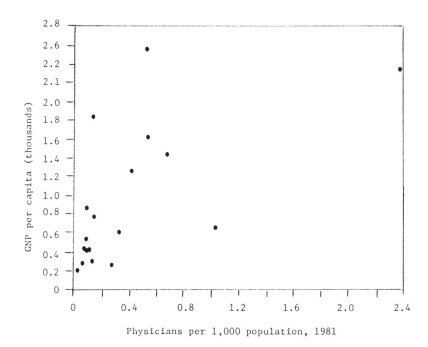

*Source:* Same as Table 1, and *World Bank Atlas,* various years.

*Figure 1.* Health Care Supply, Population, and
National Income, Physicians, 1981

reach much of the population. In some countries supply has not expanded
at all or has not kept up with the growth in population.

Figure 1 shows the changes in the supply of health care in 20 developing
countries from 1965-1983. Most countries show an increase in the supply of
physicians relative to population. A similar relationship is seen for the ratio
of registered nurses to population. In some countries, the expansion has been
quite rapid: Indonesia in terms of physicians; Brazil in terms of nurses. These
have generally been planned responses to manpower shortages or imbalances.

In the case of the hospital bed/population ratio the overall trends in supply
are not so clear. Some countries have experienced increases in hospital bed
supply relative to population (Brazil, Thailand) while others have experienced
large declines (Chile, Jordan). These declines do not necessarily represent
absolute loss of hospital beds, only the inability of supply to keep up with
population growth. Higher income developing countries such as Argentina and
Costa Rica did 'not appear to expand hospital bed supply significantly,
although they continued to add health manpower relative to population.

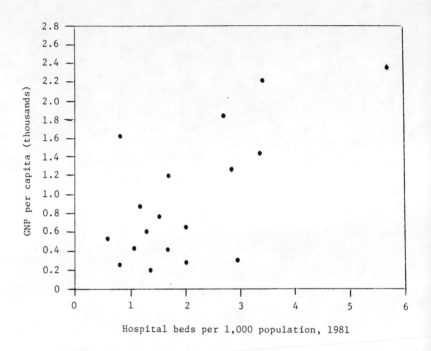

Source: Same as Figure 1, and World Bank Atlas, various years.

*Figure 2.*   Health Care Supply, Population and
National Income, Hospital Beds, 1981

In general, health care supply has been expanding. The overall level of supply is also clearly related to the level of national income. Figures 1 and 2 show the population/physician ratio and the population/hospital bed ratio plotted against GNP per capita in 1981 for a range of developing countries. A distinct relationship of increased supply with increased income is apparent, although there is considerable variability among countries.

While the supply of health care infrastructure such as essential manpower and facilities like hospitals and health centers has expanded, many countries have also allocated substantial resources to mass preventive health care programs. These include the expanded program of immunization, programs to provide major improvements in the availability of clean water, and mass family planning programs.

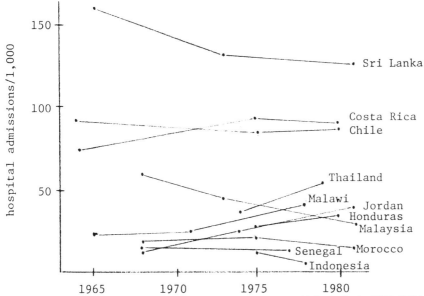

*Sources:* WHO, Statistical Annual, various years; L.A. Simenor, *Better Health for Sri Lanka,* WHO, SEA/
PHA/149, 5 Nov. '75; PAHO, Coordination de los Servicios Medicos, 1967.

*Figure 3.*    Hospital Admissions per 1000 Population c. 1965-1981

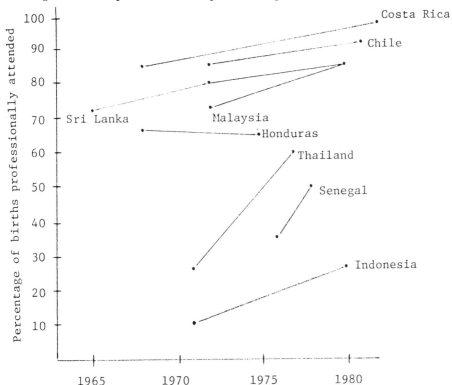

*Source:*    WHO, *The Coverage of Maternity Care: A Tabulation of Available Data,* FHE/85.1, 1985.

*Figure 4.*    Percent of Births Professionally Attended c. 1965-1981

## III.   ECONOMIC DEVELOPMENT AND THE
## STRUCTURE OF SERVICE USE AND EXPENDITURES

The expansion of health service supply just described has, of course, been accompanied by growth in the level of service use and expenditures. The growth in service use, however, has not been distributed evenly across all services and types of facilities.

Figure 3 shows changes in the number of hospital admissions per 1,000 population for 10 developing countries between 1965 and 1981. Some countries showed large increases in admissions, while others reported decreases or little change. Some countries indicating a decrease in hospital admissions have been reported elsewhere as being successful in the development of primary care networks that may be substituting for previously unnecessary hospitalizations (see, for example, Heller, 1982, on Malaysia). Unfortunately, time trend figures for primary care contacts, such as physician visits or health center contacts, are available for very few countries. Figure 4 shows a rising trend in outpatient visits per capita in four Latin American countries between 1965 and 1983.

Figure 5 presents similar time series data for the percent of professionally attended births, defined as births assisted by physicians, nurses or trained midwives. Virtually all countries report increases in the use of this type of service. Similar trends can be documented for specific preventive care services such as prenatal care as seen in Figure 6. There has also been a rapid expansion of childhood immunization levels in the last five years. Figure 7 shows the estimated current levels of immunization coverage of infants in different regions of the world. Outside of the Africa and Southeast Asia regions (these are regions as defined by WHO) immunization levels are near to or exceed 50 percent (WHO, 1985). In particular, dramatic increases have been achieved in Latin America in recent years. Vaccination coverage of children under one year against polio, for example, has risen from an average of 34 percent in 1977 to 78 percent in 1984 (WHO, 1985).

Increases in service use are reflected in increased health care expenditures, both by individuals and governments. Trends in individual expenditures are shown in Figure 8 which plots the percentage of household expenditures for health and medical care against per capita GNP. (The expenditures data are taken from national or regional household expenditures surveys.) This figure suggests a slightly increasing proportion of household resources being devoted to health care as income levels rise. Household expenditures on health range from under 1 percent to over 8 percent in the countries reported.

Trends in government expenditures on health were tabulated in a recent paper from the World Bank (de Ferranti, 1985) which presented the growth in real per capita public sector health expenditures for 47 LDCs between 1973 and 1979. Thirty-seven of the group showed real annual growth, ranging from

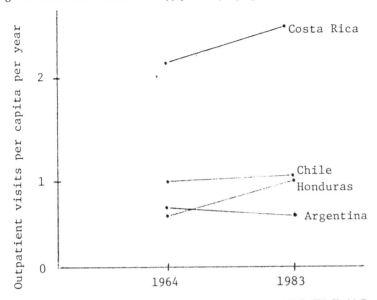

*Sources:* PAHO, Program Budget, 1986-87, PAHO document No. 187, May 1985; PAHO, Health Conditions in the Americas, 1965-68, PAHO Scientific Publication No. 107, 1970.

*Figure 5.* Use of Primary Care Services-Outpatient Visits c.1964-1983

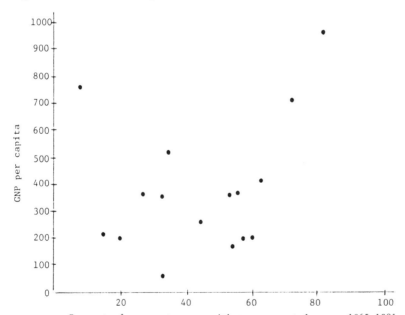

*Sources:* WHO, *The Coverage of Maternity Care: A Tabulation of Available Data,* FHE/85.1, 1985; PAHO, Health Conditions in the Americas, 1965-68, PAHO Scientific Pub. #107, 1970.

*Figure 6.* Changes in the Use of Prenatal Care Services c. 1965-1981

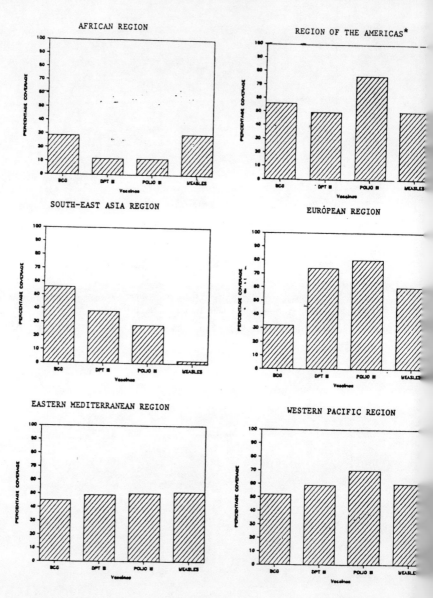

* Excluding USA and Canada.

*Source:* WHO, 1985, "Expanded Programs on Immigration: Progress and Evaluation Report by the Director-General," WHO/EPI/GEN/86/2 Anex 4, November 19, 1985.

*Figure 7.* BCG, DPT III, Polio III and Measles Vaccine Coverage of Infants, by WHO Region, Based on Data Available as of July 1985

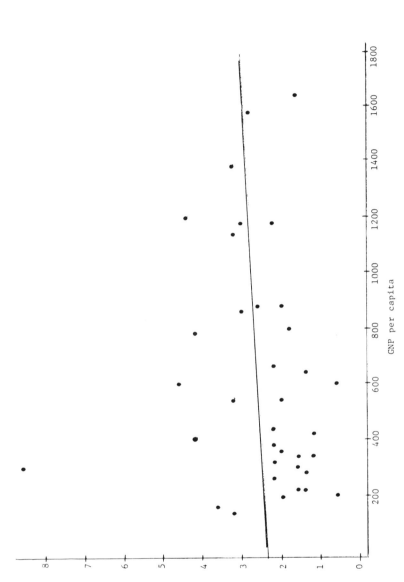

*Source:*   Shepard, D. and E. Benjamin (1986): "Mobilizing Resources for Health: User Fees and Health Financing in Developing Countries," Mimeo, Harvard School of Public Health, May 21, 1986.

*Figure 8.*   Health Expenditures as a Percent of Household Income versus GNP Per Capita

*Table 2.*   Percentage of Government Expenditures to Health

|                    | 1965 | 1980 | change |
|--------------------|------|------|--------|
| Argentina          | 3.40 | 1.70 | -1.70  |
| Bolivia            | 5.00 | 8.60 | 3.60   |
| Brazil             | 6.80 | 7.40 | 0.60   |
| Costa Rica         | 2.50 | 5.10 | 2.60   |
| Dominican Republic | 6.00 | 9.30 | 3.30   |
| Egypt              | 3.00 | 2.40 | -0.60  |
| Honduras           | 6.90 | 8.00 | 1.10   |
| India              | 5.70 | 1.80 | -3.90  |
| Indonesia          | 1.60 | 2.50 | 0.90   |
| Jordan             | 3.50 | 3.90 | 0.40   |
| Kenya              | 4.40 | 7.80 | 3.40   |
| Malawi             | 5.50 | 5.30 | -0.20  |
| Malaysia           | 6.80 | 4.50 | -2.30  |
| Morocco            | 5.70 | 3.10 | -2.60  |
| Sri Lanka          | 7.90 | 3.60 | -4.30  |
| Tanzania           | 6.40 | 5.60 | -0.80  |
| Thailand           | 3.50 | 4.20 | 0.70   |

*Sources:*   World Bank, *World Tables*
         UN, *Statistical Yearbook,* various years

negligible amounts to over 34 percent. While real spending levels are generally rising, the proportion of government spending allocated to health in the 17 countries shown in Table 2 shows no clear trend. Of these 17 countries, 5 reported increases in the budget shares devoted to health of greater than 1 percent, while the same number showed a similar decrease.

In these same countries the private sector increasingly plays an important role in providing health care. De Ferranti (1985) reported estimates of the proportion of total health expenditure accounted for by private spending in 39 countries which ranged from 12 to 88 percent. In half the countries reviewed, the majority of total health expenditure was private. It is likely that this component of health spending is growing more rapidly than public sector spending, suggesting that the rate of growth in total health expenditures is greater than the rate of growth of public expenditures alone.

## IV.  ECONOMIC DEVELOPMENT, HEALTH PROGRAMS, AND THE MIX OF HEALTH SERVICE DEMAND

To examine in more detail changes in specific types of health services, we focus on one country for which more complete data are available. First, however, it is useful to review the different types and sources of services and some of the important country characteristics that affect demand.

There are three important categories of interest in terms of the sources of service—patient-initiated care; mass programs; and traditional health care. Patient-intiated care refers to services that individuals seek on their own. This type of care is typical of the physician or health center outpatient contact, as well as hospital inpaitent services. Patient-initiated care is what is usually considered in studies of the demand for health services. It often combines both curative and preventive services, making it difficult to distinguish between them when examining health service statistics or survey data.

Mass programs are used in developing countries to provide basic services to the under-served majority—especially in rural areas. These programs emphasize preventive care, such as immunization, growth monitoring, health and nutrition education, and hygiene and sanitation. Here too the distinction cannot be made too firmly, as simple curative therapies, such as oral rehydration or routine malaria treatment for fevers, are often included as well. These services are often provided free of charge or through community financing. They are usually not considered in studies of demand, since the normal price effects of principal interest in such studies are less important. These mass programs are a significant source of increased preventive care coverage in developing countries. In addition, they may substitute for similar services provided through patient-initiated sources, thus affecting the overall level of service demand.

The third category, traditional care, is a subset of patient-intiated care. Traditional practitioners are an important source of health care in developing countries, both as competitors and complements to the modern health care sector. Such services are primarily curative, but again may be used for traditional preventive therapies.

Prices and payment mechanisms also affect demand for care. Services may be free, require personal care expenditures, or be supported through different types of personal or social insurance mechanisms. In many developing countries, public sector health care is free or very low fees are charged. Private and traditional practitioners charge for services, with large variation in prices. The role of the public sector in providing services can heavily influence the overall demand for care and the mix of care demanded. Similarly, the availability of insurance and the institutional structures governing insurance are important determinants of demand. Civil servants may be insured through government programs and, as a result, account for a large component of total health care demand. (Wheeler [1985] provides an example from Indonesia.) In Latin American countries, social insurance has been the main factor affecting the growth of demand for health services (Zschock, 1985).

An important issue in evaluating aggregate national statistics is the social differentiation within countries. Aggregate trends can disguise significant differences between regions or across income groups. Urban-rural differences in particular are large. Aggregate demand for health care may increase at a national or regional level while the coverage of specific groups in the population with basic services declines. Such differentiation should be considered where possible in looking at the national trends.

Unfortunately, detailed data on these issues are not easily available for most developing countries. The following case study on Indonesia documents trends which may be expected elsewhere.

## A.  Indonesia—A Case Study

Before the late 1960s, the development of the health sector in Indonesia had been limited. There were fewer than 3,000 physicians servicing a population of approximately 100 million or about 0.33 physicians per 10,000 population in the early 1960s. The main source of modern care for most of the population was a system of rural clinics, which was an expansion of the limited system that had been established under the Dutch colonial administration. Coverage of the population was very low. Hospitals were also in short supply, with the main facilities located in the large cities and some small hospitals located in a few district towns. Some preventive care programs were also operating, for example, immunization against smallpox and yaws, maternal and child health services provided by midwives, and food distribution programs. Funds for development and support of even this limited health system were severely curtailed by the middle 1960s as the financial crises of the late 1950s culminated in hyper-inflation in 1964-65.

Following the political cataclysm of 1965-66 and major economic reorganization, the government embarked on substantial development of social services. This endeavor was enhanced by increased exploitation of natural resources, especially petroleum, and by the subsequent explosion of oil prices, first in 1973 and again in the late 1970s. The recent fall in petroleum prices has been the first major impediment to health sector growth since that time.

Figure 9 presents a variety of data showing the development of the health care system between 1965 and 1985 in Indonesia. Population has increased over 50 percent during that period. Real per capita GNP is estimated to have risen approximately 70 percent in the decade ending in 1981.

The top two sections of the figure show indicators of health spending and health care supply. From the mid-1970s to 1980, government spending on the health sector increased dramatically, outstripping the pace of growth in national income. The figure shows growth in the development budget for health plotted against GDP growth, both indexed to 1974. Over that period, but beginning earlier, there has been a sustained increase in the supply of health care providers and facilities. While hospital bed supply has not kept up with population growth (see Table 1), the supply of trained personnel and peripheral

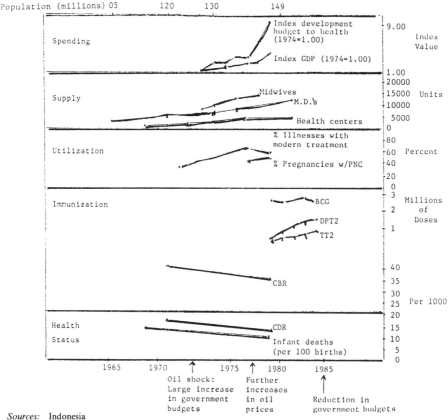

*Sources:*  Indonesia

[a] Yahya, Suyona (1985), "Health Development in Indonesia." Paper prepared for the International Symposium on Effectiveness of Rural Development Cooperation, Amsterdam, September 30 - October 4, 1985.

[b] Central Bureau of Statistics and UNICEF, *An Analysis of the Situation of Children and Women in Indonesia,* Jakarta, August 1984.

[c] World Bank, "Indonesia: Financial Resources and Human Development in the Eighties." Report No. 3795-IND, Washington, May 3, 1982.

[d] Department Kesehatan R.I., "Survei Kesehatan Rumah Tangga 1980 Data statistik." Badan Penalitian dan Pengembangan Kesehatan, Pusat Ekologi Kesehatan, Jakarta, n.d.

[e] World Bank, "Indonesia: Health Manpower Summary Report." Mimeo, Washington, D.C., n.d.

[f] McCauley, Ann P., "Health Needs and the Utilization of Health Treatment Resources in Rural Jave." Report prepared for the Health Development Planning and Management Project, Department of International Health, The Johns Hopkins University, Baltimore, Maryland, 1985.

[g] World Bank, "Indonesia: Health Sector Overview." Report No. 2379-IND, Washington, D.C., February 20, 1979.

[h] Chernicovsky, D. and O.E. Meesook, "Utilization of Health Services in Indonesia." *Social Science and Medicine,* forthcoming, 1986.

[i] UNICEF, "Statistical Profile of Children and Mothers in Indonesia." Jakarta, October 1976.

*Figure 9.*    Indonesia: Changes in Health Service Spending, Supply,
and Use and Health Status, 1960s-1980s

health facilities has grown much faster. Since 1966, the number of physicians in Indonesia has almost quadrupled, with smaller but still substantial increases for nurses and midwives. The number or rural health centers has risen from about 1,000 to over 5,000 during the same period. These peripheral units are also supported by approximately 13,000 sub-centers and an extensive system of village-level health and nutrition volunteers. These systems provide both preventive and curative care at the primary level.

Rising incomes and health care supply are reflected in increasing demand for modern services—both curative and preventive. The second two sections of Figure 9 show changes in the rates of use of modern providers for illnesses and prenatal care. These data are drawn from national household interview surveys. The proportion of illness cases consulting modern providers (physicians, paramedics, and hospitals—both public and private) has increased from about 36 percent in 1972 to between 50 and 60 percent currently as estimated by these surveys. While this latter figure is probably an overestimate reflecting survey bias, there is little question that service use has increased. In addition, these data underestimate use of modern treatment, as self-administered modern therapies purchased in local drug shops have not been counted. Increases have also been found for personal preventive care such as prenatal check-ups.

Since the late 1970s, there has also been expansion in mass disease prevention programs, such as child immunization. Following the eradication of smallpox, immunization had slowed down, with a primary focus on BCG immunizations of children to prevent tuberculosis. Indonesia is now participating in the WHO-sponsored expanded program on immunization. Levels of outreach with other antigens have been rising as a consequence. The figure shows examples of increasing coverage for DPT and tetanus toxoid vaccines.

Accompanying these increases in health programs has been dramatic expansion of the role of the private sector. In urban areas, private physician practices have increased with the overall supply of physicians. In the larger cities new comprehensive group practices are increasingly common. The private pharmaceutical sector has also expanded substantially. This expansion has included both the production of drugs in quantity and variety as well as increases in the number of small pharmacies and retail outlets. Private expenditures are currently estimated to account for over 60 percent of total health care spending.

The lower section of Figure 9 shows some measures of improvements in health status in Indonesia since the 1960s. While there have been reductions in overall death rates as well as mortality of infants and young children, these have not been as dramatic as the increases in health service supply. This reflects the bias in current patterns of health spending and service delivery on curative care for the urban population. Despite the considerable increase in activities to attack the killer diseases of childhood responsible for much of the high mortality, these programs still receive a small proportion of government funds and little emphasis in the private sector.

Thus, over the last 20 years Indonesia has seen substantial development of both health system supply and demand. Both public and private spending are up. (Public sector funds have recently been cut, however, and future increases in spending are most likely in the private sector.) Demand for both curative and preventive care is increasing. The government has been the main provider of many purely preventive services such as immunization and clean water systems. Private sources have expanded the availability of formal and informal curative services. Despite the expansion of supply and demand, aggregate health conditions remain low for a nation of Indonesia's income level. Life expectancy at birth is only 53.5 years as compared with 58.4 for all low income developing countries; infant mortality is 12 percent higher, and the crude death rate 6 percent higher than the low income developing country average (World Tables, 1983,).

## V.  HEALTH CARE DEMAND AND DEVELOPMENT VIEWED FROM THE HOUSEHOLD LEVEL

Although the unit of final consumption of health care is the individual, the decision-making unit for consumption of health care services is usually assumed to be the household. As household income rises, one would expect to see a rise in utilization of all types of services—outpatient, inpatient, and preventive, but perhaps not all equally.

In addition to the effect of rising income, economic theory predicts that utilization will be affected by the price of services. Price includes both the service fee (the money price) and the cost associated with the time it takes to travel to and from the service site, see the practitioner, and get treated (the time price). The price may differ for each household as its distance to the service varies and its monetary valuation of time varies. It also differs by type of service and practitioner as fees, travel, and waiting times are different.

In addition to the time and money prices associated with different practitioners, patients' perceptions of the quality of the care provided may vary. With rising incomes one would expect to see a shift toward services perceived as being of higher quality. Measurement of perceived quality is not easy, although it may be very important in developing countries where cultural factors play a large role.

One might expect that increased demand for health care quality and quantity would result in greater household expenditures on health care. As increased expenditure may be in cash as well as in time spent in getting services, measurement of such changes is difficult. Household expenditures on health care are aften meaasured only in terms of money outlay which is affected by changes in fees paid and travel costs. Increases in the time price of services are not captured in such measurements of expenditure. Rather, these may show up as a loss of income due to reduced work time. Rising incomes would increase the value of this time, making this unmeasured component of expenditure more important. Unless the value of the time spent in the consumption of health care is included, the money outlay by households on health gives an underestimate of actual household expenditure on health care. Valuation of this time is also problematical.

In summary, one would expect as household incomes rise that, ceteris paribus, there would be strong income response, a shift toward higher quality services, and an increase in the proportion of household income dedicated to health. Problems in measuring total prices and in defining quality of care hinder the analysis.

Predicting demand based on existing patterns of use and expenditures is risky in developing countries. With development and rising incomes the health system itself is changing. Changes in the structure of services, particularly changes in fees and geographic distribution, mean that total prices are changing, and changes in the composition of services mean that quality is changing. Health needs may also be changing with varying morbidity patterns.

Only a handful of studies have been done on household demand for health care in developing countries (see Akin, et al., 1985; Berman, 1985; or Mwabu, 1984, for an overview of these studies). These studies have run into problems of specification such as the definition of comparable services. The importance of cultural factors in determining the pattern of demand also limits their comparability across countries. Overall, the results of there studies are mixed (Berman, 1985). An income effect on demand is universally reported, although of differing strengths. Utilization of all modern services rises with income. Price effects vary. Total demand is usually shown to be inelastic with regard to price. Price is, however, an important determinant of choice among different care options, reflecting an apparent shift to higher perceived quality services with rising income. Severity of illness is a strong determinant of level and type of service demanded. There is evidence of stronger price effects for preventive services than for curative services reflecting both the greater urgency of a current illness than a possible future one and the lower perceived value of preventive care.

Studies in four countries are reviewed below: Philippines (Akin et al., 1981 and 1985); Indonesia (Berman, 1985): Kenya (Mwabu, 1984); and Malaysia (Heller, 1982). While the specific goal of each of the four studies differs, all examine the choice of treatment, given a medical complaint, in rural areas in the country concerned. All treat the household as the unit of analysis. In each of the studies a cross-section of households was surveyed and the differences in utilization across income, age and educational groups were analyzed. Changes over time with rising income are estimated from the differences among income groups. The results, while not always consistent nor strictly comparable, do

Table 3.  Summary of Four Country Studies of Household Level Demand

| | Philippines (Akin et al.) | Indonesia (Berman) | Kenya (Mwabu) | Malaysia (Heller) |
|---|---|---|---|---|
| **Income effect: with rising income** | | | | |
| Quantity | ↑ total utilization | ↑ total utilization | - - | ↑ total utilization, weak effect |
| Quality | ↑ in quality (shift to private) | ↑ in quality (shift to health centers) | ↑ in quality (illness-specific choice) | ↑ in quality (shift to modern private) |
| **Price effect: with rising price** | | | | |
| Time | ↓ utilization, strong effect | ↓ utilization | ↓ utilization | ↓ utilization, cross-price effect of travel time |
| Money | not important | - - | ↓ utilization | ↓ utilization, weak own price effect, stronger cross price effect |
| **Other effects: with increases in** | | | | |
| Age | ↑ quality | ↑ quality weak effect | ↑ quantity and quality | ↑ quantity in ages 15-45 |
| Education | ↑ quantity and quality | - - | not important | - - |
| Severity | ↑ quantity and quality | ↑ quantity | ↑ quality | - - |
| Preventive care | Mixed results - ↑ price associated with ↑ use ↑ education associated with ↑ use | - - | - - | ↑ income associated with quality and quantity of prenatal and obstetric care, strong effect |

- - Signifies that the question was not addressed.

provide a view of demand behavior under a variety of conditions. Table 3 summarizes these results.

Of the four studies, Berman alone found a strong increase in total utilization with rising income. Higher income classes in his sample used more services of all types. Akin et al., and Heller found a much weaker response. (Mwabu did not consider total utilization.) In all of the studies where perceived severity of the complaint was noted (Akin et al., Berman, and Mwabu) it was found that severity of the complaint was more important than income or price in determining whether care was sought or not.

Other factors, such as age of the patient, may influence the strength of the income response. For example, income was important in the Akin et al., study in determining levels of service use for children; demand for child health services was seen to rise with income. In the Heller study, a distinction was made between necessary and discretionary care. Rising income was shown to be associated with rising demand for discretionary care. The major effect of higher income in all four studies was a shift to higher quality services. In the Philippines the shift was toward private clinics over public clinics; in Malaysia, toward modern and private care over traditional healers and public clinics; in Kenya, toward mission clinics and hospital service; and in Indonesia, toward health centers over subcenters and village health workers.

Only Mwabu found a strong effect of money price on demand. (It is interesting to note that the differences in prices in Mwabu's study area were greater than in the other studies.) In the Berman study, money price was not considered since it was the same at all the facilities studies. Akin et al. found money price to have an insignificant effect on demand and omitted it from their analysis. Heller found total demand to be inelastic with respect to money price but found that money price differences among providers were important; that is, the cross-price elasticities were significant. In other words, the money price of service did not have much effect on the decision to seek care or not. Once it was decided to seek care, however, price was important in determining which provider was chosen.

The time price component of total price was shown to have a much more important influence on health care consumption than did money price. Akin et al. found both own and cross-time price (between different providers) elasticities to be important in the decision of whether and where to seek care. In the Indonesia study this effect was particularly important for the poorer segments of the population. Heller considered travel, waiting, and treatment time separately. He found that increased travel and treatment time were associated with lower utilization, but that expected waiting time was not a deterrent to seeking care. He hypothesized that there were opportunities for socializing that made waiting time less onerous. Mwabu considered the possibility that the effect of travel time might be mitigated if there were other tasks to be performed in the area of the clinic and his analysis confirmed this hypothesis.

The distinction between curative and preventive care utilization was made by both Akin et al., and Heller. Heller found that increased incomes led to increased utilization of preventive care. The results from Akin et al. were less clearcut. Higher educational level was associated with greater utilization of preventive care, as would be expected. Other results are counter-intuitive. Use of preventive services increased with both time and money price. One possible explanation offered by Akin et al. was a quality effect, but the data do not allow testing of this hypothesis.

Other findings of these studies support the notion that health care is seen as an investment in economic productivity. The likelihood of treatment and the quality of treatment were shown to be higher in the productive years in the three studies that considered age of the patient as a variable (Akin et al., Heller, and Mwabu). Akin et al. also found that both quantity and quality of care increased with educational level. This finding could be interpreted as suggesting either that the benefits of higher quality care were better understood or that better educated patients had more of an investment to protect. Mwabu, on the other hand, did not find educational level to be an important variable.

An interesting feature of the Mwabu study is his consideration of the differences in choice of provider for different visits in the treatment of the same illness episode. His results show that there is a learning process in the search for care. In addition, as the number of visits that will be necessary to cure a particular complaint increases, the price of care becomes more important in determining whether and where care is sought. It might, therefore, be preferable to calculate elasticities with respect to total expenditures per episode rather than the price of a single treatment visit.

It is important to recognize some important factors that are not addressed in economic analyses such as the four studies considered here. First, the cultural context of health care decisions by the household cannot be ignored. Traditional beliefs about the nature and causes of diseases influence demand for modern medical care. The existence and importance of traditional health systems affect utilization of modern services. The strength of traditional belief systems may be mitigated by rising educational levels associated with development. Second, health policy, particularly fee structure and service distribution, influences the pattern of demand. It is interesting to note that the money price response was greatest in Kenya where the range of prices was greatest. Time price response was lowest in Malaysia where the density of the service delivery system made differences in distance to services lowest. Other policies and programs may also influence the pattern of demand such as health education programs and vertical service delivery campaigns such as the expanded program for immunization. Finally, seasonal patterns of morbidity as well as the seasonal distribution of income and the demand for labor may affect the choice of treatment.

## VI.  CONCLUSION

The aggregate data show a strong trend of increasing health care expenditures as income increases, both at the household and national level. Demand for health care tends to rise faster than the increase in income.

While it is difficult to distinguish curative from preventive health care, curative services predominate in overall demand. This reflects their higher cost as well as more immediate value to consumers. In addition, there are often (perverse) incentives built into the financing of health care that encourage use of curative care, even to the point of substituting for preventive services.

As national incomes rise, government expenditures on health also tend to rise, often more rapidly than aggregate income. Except in countries where public sector health care is overwhelmingly dominant, private health expenditures may rise at a faster rate than public expenditures. This reflects the tendency for the private sector to pick up the higher value components of health care demand as well as to respond more rapidly to changes in consumption patterns in the population as incomes rise. For example, many countries have experienced very rapid growth in private sale and consumption of pharmaceuticals.

What guidelines might we derive from past experience? First, health planners must anticipate the rapid increase in the demand for health care, both in terms of quantity and quality, as incomes rise. Overall, this increase will emphasize curative care, even though aggregate health needs may still require that priority be given to preventive programs. The increased demand for health care may have a significant effect on general consumption. Health care demand can also increase the need for foreign exchange to procure imported equipment and drugs. Once countries have invested in health facilities, the recurrent cost requirements to maintain these facilities may be substantial. In times of fiscal austerity this can create problems. Governments will probably still need to play the major role in providing preventive care services.

Second, despite the emphasis in many developing country governments on people's right to free or inexpensive health care, there is evidence of the potential to finance increasing health care demand from users. In government systems, this might be accomplished through public revenue collection or user fees, with proceeds used to finance increased coverage for basic services, or where services are already available, to improve their quality. User fees, however, must be carefully designed to provide the right incentives to users in terms of appropriate use. Care should also be taken to understand the effects of fees on low income or specially targeted users. In some cases fees may be counterproductive. Financial incentives for the use of certain "public goods" services such as immunization or family planning may also be appropriate.

Third, with increasing demand, the private sector seems ready and well-suited to provide many services previously provided by the government. In mixed systems, governments should consider how to best encourage the participation of the private sector, where appropriate, to relieve the state of the burden of financing and managing selected services. Unless government is prepared to continue to bear rapidly rising costs, a greater role for the private sector in the provision of some services will be a useful option.

Fourth, the experience of higher income countries with runaway health care costs provides a warning to developing countries about the dangers of developing institutional arrangements with perverse and distorted incentives affecting efficiency. In particular, social and private insurance must build in incentives to promote cost containment and appropriate use. Early missteps in this area may be difficult to correct as it is easier to expand benefits to promote usage than to contract them once errors have been made.

As incomes rise in developing countries, there will no doubt be a fascinating range of experiments and innovations to expand the benefits of modern health care. The scarce resources and greater health needs of many poor countries require that these be done wisely, assuring that the rewards of modern technology are allocated as effectively, equitably, and efficiently as local conditions permit.

# REFERENCES

Akin, J.S., Guilkey, K.K., and Popkin, B.M. (1981). "The Demand for Child Health Services in the Philippines," *Social Science and Medicine,* Vol. 15C.

Akin, J.S., Griffin, C.C., Guilkey, D.K., and Popkin, B.M. (1985). *The Demand for Primary Health Services in the Third World,* Rowman and Allanheld.

Berman, P. (1985). *Equity and Cost in the Organization of Primary Health Care in Java, Indonesia,* Ph.D. Dissertation, Cornell University, Department of Agriculture Economics, A.E. Research 85-5, Ithaca, New York.

DeFerranti, D. (1985). *Paying for Health Services in Developing Countries,* World Bank Staff Working Paper No. 721.

Grossman, M. (1972). *The Demand for Health: A Theoretical and Empirical Investigation,* National Bureau of Economic Research Occasional Paper No. 119, New York.

Heller, P.S. (1982). "A Model of the Demand for Medical and Health Services in Peninsular Malaysia," *Social Sciences and Medicine,* Vol. 16.

Hinman, A. et al. (1982). "Health Services in Shanghai County," *American Journal of Public Health,* Supplement, Vol. 72, September.

Kravis, I., et al. (1982). *World Product and Income: International Comparisons of Gross Product,* Baltimore: Johns Hopkins University Press.

Mushkin, Selma. (1965). "Health As Investment," *American Economic Review* .

Mwabu, G.M. (1984). *A Model of Household Choice among Medical Treatment Alternatives in Rural Kenya,* Ph.D. Dissertation, Boston, MA: Boston University.

Wheeler, M. (1980). "Health Financing in Indonesia, A Report to H.E. the Minister of Finance,
      Government of Indonesia," Development Administration Group, Institute of Local
      Government Studies, University of Birmingham, mimeo, December.
World Bank. (1983). *World Tables* (3rd edition), Baltimore: Johns Hopkins University Press.
World Health Organization. (1985). "Expanded Programme on Immunization: Progress; An
      Evaluation Report by the Director General," WHO/EPI/GEN/86/2, Annex 4, November
      19.
Zschock, D.K. (1985). "Medical Care under Social Insurance in Latin America," *Latin America
      Research Review,* 20:3.

# PART III


# CASE STUDIES IN PUBLIC HEALTH
AND DEVELOPMENT

---

# HEALTH CARE IN INDONESIA:
## DEALING WITH DIVERSITY

William A. Reinke

The 165 million people of Indonesia make it the fifth most populous country in the world. Moreover, the population is very unevenly distributed over 3,000 islands. More than 60 percent of Indonesians live on the island of Java, which has less than 7 percent of the nation's land area. In contrast to the population density of 691 persons per sq. km. on Java, the much larger island of Kalimantan contains 12 persons per sq. km. The distribution of health resources likewise varies but not necessarily in accordance with population density or need. In sharp contrast to this diversity is the highly centralized pattern of political control. Nevertheless, the commitment to equitable satisfaction of the varied health and developmental needs of the country is apparent to the most casual observer.

Our main purpose is to elaborate current health policy as a reflection of that commitment. To understand the policies that have evolved, however, we need a contextual backdrop and some historical perspective. The discussion begins, therefore, with an overview of Indonesia's socioeconomic conditions

**Research in Human Capital Development, Vol. 5, pages 175-191.**
**Copyright © 1988 by JAI Press Inc.**
**All rights of reproduction in any form reserved.**
**ISBN: 0-89232-508-9**

in general and its health conditions in particular. This is followed by a description of the political and bureaucratic structures within which health policy is formulated, planning takes place, and services are delivered. The next section reviews the progress made since independence in the development of health resources and the organization of service programs. This then permits more meaningful presentation of the Long Term Health Development Plan that has been adopted for policy and programmatic guidance during the remainder of this century. The present Fourth Five-year Plan for 1984-1989 has been developed within that framework. Having established the main directions in health development being pursued by the Government of Indonesia, we underscore in a concluding section a few of the principal issues and challenges to be faced in policy implementation.

# I.   THE SETTING

The 1980 census in Indonesia showed that the population had grown in the preceding decade from 119 to 147 million. The annual growth rate of 2.3 percent reflected a higher than expected reduction in the crude death rate from 18.7 to 12.4 per 1,000 population. Meanwhile, an active family planning program had succeeded in bringing the crude birth rate down by 21 percent to a level of 35 per 1,000. During the same period GNP is estimated to have increased by 7 percent annually, and by 1983 had reached $530 per capita. As a result, Indonesia is now classified by the World Bank as a middle-income country.[13]

The country is notable for having invested much of its rapid growth in rural development, considering that 78 percent of the population is rural. Moreover, priority attention has been given, with limited success to date, to the transmigration program designed to enhance development of the other islands and concurrently to decrease population density in Java and Bali.[10]

The literacy rate has reached 72 percent overall, 50 percent for females, and primary school participation is near 100 percent. Junior secondary graduates represent one-third of eligibles and about one-fourth of those of secondary school age successfully complete their education.[7] While the proportions are not especially impressive, the numerically large and rapidly growing pool of graduates with questionable qualifications is raising serious questions regarding their absorption into the workforce. By the year 2000 the workforce is expected to grow from 55 million to 87 million.[10] The Ministry of Health in particular is considering the advisability of creating new roles for these school leavers in an effort to improve the coverage and strengthen the management of primary health care in remote areas.

During World War II Indonesia suffered under Japanese occupation and wartime conditions. Following independence in 1945, a period of turmoil and economic stagnation ensued under the Sukarno regime leading to overthrow

*Table 1.* Current and Projected Levels of
Selected Health Indicators For Indonesia

| Indicator | Current | Year 2000 |
|---|---|---|
| Life expectancy (years) | 56 | 68 |
| Infant mortality (per 1,000 live births) | 100 | 35 |
| Birthweights under 2500 gms. (%) | 14 | 7 |
| 3-year-olds weight under 11.5 kg. (%) | 30 | 15 |
| Neonatal tetanus incidence (per 1,000 live births) | 11 | 1 |
| Immunization coverage (% children < 14 mo. immunized) | 40 | 80 |
| Deliveries by trained birth attendants (%) | 40 | 80 |
| Clean water supply - rural (%) | 18 | 100 |
| Clean water supply - urban (%) | 40 | 100 |

*Source:* Long-Term Main Development Programmes Plan, Ministry of Health, Indonesia, 1983, pp. 192-195.

in 1966. Only in the late sixties did a period of sustained development begin. The First National Development Plan covered the years 1969-1974. This was followed by successive five-year plans to the present plan for 1984-1989.

Despite rapid progress in recent years, therefore, indicators of health in Indonesia remain below those of neighboring countries. In 1981, for example, life expectancy in Indonesia was estimated to be 56 years, compared to 61 in Thailand and 63 in Malaysia. Roughly 10 percent of births lead to death in infancy, mainly due to diarrheal and respiratory diseases and neonatal tetanus. Forty-six percent of all deaths occur in children under the age of five.[10] Diarrhea alone claims 600,000 lives annually. Four types of malnutrition seriously affect health status at all ages: protein-energy malnutrition, iron deficiency anemia, vitamin A deficiency and iodine deficiency.[13] Thirty percent of pre-school children suffer from protein-energy malnutrition;[5] 9 million school children are anemic;[13] 12 million persons have goitre.[10] Although malaria is no longer a serious problem in Java and Bali, incidence elsewhere is estimated to be as high as 100-200 per 1,000 population.[10] Table 1 lists selected indicators of recognized importance, along with improvements targeted for the year 2000 in the Long Term Health Development Plan.[10]

## II. THE PHILOSOPHY AND STRUCTURE OF GOVERNMENT

The country is organized into 27 provinces, 315 districts and 3,350 subdistricts. Since 1969 the number of health centers has increased five-fold to total more than 5,000. At present, therefore, virtually every subdistrict has a health center and most are staffed by a physician. In addition, there are several subcenters staffed by paramedics to serve the 20 or so villages typically situated within a subdistrict. Hospitals are located at district level, but they tend to have low occupancy rates. In contrast to the growth in ambulatory services, the number of hospital beds has increased by only one-fifth since 1969, now totaling just over 100,00. Because of the corresponding growth in population during this period the population/bed ratio has worsened from 1,300 to 1,500.[13]

Clearly there has been a dedicated effort to expand health services at the periphery. This has taken place within the framework of a highly centralized government decision making apparatus, uniquely coupled with a long tradition of village leadership and mutual self-help within the community. It is necessary, therefore, to comment upon the philosophy of governance as well as its structure.

## A.   Philosophy Regarding Authority

The Indonesian constitution is firmly founded on the five-fold philosophy of Pancasila, which embraces belief in: God, democracy, nationalism, human worth, and social justice. It is noteworthy that in a largely Muslim society this ideology is meant to supersede strictly religious teachings. Recently the Indonesian Parliament has extended the concept of the secular state to all mass organizations, thereby frustrating any attempt to create an Islamic state.

Against this expression of the dominance of the secular state is an ancient Javanese moral concept that is not easily translated but has been elaborated as follows.

> It suggests that a leader must qualify himself as a catalyst to stimulate the community, a personality whose guidance is to be respected, and who is able to develop self-respect and self-reliance among the community forces. His task is to encourage people, to show them the way how to do, but once they are able to assume responsibilities of their assignment, he should step aside and keep on assisting. This concept has been applied in the strategies of community health, including the family nutrition improvement programme (UPGK), and the village family planning programme in the rural and the urban areas.[13]

Closely related is the concept of "gotong royong." This, too, is difficult to translate but has the connotation of a community joining forces to support the special needs of its members. The consequent tensions regarding the locus of decision making are manifest in policies that reflect central government initiative in planning, organizing and funding equitable access to health care, coupled with encouragement to private enterprise and community participation.

## B.   Formal Structure of Government

In principle the National Parliament selects the President, who in turn selects provincial governors from lists of nominees provided by the provincial legislatures. Corresponding administrative structures exist at lower levels of government. Each includes a health official. Thus, the chief of provincial health services comes under the governor.

Parallel to the administrative chain of command, a technical hierarchy exists through the central Ministry of Health. While the Minister's representative at the provincial level wields little or no formal authority, he holds a position of significance inasmuch as most health policy and funding originate with the central Ministry of Health. To the extent that local funds are tapped, however, priorities are mainly established through administrative, not technical, channels.

Fortunately, arrangements are generally made for the same person to fill both the administrative and technical health positions at provincial and district levels. This simplifies decision making somewhat, but the health officer must learn to serve two masters effectively.

## C.  Development of Planning Capability

Much of the sustained progress in Indonesian development in recent years has been attributed to effective planning. Several unsuccessful attempts were made under President Sukarno to establish planning bodies. The last of these, formed in 1963, was named the National Development Planning Agency and has come to be known by its Indonesian acronym, Bappenas. When Suharto ascended to power in 1966, he gathered around him several economic advisors from the faculty of the University of Indonesia. Two of the closest advisors were appointed to leadership in Bappenas in 1967 and asked to prepare a five-year development plan to begin in 1969.

Granted 2 years lead time, a serious planning effort could be undertaken. That effort has been maintained, and even accelerated, in the years since completion of the first plan. In 10 years the number of multidisciplinary professionals in Bappenas more than tripled to exceed 100. Each of the 4 plans that have now been prepared has served as a realistic base for development in Indonesia, in large part because of "the bringing together of the planning process with the budgetary process, both institutionally and functionally, so that joint Bappenas/ Finance Ministry teams can give aspects of the national plan periodic and concrete expression in the annual development budget."[6]

Within the Ministry of Health a Bureau of Health Planning was created in 1975. Since its formation, the Bureau has established a good working relationship with Bappenas and has gained recognition it its own right as a competent planning body. It is mainly responsible for the well-conceived Long Term Health Development Plan[11] and the Fourth Five-Year Health Development Plan[5] described later.

Two other Ministry of Health entities are worth noting for their contribution to plan development and implementation. The National Institute of Research and Development has an especially active unit devoted to health services research, an obvious contributor to planned change. The National Center for Education and Training has responsibility for all Ministry in-service training and for the pre-service training for technical and other nonprofessional staff. Its role in manpower planning and development is therefore crucial.

## III.   ACHIEVEMENTS DURING PLAN PERIODS I-III

Considering the state of affairs prior to the First Plan, remarkable progress has been made since then. The few facilities that had been constructed earlier had been developed in the absence of clear policy guidelines. Medical care and disease control programs had been mounted from place-to-place on a largely ad hoc basis. Clinics and hospitals providing curative services were separate from preventive Centers for Mother and Child Welfare. Public health staff engaged in sanitation activities formed yet another unit.

The First Plan period was mainly one of consolidation and strengthening of existing services, as well as health education. Intended expansion of services was thwarted by resource limitations, notably personnel shortages, and no new clinic facilities were built.[13]

The momentum generated during the First Plan carried over into the Second with more tangible results. In addition, the health sector was benefited in the Second Plan period (1974-79) by special funds dispensed under the heading "Presidential Instruction" (INPRES). According to this mechanism, extrabudgetary funds are made available from the Center for specially designated purposes, and in the case of health have mostly gone directly to rural districts for infrastructure development. Beginning in 1974 new health centers were built under INPRES, indicating that health had become a national priority equivalent in importance to education and agriculture.[13] About one-third of the central-level funding during the Second Plan was derived from INPRES, and the pattern has continued since.[3]

An enhanced training capacity began to bear fruit during the Second Plan as well. All categories of health workers approximately doubled in number during that period. The number of health centers staffed by doctors grew even more rapidly during the Third Plan period.[5] Whereas the annual number of medical college graduates approximated 850 during the Second Plan, this increased to about 1,500 during the Third Plan, and nearly two-thirds of the latter took positions in government health centers.[10] Nearly all also engage in private practice. Although the 13 public and 8 private medical colleges experience dropout rates that average nearly 30 percent, those who graduate generally remain in service for many years; the virtual absence of a brain drain makes Indonesia quite unique among developing countries.

Apart from physicians, recent manpower priorities have shifted from quantitative concerns to the quality of training and the rationalization of roles. The number of nurse training categories, for example, has been reduced from 24 to 2 to emphasize the distinction between hospital and community nursing. More than 13,000 in the latter category were trained during the Third Plan, but this is still considered grossly inadequate in light of future priorities in primary health care.[5]

The rate of expansion in health development is seen most dramatically in budgetary figures. The Second Plan exhibited a ten-fold increase in budget over the First. Average annual increases during the Third Plan amounted to 38 percent. Throughout the Second and Third Plan periods, central government routine, development and INPRES health budgets combined grew by 16 percent per year in real terms.[2] About 80 percent of the Third Plan funds came from the central government: 8 percent were derived from provincial levels, and 12 percent came from the districts. To keep these figures in perspective, the vast increases in development activity generally in Indonesia should be noted. As a result, the 1983 health budget was only about 4 percent of the total government budget.[10]

## IV.  PRESENT CONDITIONS AS THE BASIS FOR EMERGING POLICY

Having portrayed the dynamics of health development in Indonesia over the past 15 years, we should pause briefly to examine more closely where the country has come, so that we may see more clearly the main issues that are now attracting the attention of policy makers and planners.

It is estimated that in 1980 about 2 billion dollars, or $13 per capita was being spent on health. Less than 3 of the $13 was attributable to the Ministry of Health. About $2 came from other government agencies and more than $8 represented transactions in the private sector. Within the government health sector, about one-third of the expenditures were in the routine budget, the rest coming from the development budget and INPRES.[7] About 38 percent of development funds went to the hospital sector, 28 percent to health centers, and 17 percent to community activities, including communicable disease control and environmental sanitation.[11]

Though the bulk of expenditues come from the Center, as much as 8 percent of district revenues are used for health services, the majority (60 percent) of district health expenditures relating to hospital care. About one-third of total hospital costs are met out of district funds.[4]

To summarize, although the central government has exhibited a clear bias in favor of expanding access to government services at the periphery, the private sector remains dominant. Moreover, a substantial portion of government funds continues to be allocated to costly hospital care (though the situation is not as extreme as in many countries), and much of the burden of hospital costs falls upon local jurisdictions.

Considerable thought is being given to possible ways of mobilizing private resources more effectively in the public interest. The government has endorsed the principle of health insurance and various mechanisms for implementation are under review. Roughly 6 million government employees are already covered by one plan, and a contributory program of expansion to other workers could be in the offing. In addition to the advantages of risk-sharing, this approach could channel private revenues into publicly regulated (if not publicly provided) services of acceptable quality.

Private expenditures on pharmaceuticals are a matter of special concern to the government. Of the $8 per capita in private expenditures on health noted above about $3 went into drug purchases.[2] Although 98 percent of the drugs consumed are manufactured in Indonesia, 95 percent of the raw materials are imported. Moreover, only about 10 percent in value of this half-billion dollar industry is managed by the government. The aim is to increase this to 20-30 percent by the year 2000.[10]

Since the beginning of the First Plan in 1969, the number of doctors has tripled to reach 16,000, and an eight-fold increase in nurses has been achieved to reach a total in excess of 40,000.[13] Even so, the ratio of one doctor per 10,000 population in Indonesia is somewhat below that of neighboring Thailand and much less than half that found in Asian countries like India, Pakistan and the Philippines. Moreover, nearly one-fourth of Indonesian physicians are located in Jakarta, and another third reside in 10 other urban centers.[8]

Although most health providers engage in private activities, the majority have government positions as well in one of the 1,200 hospitals, 5,000 health centers or 14,000 subcenters. Half of the hospitals are private, but they contain only 30 percent of the beds.[12] Although there is only one bed per 1,500 population on average, occupancy rates are typically below 60 percent. The large expansion of health centers and subcenters in recent years has meant that each health center serves 30,000 people on the average, and there is one subcenter per 12,000 population.[5] Villages are also served by part-time health posts, mobile units, volunteer health and nutrition cadres, and salaried village malaria workers. The most remote islands are only reached by boat at present, but modern technology, including the Palapa satellite, is bringing about rapid improvement in communications and is having a consequent unifying effect.[10]

Facilities counts at the end of the Third Plan are summarized in Table 2, along with increments projected during the Fourth Plan period. Indonesian policy is clearly oriented toward a relatively lean health care configuration. Great emphasis in the past has been placed upon adding facilities at the periphery and training less sophisticated and costly staff, and continuation of this policy is evident, at least in the near term.

*Table 2.* Current and Projected Numbers of Health Facilities in Indonesia

| Type Facility | No. in 1984 | Projected Additions to 1989 | Percent Increase |
|---|---|---|---|
| Health centers | 5,353 | 500 | 9 |
| Subcenters | 13,636 | 6,000 | 44 |
| Mobile centers | 2,479 | 1,521 | 61 |
| Government and private hospitals | 1,246 | 83 | 7 |
| Hospital and health center | 103,505 | 15,880 | 15 |

*Source:* Fourth Five-Year Health Development Plan, 1984-89, p. 24.

As recently as the 1960s dispensaries, MCH clinics, and environmental services were quite separate. Now, however, the health center is recognized as a comprehensive care facility with 13 clearly designated functions as follows:[10]

1. promotion of maternal and child health;
2. promotion of family planning;
3. improvement of nutrition;
4. promotion of environmental health;
5. disease prevention and control through immunization and epidemiological surveillance;
6. health education;
7. treatment of diseases and accidents;
8. community health care;
9. promotion of school health service;
10. promotion of dental health;
11. promotion of mental health;
12. simple labortory examinations; and
13. recording and reporting.

Success in these efforts to date has been modest at best. A 1977 survey showed that only 45 percent of respondents had ever seen a physician, and 16 percent of residents living within one kilometer of a health center had actually used it.[8] More recent studies tend to show that about one-fifth of all illnesses are treated at the health center.[1] Approximately 40 percent of pregnancies receive ante-natal care, and a similar proportion are delivered by trained personnel, mostly from the health center.[5] Largely through INPRES intiatives, one-third of rural residents have safe drinking water and one-fourth have access to sanitary toilets.[5]

## A.  Special Programs to Encourage Services Access and Utilization

Partly as a result of frustrations in encouraging health center acceptance, a number of special programs have been introduced from time to time to reach villages with family planning, nutrition services, and primary health care generally. Three such programs are especially noteworthy as reflections of government policy.

### 1.  Family Planning

The Government of Indonesia was among the first to endorse a policy of family limitation. Moreover, almost from the beginning it was recognized that family planning success required a broad base of support not limited to health. In 1970, therefore, and intersectoral Family Planning Coordinating Board (BKKBN) was formed to oversee a vigorous program of Family Planning services. Although the BKKBN has become increasingly involved over the years in service delivery, largely through health units, it remains organizationally outside the Ministry of Health. It has been well-funded and has established a large, tightly structured organization that extends to the village grassroots. BKKBN has gained a reputation for *esprit de corps* and has acquired a generally high status that cannot be attributed solely to its limited accomplishments in reducing the birth rate. Rather, its success seems largely attributable to an excellent communications network that, for example, produces monthly reports from the field and prompt feedback of comparative performance, coupled with a decentralized system of financial management that permits budgeting for local needs. Through this impressive network to the villages of Indonesia, BKKBN is now vigorously extending its scope of activities to immunization and nutrition services, including growth monitoring and nutrition education.[13]

### 2.  Family Nutrition

In 1974 another intersectoral Family Nutrition Improvement Program (UPGK) was organized to deal with the nutritional problems of preschool children and mothers. The program involving 10 ministries and intersectoral nutrition improvement boards at national, provincial, district and subdistrict levels grew out of the recognition that the serious problem of malnutrition had been inadequately handled by a narrow health sector approach. The program initially focused on nutrition education and monthly baby weighing but has grown to include other nutrition activities, such as the distribution of vitamin A capsules and iron tablets, and related functions, e.g., promotion of breastfeeding and use of oral rehydration for diarrhea.[13]

During the recently concluded Third Plan period, UPGK reached 36,500 of Indonesia's 62,000 villages with its weighing program and distributed over 10 million vitamin A capsules and 1.7 million iron tablets.[5] Actual impact on malnutrition is less apparent and admittedly more difficult to assess.

### 3. *Primary Health Care*

As already noted, the Ministry of Health several years ago became concerned with the confusing array of nursing positions in existence and attempted to streamline the system, giving greater emphasis to community nursing. In 1975 the Ministry began a village outreach program to be based upon over 20,000 primary health nurses (PK) to be trained by the Ministry. There were to be six PK per health center and one per subcenter. Each would look after 5-7 village health promoters who in turn would be responsible for 15-20 households each. Recalling that the program was launched three years before the Conference at Alma-Ata focused overriding attention on primary health care, it is perhaps not surprising that it foundered for lack of funds and government commitment.[8]

Two years later the Village Community Health Development Program (PKMD) was tried out in five provinces to provide a broad range of community-based health promotion activities, as well as basic care of common illnesses and referral as necessary. Based upon the mutual self-help concept of "gotong royong," this locally sponsored inter-sectoral approach has expanded and gained wide acceptance, but it, like primary health care generally, labors under the difficulty of providing competent decentralized management of a broad range of basic services.

A common theme runs through these separate program experiences. In a nation as large, diverse and bureaucratically centralized as Indonesia, it is extremely difficult to establish a network of services that effectively reaches 60,000 scattered villages. While the difficult task might be accomplished in a specific field like family planning, cognizance must be taken of the fact that the health problems are closely interrelated and subject to multi-sectoral causalities, as well as solutions. How can such complexities be taken into consideration without a dissipation of efforts that dulls their impact to intolerably low levels?

The challenge is especially timely and real now that the Fourth Development Plan for Health, building upon the PKMD approach, has assigned top priority to the Program of Integrated Services (YANDU) designed to link five key programs: maternal and child health; family planning; nutrition; immunization; and diarrheal diseases control. The integration is to be achieved through the existing health infrastructure of health centers, subcenters and mobile units, but BKKBN and other resources are to be fully utilized.[13] The aim, of course, is to coordinate efforts synergistically rather than simply to provide duplication. This is difficult in any bureaucracy, including that of Indonesia supported by its tradition of gotong royong. The issue must be faced within the broader framework of future policy developed in the next section.

# V. A LOOK AHEAD

The 1978 International Conference on Primary Health Care led to the Declaration of Alma-Ata, which was endorsed by the Government of Indonesia as the future basis for health policy. A long-term restructuring of the National Health System was mandated to embody the features of primary health care. The National Health System (SKN) statement (in excess of 100 pages) of 1982 is a three-part elaboration of direction and strategy for health development to the year 2000. The three parts cover: Basic Policies for the National Health System; the Long-Term Health Development Plan; and Basic Structure of the National Health System. The Development Plan is the heart of the document and is further detailed in the Long-Term Health Development Programmes Plan. There are, in fact, 15 programs to be carried out within five priority areas to satisfy five defined objectives. The program descriptions outline the progress to be made under each of the successive five-year development plans to be carried out until the year 2000. Indeed, the Fourth Five-year Development Plan does closely follow the objectives and programatic guidelines of the Long-Term Plan.

Table 3 lists the policies, plan objectives, priorities and programs laid out in SKN. It is unnecessary here to describe each program in detail, but selected highlights and commentary are in order.

*Table 3.*   Policies of the National Health System and Main Features of the Long-Term Health Development Plan

---

*Policies*
1. Comprehensive, integrated services accessible and acceptable to all to be provided with community participation.
2. Priority to poor, infants, children, mothers and laborers.
3. Services to employ appropriate technology at affordable cost.
4. Collaboration with other sectors.
5. Both regional and national approaches called for.
6. Rational use of resources stressed to give optimal results.
7. Programs to be adjusted to local needs.
8. Local management to be gradually improved.
9. Community, including private agencies, to be properly directed to ensure adherence to government policy.
10. Importance of health education acknowledged.

*Long-Term Plan Objectives*
1. Promotion of community capacity for self-help.
2. Improvement of the environment.
3. Improvement of nutritional status.
4. Reduction of morbidity and mortality.
5. Development of healthy and prosperous families with increasing acceptance of the small family as norm.

*Table 3 (continued)*

| Priority Tasks | Programs |
|---|---|
| 1. Promotion and strengthening of health efforts | 1a. Improvement of health center performance. |
| | 1b. Strengthening of referral system |
| | 1c. Prevention and control of diseases |
| | 1d. Promotion of occupational health |
| | 1e. Health education |
| 2. Health manpower development | 2a. Education and training |
| | 2b. Personnel management |
| 3. Food and drug control | 3a. Supplies distribution and control |
| | 3b. Control of hazardous substances |
| 4. Improvement of nutrition and promotion of environmental health | 4a. Nutrition improvement |
| | 4b. Promotion of environmental health |
| 5. Strengthening of management and legislation | 5a. Improvement of management procedures |
| | 5b. Facilities improvement |
| | 5c. Improvement of health information systems |
| | 5d. Health services research and development |

*Source:* National Health System, Ministry of Health, Indonesia, 1982.

## A. Principles and Policies

The 10 basic policies enunciated by SKN are based upon eight stated principles of health development. While most of these are general endorsements of national welfare, the value of human life, equity and health as a basic right, two of the principles are worth singling out for quotation:

> The government as well as the community are responsible for the health of the people.

> The government is primarily responsible for the national health development, which shall be jointly executed by the government and the entire community, including the private sector. The health program shall be implemented on the basis of the primary health care concept, emphasizing the integrated promotive, preventive, curative and rehabilitative approach.[11]

The search for a proper balance between public and private endeavors and between government responsibility and control on the one hand, and community participation and mutual self-help on the other reflects a tension that appears repeatedly in the statements on principle, policies and programs.

Two other features of the policy statement deserve special attention: acknowledgement of the importance of inter-sectoral collaboration; and recognition of regional differences and the need for decentralized management. How these policies will fare in practice makes for interesting speculation, given some of the unfulfilled promises of the past.

Overall, the SKN is notable for its emphasis on simple care, prevention and improved coverage to the traditionally disadvantaged. On this score there is room for optimism, for this is an extension of policy that has been evident for some time.

## B.   Priorities and Programs

The list of priorities and programs covers the typical range of concerns, and the proposed actions are for the most part what might be reasonably expected. Sometimes the flavor of a proposal is rather striking, however. As various service needs are put forth, the repeated reference to primary health care through the Village Community Health Development (PKMD) approach sets an unmistakable tone.[10] Even the occupational health program is to develop some form of work-risk insurance to be financed with participation of the community.[10]

Increased reliance on community financing in general is encouraged. For example, one of the proposed steps toward improved quality of health center services is creation of a Community Health Fund.[10] Interestingly, it is anticipated that:

> Funds coming from the Government will be utilized primarily for preventive and rehabilitative health efforts, while those from the community will mainly be used for curative and promotive health efforts. In order to harmonize the utilization of the funds coming from the Government and those coming from the community a special body is needed.[10]

The need is expressed for systematic supervision of the private sector as well.[10]

One dissonant chord is sounded in the call for community based services. In the discussion of education and training it is pointed out that the future need (unexplained) for applicants with a higher basic education, coupled with the increasing pool of secondary school graduates, will lead to an upgrading of training and the consequent qualifications needed for trainers.[10]

The proposed service improvement programs are arranged in a curious way. Disease control and occupational health are combined with the improvement of health center services, referrals and health education under the general priority heading Promotion and Strengthening of Health Efforts. Nutrition and environmental health, in contrast, are combined under a separate priority heading. It is hard to see the significance of this arrangement.

What is clearly significant, however, is that all of the remaining programs deal with management and support of services rather than their delivery. Even the first program of health center improvement is largely devoted to strengthening of health center management.[10] Personnel management receives major attention under Health Manpower Development and improvements in management information and procedures are separately and prominently called for.

The production and distribution of drugs is another area that the planners have tackled forcefully. Concerned about the urgent need for wider availability of essential drugs to persons at all income levels, the plan stresses the importance of reduced reliance on importation and looks to development of Indonesian raw materials and both government and private production of items of targeted priority.[10] Increased research on the therapeutic value of widely used traditional drugs is also proposed.

Health services research in general receives programmatic attention. The Ministry of Health in Indonesia is already rather unique in having its own research institute of recognized competence. The plan calls for further strengthening of career ladders for researchers.[10]

## C. The Dilemmas Remain

No policies and programs can guarantee resolution of troublesome issues. Dedicated commitment to stated aims is required, and in some cases altogether new programs may be necessary. In this closing section we underscore some of the more perplexing problems that are likely to challenge Indonesian policy-makers and planners for years to come.

Underlying many of the issues is the reality that universal access to opportunities for health improvement cannot possibly be realized without the resources and devoted effort of government, the private sector and the lay community. Determination of the contribution needed from each group to achieve the proper balance of curative, preventive, promotive and rehabilitative services is a concern that has been raised by Indonesian planners and will surely continue to be discussed.

With regard to the public/private dilemma, the Long-Term Health Development Plan encourages expansion of private curative services so that the government can focus on disease prevention and health promotion. In particular, the Plan calls upon the private sector to foster hospital expansion, claiming public responsibility instead for improving access to basic services at the periphery. The Plan then voices concern about the regulation of private initiatives to ensure that public interests are satisified.[10] It is silent, however, about an equally troubling aspect of the public/private dilemma. Government salaries in Indonesia are notoriously low, and medical and paramedical workers alike typically receive the bulk of their income from private endeavors. This raises questions of divided loyalties and possible effects on the quality of government services. On the other hand, private earnings are effectively subsidizing public service, and removal of the subsidy could place an intolerable burden on government finances. The private practice issue is common to many countries, but it is probably nowhere as extreme as in Indonesia.

Relations between government and the community create another set of economic issues. The strong support expressed in the Plan for the PKMD approach to primary health care[5] includes community financing through insurance mechanisms, community health funds, etc.[10] While the merits of this in reaching and involving previously underserved populations are apparent, it is also possible that the poor will end up paying for services that more affluent working groups receive free from government- or employer-financed insurance schemes. Considerations of equity are inherently difficult and delicate!

Apart from purely economic considerations, attempts to improve services coverage at the periphery raise a number of organizational and management issues as well. Health centers are asked to provide more services and, in addition, to supervise community activities.[5] One might question whether the community should not supervise its own efforts; collaboration with the formal health system would seem more appropriate than supervision by it.[9] Be that as it may, there is a real danger that a highly "successful" community services program might, in fact, overload peripheral workers and create a consequent imbalance in clinical, outreach and supervisory activities.[10] Where there is not time to do everything, clinical functions invariably are given priority.

The push for decentralization raises management questions at the district level as well as at the point of service delivery. District managers are poorly trained for carrying out the most basic management functions related to personnel, supplies and finances. What is called for is an analysis of both service and management functions leading to more rational allocation of those functions among staff, coupled with a training program to prepare staff for revised roles.[2] The Ministry of Health has, in fact, begun such a study on a pilot basis through the University of Indonesia, with consultation from The Johns Hopkins University.

More broadly, there is the omnipresent issue of the relationship between health and development. The relationship has a special twist in Indonesia through the transmigration program aimed at more even population distribution and development throughout the islands. Although the program has not yet been successful in altering the concentration of population in Java,[11] serious efforts continue. Areas to which transmigrants and development activities are targeted receive priority attention in malaria control and environmental improvement. It is hoped in turn that population redistribution and diversification of development will produce health benefits.

We have hardly exhausted the list of important issues faced by Indonesian policymakers as they seek Health for All by the year 2000. Even the partial list assembled is enough, however, to keep them fully occupied for much of the remainder of the century.

# NOTES AND REFERENCES

1.  Berman, Peter. (1984) *Equity and Cost in the Organization of Primary Health Care in Java, Indonesia*, Ph.D. Dissertation, Cornell University, Department of Agricultural Economics, A.E. Research 85-5, Ithaca, New York.

2.  Department of International Health of The Johns Hopkins University. (1976). *The Functional Analysis of Health Needs and Services*, London: Asia Publishing House.

3.  Ferster, G. (1979). "Expenditure Pattern of Special Presidential Funds During the Second Five-Year Development Plan Period," Ministry of Health, Indonesia.

4.  Ferster, G., Komarini, A., and Arief, J. (1979). "Review of Public Financing in the Health Sector," Ministry of Health, Indonesia.

5.  *Fourth Five-Year Development Plan.* (1984). Chapter 23: "Health," Republic of Indonesia.

6.  Hoadley, J. Stephen. (May 16, 1976). "The Politics of Development Planning Agencies: The Evolution of Indonesia's Bappenas," Unpublished paper presented before New Zealand Political Studies Association Conference, Wellington, New Zealand.

7.  *Indonesia Financial Resources and Human Development in the Eighties.* (1982). World Bank Report No. 3795-ND.

8.  *Indonesia Health Sector Overview.* (1979). World Bank Report No. 2379-ND.

9.  Korten, David C. (ed.). (1979). *Population and Social Development Management*, Caracas, Venezuela: Population and Social Development Management Center.

10. *Long-Term Main Development Programmes Plan in the Field of Health, 1983/4-1998/9.* (1983). Ministry of Health, Indonesia.

11. *National Health System.* (1982). Ministry of Health, Indonesia.

12. *Report of the Department of Health.* (1983). Republic of Indonesia.

13. Surjaningrat, Suwardjono. (1983). *The Development of Integrated Health, Nutrition and Family Planning Programme in Indonesia*, Ministry of Health, Indonesia.

# URBAN-RURAL FOOD AND NUTRITION CONSUMPTION PATTERNS IN INDONESIA

Dov Chernichovsky and Oey Astra Meesook

## INTRODUCTION

As is the case for many other developing economies, urbanization is one of the basic characteristics of Indonesia's modernization and changing socioeconomic scene. Indonesia's urban population grew 4.5 percent annually between 1970 and 1980, compared with a 2.3 percent growth rate for the total population during the same period. Twenty-two percent of Indonesia's population was considered to reside in urban areas in 1982 (World Bank, 1984).

A critical element in the welfare of urban dwellers, newcomers from rural areas in particular,.is their diet; this is of particular concern in a rapidly growing urban population for a number of reasons. First, food prices are likely to be higher in urban than in rural areas where most foods are produced. Hence,

Research in Human Capital Development, Vol. 5, pages 193-205.
Copyright © 1988 by JAI Press Inc.
All rights of reproduction in any form reserved.
ISBN: 0-89232-508-9

for identical levels of income, urban dwellers may be worse-off than rural residents. Second, the relative prices of different foods are likely to differ between the two areas. This may upset customary diets which have been established over generations. Third, for any given level of income, city life offers more options which compete with food consumption for household income, and hence may be detrimental to the diet. Fourth, there is nothing in the urban environment that can support one's diet, whereas food gathering is common in rural areas where people are close to food sources.

The objective of this paper is to examine general patterns of urban-rural food consumption and diet in Indonesia with the above hypotheses in mind. It would be preferable to have panel data showing changes in the diets of families when they migrate from rural to urban areas. Unfortunately, we do not have such data. Instead, we infer likely situations by observing differences in diets in urban and rural areas. The paper focuses on two related questions. First, what would the average rural family face in a town in terms of their diet, given differences in food prices? Second, is the urban or rural family more at risk of malnutrition when incomes and prices in the two areas change?

The data used are from the 1978 National Socioeconomic Survey (SUSENAS) which has already been used in a similar analysis focusing on poverty (Chernichovsky and Meesook, 1984)

# I.  DISTRIBUTION OF POVERTY
# IN URBAN AND RURAL AREAS

Food consumption and, in particular, its composition are related to income, relative prices and other household characteristics. We look therefore at the urban-rural incidence of poverty in Indonesia as a basic predictor of food consumption and diet patterns in Indonesia.

We do not attempt to define objectively a poverty line for Indonesia since we feel that such a line, however carefully defined, necessarily incorporates many arbitrary assumptions. For purposes of comparing different groups of the population, we classify households into three groups according to their levels of per capita consumption expenditures. The "poor" will refer to the two lowest quintiles (or 40 percent) of the distribution of the population ranked by their household's level of per capita consumption expenditure; "the better-off" will refer to the next two quintiles; and "the rich" will refer to the top quintile (or 20 percent). A household or an individual is said to be in poverty if it or he belongs to the "poor" group.

Table 1 gives the incidence of poverty, the proportion of households classified as poor, for urban and rural areas of Indonesia. By this definition, the overall urban incidence of poverty is 14 percent compared with 42 percent for rural households.

*Table 1.*   Incidence of Poverty, and the Distribution of Households and of the Population by Household Per Capita Consumption Level, By Area of Residence, Indonesia, 1978

|  | *Percent* | | |
|---|---|---|---|
|  | *Urban* | *Rural* | *Urban & Rural* |
| *Incidence of Poverty* | 14.1 | 41.7 | 37.1 |
| *Share of Households* |  |  |  |
| Poor | 6.3 | 93.7 | 100.0 |
| Better-Off | 15.3 | 84.7 | 100.0 |
| Rich | 36.6 | 63.4 | 100.0 |
| All | 16.6 | 83.4 | 100.0 |
| *Share of People* |  |  |  |
| Poor | 7.3 | 92.7 | 100.0 |
| Better-Off | 18.1 | 81.9 | 100.0 |
| Rich | 42.1 | 57.9 | 100.0 |
| All | 18.6 | 81.4 | 100.0 |

*Source:*   Data tapes of SUSENAS 1978 (May round), Biro Pusat Statistik, Jakarta.

Rural households constituted 83 percent of all households in Indonesia at the time of the survey. Combined with the higher incidence of poverty among them compared with urban households, this means that nearly all, 94 percent, of poor households are found in rural areas according to the definition of poverty used here.[1]

## II.   FOOD CONSUMPTION PATTERNS AND FOOD PRICES

Not surprisingly, rural households spend on average a higher share of their total reported monthly expenditures on food consumption compared with their urban counterparts, about 70 percent compared with 60 percent (Table 2), and a smaller proportion on goods and services, housing, schooling and health. These differences reflect both the income differentials between the two locations and differences in opportunities.

Within the food basket, a higher share is spent on rice, corn and cassava in the rural areas, while urban residents spend higher proportions on meat and poultry, eggs, dairy products, vegetables, legumes and "other items," which include oils, and many other ready-made foods (see Table 3).[2]

*Table 2:* Proportion of Monthly Expenditures Allocated to Major
Consumption Categories, by Location, Indonesia, 1978 (Percent).

| Consumption Category | Location | |
|---|---|---|
| | Urban | Rural |
| Food | 57.30 | 68.20 |
| Alcohol & Tobacco | 5.14 | 4.73 |
| Housing & Fuel | 16.72 | 11.08 |
| Clothing & Footwear | 4.77 | 5.02 |
| Goods & Services | 8.17 | 3.36 |
| Schooling | 2.31 | 0.82 |
| Health | 1.52 | 0.97 |
| Durable Goods | 1.74 | 1.83 |
| Taxes & Insurance | 1.09 | 1.19 |
| Parties & Ceremonies | 1.24 | 2.79 |

*Source:* SUSENAS 1978 data tapes, Biro Pusal Statistik, Jakarta.

A general comparison of urban and rural diets shows that they are not that different in terms of average quantities (Table 3). In fact, the quantities of food reported as being consumed in the rural areas are higher than in the urban areas; 996 grams of food per capita per day (excluding eggs) compared with 925 grams.

Some qualitative differences emerge, however. The rural diet is richer in staples, notably in corn and cassava, which make up the bulk of the difference between the areas. These are relatively rich in calories and carbohydrates. The urban diet contains more meat and poultry, dairy products and legumes which are relatively rich in proteins and fats. It is important to note that much of this differential is created by the numbers of households reporting some consumption of certain foods (second panel, Table 3). On the whole, the urban population has a more varied diet.

Food consumption patterns reflect, among other things, the effects of relative prices in the two areas. For the time being, we shall ignore income differentials and their potential effect, and focus on differences in relative prices which affect the well-being of households with identical incomes in the two areas. The effect of income is derived from the price effects which are postulated to increase some of the observed differentials in consumption patterns.

The data in Table 4 show that the rural average per capita daily food basket costs about 60% [ = (262.28/163.14 − 1) × 100] more in urban than in rural areas. Urban prices are higher across the board, notably for potatoes, vegetables, and "other items."[3] The data in the last panel in Table 4 show the ratio of urban and rural prices of each food group expressed in terms of the ratio of the prices of rice. Relatively speaking, prices of legumes, dairy products and meats are lower in urban areas, and staples in rural areas. That is, we

*Table 3.* Proportion of Food Budget Allocated to Food Groups, Proportion of Population Reporting Consumption, and Per Capita Consumption by Area of Residence, Indonesia, 1979

| Food Group | Proportion of Food Budget Allocated to Food Group (percent) | | Proportion of Households Reporting Consumption of Food (percent) | | Per Capita Daily Consumption (in grams) | |
|---|---|---|---|---|---|---|
| | Urban | Rural | Urban | Rural | Urban | Rural |
| Rice | 27.89 | 35.11 | 99.59 | 93.32 | 322.85 | 321.49 |
| Corn | 0.40 | 4.31 | 9.63 | 26.43 | 8.83 | 59.36 |
| Wheat | 0.25 | 0.68 | 12.44 | 7.47 | 4.04 | 5.86 |
| Cassava | 0.50 | 2.16 | 33.18 | 47.17 | 26.01 | 89.72 |
| Potatoes | 0.53 | 0.78 | 32.50 | 22.18 | 14.95 | 27.81 |
| Fish | 6.90 | 6.50 | 83.52 | 81.45 | 41.34 | 34.37 |
| Meat/Poultry | 3.91 | 2.19 | 42.74 | 17.55 | 11.67 | 6.11 |
| Eggs | 2.03 | 0.87 | 54.99 | 26.29 | 0.11(units) | 0.05(units) |
| Dairy Products | 2.03 | 0.45 | 38.25 | 9.13 | 28.00 | .62 |
| Vegetables | 7.20 | 7.32 | 97.21 | 97.49 | 132.59 | 146.33 |
| Legumes | 3.85 | 3.02 | 81.48 | 62.46 | 51.82 | 28.79 |
| Fruits | 3.39 | 2.36 | 68.41 | 51.58 | 66.49 | 52.20 |
| Other Items | 41.12 | 34.25 | 99.24 | 99.70 | 235.50 | 222.73 |
| Total | 100.00 | 100.00 | | | 924.92* | 996.34* |

* Excluding eggs.
*Source:* SUSENAS 1978 data tapes, Biro Pusal Statistik, Jakarta.

indeed observe the expected effects of relative prices on the patterns of food consumption in the two areas; people consume relatively more of those foods which are relatively inexpensive in their locations. The noteworthy exception is "other items" which include many ready-made foods and soft drinks common in urban areas.

The above data suggest that, on the average, urban incomes are insufficient to offset price differentials between urban and rural areas. The average person in the urban areas eats somewhat less than his rural counterpart, and opts for those food commodities which are relatively inexpensive in the urban areas. The effect of income thus appears to be insuffient to outweigh the effect of higher prices as far as food consumption is concerned.

*Tables 4.* Prices\* Per Kilogram of Food (Except for Eggs), Rural Food
Baskets in Urban Prices, and Relative Prices, Indonesia, 1978

| Food Group | Price Per Kilo- gram (Rp) | | Rural Per Capita Food Basket in Urban and Rural Prices | | Ratio of Urban to Rural Price Expressed in Terms of Ratio of Rice Prices |
|---|---|---|---|---|---|
| | Urban | Rural | Urban Prices | Rural Prices | |
| Rice | 153 | 139 | 49.40 | 44.88 | 1.00 |
| Corn | 82 | 65 | 0.72 | 0.57 | 1.15 |
| Wheat | 142 | 118 | 0.57 | 0.48 | 1.09 |
| Cassava | 36 | 27 | 0.94 | 0.70 | 1.21 |
| Potatoes | 111 | 62 | 1.66 | 0.93 | 1.63 |
| Fish | 462 | 341 | 19.10 | 14.10 | 1.23 |
| Meat & Poultry | 1071 | 914 | 12.50 | 10.66 | 1.06 |
| Eggs (Units) | 45 | 36 | Nil | Nil | 1.14 |
| Dairy Products | 759 | 731 | 6.68 | 6.43 | 0.94 |
| Vegetables | 151 | 96 | 20.02 | 12.73 | 1.43 |
| Legumes | 198 | 174 | 10.26 | 9.02 | 1.03 |
| Fruits | 157 | 100 | 10.44 | 6.65 | 1.43 |
| Other Items | 552 | 242 | 129.99 | 56.99 | 2.07 |
| Total | | | 262.28 | 164.14 | |

\* For the definition of prices, see Chernichovsky & Meesook (1984).

## III.  CONSUMPTION OF NUTRIENTS AND NUTRITIONAL DEFICIENCIES

Minimal nutritional requirements, average levels of nutrient consumption, and proportions of the population deficient in different nutrients as derived from food consumption data are show in the three panels in Table 5.

Minimal nutritional requirements adjusted for the household's age composition for the urban and rural populations are practically identical (Chernichovsky and Meesook, 1984). This indicates that the demographic make-up of the two populations is not sufficiently different to produce any differences in average nutrional requirements.

Daily consumption levels of nutrients differ, however. The urban population reports consumption of fewer calories and all other micronutrients except calcium than the rural population. The opposite is true for proteins and fats.

Average figures thus tend to suggest that, in spite of lower average levels of expenditures, the rural population is not nutritionally worse-off than the urban population. In fact, relatively high levels of protein combined with fat (from meats and oils), one of the common nutritional signs of urbanization,

*Table 5.* Minimal Nutritional Requirements, Per Capita Nutrient Consumption and Proportions Deficient in Nutrients

| Nutrients | (units) | Estimated Minimal Per Capita Daily Requirements | | Per Capita Daily Consumption of Nutrients | | Proportion of Population with Nutritional Deficiency (percent) | |
|---|---|---|---|---|---|---|---|
| | | Urban | Rural | Urban | Rural | Urban | Rural |
| Calories | (calories) | 1929.00 | 1939.00 | 1912.00 [2.7] | 2002.00 [1.6] | 57.90 | 53.59 |
| Protein | (grams) | 40.41 | 40.43 | 53.91 [4.6] | 50.34 [2.7] | 33.05 | 41.09 |
| Fat | (grams) | — | — | 37.07 | 29.27 | — | — |
| Carbohydrates | (grams) | — | — | 344.00 | 388.00 | — | — |
| Calcium | (mg.) | 0.56 | 0.56 | 308.00 | 286.00 | 0.11 | 0.50 |
| Iron | (mg.) | 13.78 | 13.75 | 9.44 | 9.79 | 83.23 | 81.54 |
| Vitamin A | (Intl. units) | 3291.00 | 3291.00 | 5361.00 [6.3] | 5754.00 [9.3] | 39.47 | 47.21 |
| Thiamin | (mg.) | 0.78 | 0.79 | 0.90 | 0.89 | 47.25 | 49.31 |
| Riboflavin | (mg.) | 1.10 | 1.10 | 0.70 | 0.70 | 85.26 | 86.74 |
| Niacin | (mg.) | 12.82 | 12.84 | 14.00 | 14.90 | 49.61 | 47.50 |
| Vitamin C | (mg.) | 28.60 | 28.54 | 141.00 [7.2] | 157.00 [4.8] | 12.17 | 11.72 |

*Note:* The skewness measure for the distribution is shown in parentheses.
*Source:* SUSENAS 1978 data tapes, Biro Pusal Statistik, Jakarta.

may be a mixed blessing for the urban dwellers because these diets may a precursor to cardiovascular problems common in other urban societies.

The final panel in Table 5 gives estimated proportions of the population with nutritional deficiencies. There is a higher probability of an individual being calorie-deficient in the urban areas and protein-deficient in the rural areas. Among the micronutrients, there is a higher likelihood of being deficient in vitamin A in rural areas than in urban areas.[4]

However, the situation for urban areas is on the whole less favorable than these averages imply. Focusing on the actual distributions of four nutrients, namely calories, protein, and vitamins A and C, the skewness measures (shown in parentheses in Table 5) show that, except for vitamin C, the urban distribution is much more skewed (to the left) than the rural distribution. Hence even for proteins, the chances of being deficient may actually be higher in urban than in rural areas.

For both areas of residence it is clear that there is a distributional problem; while the average figures do not suggest a high likelihood of deficiencies when compared with requirements, the likelihood of being deficient in a particular nutrient is in fact quite high, particularly in urban areas.

## IV.  CHANGING INCOMES AND PRICES AND THE RISK OF MALNUTRITION

It is clear from the discussion thus far that the transition from rural to urban areas may entail, on the average, a change in the diet because both absolute and relative food prices differ between the two settings. These differences appear not to be compensated by higher average incomes for urban dwellers. The risk of malnutrition is still serious in both rural and urban areas, but perhaps more so in the latter in spite of its relatively higher incomes.

The next question is how precarious is the nutrional status of the two populations as incomes and prices of particular foods change? Such a change could be the result of government policy concerning particular foods or of changes in production and import costs.

Ultimately, the sensitivity of consumption of any nutrient depends on two parameters: the sensitivity of particular foods to changes in incomes and prices, i.e., pertinent income and price elasticities, and the contributions of these foods to the consumption of different nutrients (Chernichovsky and Meesook, 1984). We now focus on these parameters.

Table 6 shows the relative contributions of various food groups to the consumption of calories, proteins and vitamins A and C in urban and rural areas. Rice is a dominant factor in the consumption of both calories and proteins; vegetables in the consumption of vitamins. Moreover, the contributions of the two food groups are similar in the two areas. This may

*Table 6.*     The Contributions of Food Groups to the Consumption of
Calories, Protein, and Vitamins A and C.

| | | *(Percent)* | | | |
|---|---|---|---|---|---|
| Food Groups | | Calories | Protein | Vitamin A | Vitamin C |
| Rice | Urban | 61.79 | 45.32 | 0.00 | 0.00 |
| | Rural | 57.83 | 45.45 | 0.00 | 0.00 |
| Corn | Urban | 3.93 | 0.85 | 2.17 | 0.31 |
| | Rural | 12.80 | 5.33 | 8.54 | 2.87 |
| Wheat | Urban | 0.60 | 0.78 | 0.06 | 0.00 |
| | Rural | 0.99 | 1.07 | 0.49 | 0.00 |
| Cassava | Urban | 1.94 | 0.61 | 0.00 | 6.33 |
| | Rural | 8.80 | 2.96 | 0.00 | 11.54 |
| Potatoes | Urban | 0.79 | 0.48 | 6.10 | 2.33 |
| | Rural | 1.56 | 1.03 | 8.02 | 3.73 |
| Fish | Urban | 2.61 | 15.15 | 2.23 | 0.00 |
| | Rural | 2.43 | 15.99 | 2.26 | 0.00 |
| Meat/Poultry | Urban | 1.08 | 3.22 | 0.34 | 0.00 |
| | Rural | 0.51 | 1.63 | 0.27 | 0.00 |
| Eggs (Units) | Urban | 0.45 | 1.75 | 1.82 | 0.00 |
| | Rural | 0.16 | 1.06 | 0.82 | 0.00 |
| Dairy Products | Urban | 1.43 | 4.20 | 1.44 | 0.37 |
| | Rural | 0.52 | 1.37 | 0.23 | 0.03 |
| Vegetables | Urban | 3.78 | 7.44 | 72.48 | 75.64 |
| | Rural | 4.11 | 9.08 | 69.52 | 71.20 |
| Legumes | Urban | 4.67 | 15.40 | 0.87 | 0.68 |
| | Rural | 3.21 | 10.54 | 0.70 | 0.44 |
| Fruits | Urban | 1.60 | 0.80 | 9.69 | 11.67 |
| | Rural | 1.20 | 0.58 | 7.40 | 7.85 |
| Others | Urban | 19.08 | 6.89 | 2.80 | 1.43 |
| | Rural | 14.16 | 5.62 | 1.75 | 1.18 |

*Source:*   SUSENAS 1978 data tapes, Biro Pusal Statistik, Jakarta.

reflect among other things the impact of tradition on diets; the two food groups represent the core of the average Indonesian diet and hence any rise in their prices may have a substantial impact on nutritional levels across the different areas. In this regard it is important to note the importance of fish in protein consumption in the two areas.

Significant differences in consumption patterns between the two areas exist, however. The urban population relies relatively more on meat and poultry, eggs and dairy products; the rural population relies more on corn, cassava and potatoes.

The above information is included in direct estimates of pertinent income and food price elasticities of demand for calories and protein (controlling for family size).[5] These estimates, obtained separately for urban and rural areas, were used to predict the additional population which might become calorie-

*Table 7.* Likely Changes is Proportions of
Population Deficient in Calories and Protein

| | Percent | | | |
| --- | --- | --- | --- | --- |
| | Calories | | Protein | |
| 10% points change in (direction of change) | Rural | Urban | Rural | Urban |
| Household Monthly Expenditure (−) | 5.0 | 2.7 | 4.8 | 2.7 |
| Price of | | | | |
| Rice | 1.6 | 2.0 | 1.6 | 1.2 |
| Corn | 0.4 | * | −0.4 | 0.0 |
| Wheat | −2.0 | * | −1.2 | * |
| Cassava | −0.4 | * | * | * |
| Potatoes | * | * | * | * |
| Fish | * | 0.4 | 0.8 | 0.8 |
| Eggs | * | −0.8 | −0.4 | −0.4 |
| Meat & Poultry | 0.8 | 0.4 | 0.8 | 0.4 |
| Dairy Products | 0.8 | * | 0.8 | 3.9 |
| Vegetables | * | * | 0.4 | * |
| Legumes | * | * | 0.4 | 0.8 |
| Fruits | −0.4 | 0.4 | 0.4 | 0.4 |
| Other Items | −0.8 | 1.2 | 0.8 | 1.2 |

* Nil or statistically insignificant effect.

and protein-deficient with a 10 percent drop in monthly expenditures, a proxy for income, or a 10 percent increase in prices of different foods.

The results are reported in Table 7.[2] They show that a change in expenditures and prices will have an impact on the two populations for different reasons; income changes are more critical in rural areas, prices in urban areas. A drop in expenditures will cause a 5 percent addition to the population deficient in calories in rural areas, and only 2.7 percent in urban areas. The results are identical for protein. This suggests that a 10 percent change in expenditures, in conjunction with heavy reliance on particular foods, namely rice and vegetables, leads to an across-the-board change in food consumption affecting at least these two nutrients in a similar fashion in each area.

Changes in prices affect calorie and protein consumption differently and have a different impact in each area. With regard to calories, the urban population is more sensitive than the rural population to a change in the price of rice. A 10 percent increase in its price is likely to increase the calorie deficient population by 2 percent in urban areas, and by 16 percent in rural areas. Another notable item differentiating the two populations in this regard is "other items," the change in price of which affects the urban population more. With regard to protein, changes in the price of rice are likely to affect the rural areas more than the urban. On the other hand, changes in the prices of dairy products and "other items" are relatively more critical for the urban population.

# V.  CONCLUSION

In an attempt to establish dietary and nutritional patterns associated with urbanization in Indonesia, we compare levels of expenditures as well as food and nutrition consumption in urban and rural areas.

In spite of the relative affluence of the urban population, it does not fare better than the rural population in terms of diet. Urban diets are more expensive in absolute terms; relative prices also bias consumption away from grains which are rich in carbohydrates towards other foods which are rich in protein and fat. Price differentials between the areas appear to outweigh the income differentials as far as food consumption is concerned.

As a result, the urban population is on average better-off in terms of the consumption of protein and vitamin C, and worse-off in terms of calories and other micronutrients.

In part because of a more severe distributional problem in urban areas, the urban population may be more at risk of malnutrition than the rural population, especially if incomes or prices change adversely. This situation may represent one of the more basic problems associated with urbanization in Indonesia.

# ANNEX:   GROUPING OF FOODS

(1)  *Rice* includes free-market, self-produced, and glutinous rice, as well as rice byproducts (such as rice flour).

(2)  *Corn* includes both fresh and dried corn on the husk, shelled corn, and corn meal.

(3)  *Wheat* includes wheat flour and other grains.

(4)  *Cassava* refers to fresh and dried cassava, and cassava meal.

(5)  *Potatoes* cover sweet potatoes, potatoes, taro and sago. (The latter two are starchy plants similar to potatoes.)

(6)  *Fish* includes fresh ocean and inland fish, salted and dried fish, canned fish, shrimp, and shellfish.

(7)  *Meat and poultry* covers beef from cattle and carabao (water buffalo), mutton, pork, preserved meat, veal, chicken, and turkey.

(8)  *Eggs* are treated separately because of the difficulty of combining this item with any other.

(9)  *Dairy products* cover fresh milk, evaporated milk, powered milk, and cheese.

(10) *Vegetables* include spinach, kangkung spinach, cabbage, mustard greens, beans, peas, strong beans, tomatoes, radishes, carrots, cucumbers, cassava leaves, eggplant, bean sprouts, squash, red and white onions, red and cayenne peppers, and papaya leaves.

(11) *Legumes* refer to peanuts, green and red beans, soybeans, tunggak beans, bean curd, soybean cake, tauco, peanut cake, and lamtoro.

(12) *Fruits* include citrus fruits, mangoes, apples, avocados, rambutan, dukuh, durian, salak, pineapple, bananas, papaya, jambu, guava, sawo, belimbing, kedongdong, and watermelon.

(13) *Other* includes salt, pepper and other spices, fish paste, ketchup, coconut, cooking oil, butter, lard, brown and granulated sugar, tea, coffee, cocoa, fried fish sticks, noodles, monosodium glutamate, lemon syrup, bottled drinks (lemonade, cola, orange soda, etc.), bread, beer, and alcohol.

For computational purposes, those foods given in units other than kilograms were converted to kilograms. All items in food groups 1-6 and 10-12 were given initially in kilograms; conversion for foods in the remaining groups are given below.

Group 7 contains chicken and turkey, each given in units of one bird. A chicken was assumed to weigh one kilogram; a turkey was assigned a weight of 4.5 kilograms.

Group 8 comprises only eggs; therefore, no conversion was necessary.

Group 9, the item "fresh milk" was given in liters. One liter of fresh milk has a weight of 1.032 kilograms.

Because of the diverse nature of group 13, the foods it contains are presented in several different units. Fried fish sticks, noodles, and bread were the only items given in kilograms. A number of items were units of 100 grams which have been converted into kilograms. These items are salt, pepper and other spices, fish paste, butter, lard, brown sugar, granulated sugar, tea, coffee, cocoa, and monosodium glutamate. A bottle of ketchup was assigned a weight of 500 grams; likewise, a coconut was assumed to weigh 500 grams. Cooking oil, lemon syrup, and bottled drinks were each given in liters; the first has a weight of 0.93 kilograms per liter, while the latter two each weigh 1.04 kilograms per liter. A 12-ounce bottle of beer has a weight of 0.36 kilograms; a "shot" of alcohol containing one and a half ounces weighs 0.042 kilograms.

# NOTES

1. The choice of a different definition would give quantitatively different figures, but the results would be qualitatively no different from those reported in this paper.
2. See the Annex for the definition of food groups.

3.   These differentials also reflect qualitative variations in foods; for example, the difference in the price of rice (which is regulated) reflects consumption of improved varieties in the urban areas. This in part reflects the effect of relatively higher incomes there.

4.   The reader is reminded that these figures should not be taken at face value; rather, they should be taken as indicators of the likelihood of becoming deficient given the characteristics of the distribution.

5.   The estimates are available upon request from the authors.

6.   These estimates are based on a theoretical log-normal distribution with the same mean and standard deviation as the actual distribution.

# REFERENCES

Chernichovsky, D., and Meesook, O.A. (1984). "Patterns of Food Consumption and Nutrition in Indonesia," World Bank Staff Working Paper No. 670.

World Bank. (1984). *World Development Report, 1984*. Oxford University Press, New York: Tables 19 and 22, pp. 254, 260.

# HEALTH SYSTEMS OF KOREA

Seung-Hum Yu

## INTRODUCTION

Korea is a peninsula with an area of 221,000 square kilometers (including North Korea), which is connected to China and Russia at the northern end, and situated to the west of Japan. It is located in the temperate zone, and thereby has four seasons of three months each.

Korea has a long history of more than 5,000 years and steeped in tradition. It has its own alphabet, a phonetic alphabet invented more than 500 years ago. In addition, to some extent, Koreans have used Chinese characters in writing, pronouncing them differently from the way they are pronounced in China. Koreans are a single ethnic group. Korea has had skilled artists, many of whom were taken to Japan.

Since the fourteenth century, Koreans have lived under the influence of Confucianism, and still conservative Oriental thinking is not uncommon although attitudes are rapidly westernizing. Buddhism was introduced in the fourth century and it is still a prosperous religion in Korea today. Catholicism was introduced 200 years ago and Protestantism 100 years ago.

Research in Human Capital Development, Vol. 5, pages 207-217.
Copyright © 1988 by JAI Press Inc.
All rights of reproduction in any form reserved.
ISBN: 0-89232-508-9

At the end of World War II, the Korean peninsula was divided at the 38th parallel into two countries: the north, communist, and the south, democratic. Since the disarmament treaty was put into effect immediately following the Korean War (1950-1953), South Korea has been bounded on the north by the demilitarized zone, which is 155 miles wide. (Hereafter, Korea denotes South Korea [the Republic of Korea]).

South Korea has a total area of 99 square kilometers and a population of forty million. The Korean economy has been rapidly improving from the time the country lay in ruins after the war: a succession of five-year economic development plans started in 1962 when the per capita GNP was 82 U.S. dollars, and by 1984 the per capita GNP had grown to 2,000 dollars. Since the fourth five-year plan (1977-81), social development, including the development of health services, has received greater emphasis. The title of the fifth five-year plan included the word social rather than merely the words Economic Development Plan as previous plans had, an addition which implied more emphasis on education, health and welfare.

In the 1960s, about 70 percent of the population lived in the rural areas; however, now nearly 70 percent of the population lives in the cities due to rapid industrialization. Korea is no longer recognized as an agricultural country, although it is self-sufficient in rice production. The level of education is very high and the illiteracy rate is negligible: outside those who are very old, an illiterate person is seldom seen.

## II.   SOME HEALTH CARE INDICATORS AND RESOURCES

### A.   Some Health Indicators

The crude birth rate is 23.0, the crude death rate is 6.2, and the natural increase rate is 16.8 per 1,000 persons (1984). A nationwide family planning program was started in the early 1960s, which was regarded worldwide to be very successful. Both the government and private sector, through the Planned Parenthood Federation of Korea, have been pushing the population policy for the last quarter century.

The infant mortality rate has been decreased from about 60 in the late 1950s to about 30 per 1,000 live births in the 1980s. The main causes of infant death in the 1970s were gastritis, pneumonia, and neonatal diseases; however, congenital anomaly became the leading cause of death in the 1980s, with pneumonia and perinatal diseases next in line.

The morbidity pattern has been changing. Chronic diseases such as pulmonary tuberculosis were one of the health problems in the 1950s and 1960s, however, both incidence and prevalence of them have dropped significantly in the 1980s. Acute communicable diseases such as cholera and typhoid fever were no longer a problem after the mid-1970s since environmental hygiene and public health programs were developed.

The main causes of death have obviously been changing: pneumonia and bronchitis, tuberculosis, and gastritis were the main causes of death in the 1950s, but cerebrovascular diseases, malignant neoplasm, and other circulatory diseases are main causes in 1980s. The disease pattern is becoming like that found in developed countries.

Life expectancy at birth was 45 for men and 50 for women in the late 1940s, but it increased to 63 for men and 69 for women by the late 1970s. Life expectancy at the age of 60 was 13 years for men and 18 years for women in the late 1970s, which means that in the future Korea will be facing health care problems of the elderly who now comprise about 6 percent of the total population.

Nutritional status is fairly good; malnutrition is very rare, although nutritional imbalance is seen in some rural areas. Obesity is becoming a problem especially in the big cities. Parasite eradication has been successful and parasitic infection is rare. Pollution due to rapid industrialization has become one of the most important public health problems.

## B.   Health Care Resources

Western medicine was introduced into Korea a century ago by an American medical missionary, but German medicine, in particular, was an influence during the period Korea was under Japanese rule (1910-1945). Since World War II, American influence has again become dominant in the field of medicine and health.

### 1.   Health manpower

There were only 8 medical schools in Korea until the 1960s and about 800 medical graduates were produced each year. However, more than 4,000 physicians went to the United States for residency training in the 1960s and early 1970s and did not return. This resulted in a serious physician shortage.

Since the dawn of the 1970s, the demand for medical care has been rapidly increasing due to rapid economic growth. The number of medical schools increased to 28 in 1985, and about 2,000 new medical graduates are produced annually; this number is expected to rise to 3,000 when all 28 medical schools are running at full capacity. At present there are more than 20,000 medical doctors in practice in Korea. There are 10 dental schools currently turning out over 700 new dentists annually. At present there are 5,000 working dentists. A total of 29,000 pharamcists are licensed. There are 4,500 nurse graduates annually from 43 three-year junior colleges of nursing and 17 four-year colleges of nursing. A shortage of nurses was evident in the late 1960s and early 1970s because of emigration to West Germany and the United States. In order to compensate for this, the number of nursing schools was increased, and nurses are no longer in short supply.

## 2. Medical Care Facilities

There are 500 hospitals of various sizes, and about 70,000 beds; the bed/population ratio is 2 beds per 1,000 population. There are about 8,000 clinics, with a total of about 2,500 beds. It is quite common for the clinics to have several beds for short-stay inpatient care.

Medical facilities are unevenly distributed geographically, and accessibility to them in rural areas is not as good as in urban areas, as is the case, of course, in any other country. In order to solve the problem of inaccessibility of medical care, the government stations doctors in each township and community health practitioners in the more remote areas.

Of the facilities available, the public sector has about 20 percent of the hospitals and hospital beds; since the government has not invested enough in medical care facilities, the private sector has the major portion. Among those found in private sector, the majority are run by physicians and these hospitals have 100 to 200 beds each. Community hospitals are not common.

About 4 percent of the GNP is spent on health care. A total of 255,000 won (285 United States dollars), or 5.9 percent of total consumption expenditure in the rural households was spent for health care in 1984.

## III.   HEALTH CARE DELIVERY SYSTEM

### A.   Personal Medical Care

Until the mid-1970s, an individual's medical care was his own responsibility, except in the case of the indigent who was cared for by the government. Many persons visitied the herbalist or drugstore, a not uncommon practice.

The government started the Workmen's Compensation Program and voluntary medical insurance in 1963. This was the time when many Korean medical graduates were going to the United States for further training and not returning. Also, Korean nurses were finding good employment opportunities in other countries. Thus, there was a general shortage of medical personnel, but it was most severe in rural areas. At the time these government programs were initiated, some philanthropic institutions, mostly religion-related hospitals, were offering charity care, to some extent, and public hosptials were caring for nonpaying patients in part. Some efforts made by voluntary organizations to provide charity care on a mobile basis in medically underserved areas were common until the late 1960s.

At the beginning of the 1970s, the demand for medical care was rapidly increasing as a result of the growth of the economy. The number of medical and nursing schools and, hence, the number of graduates increased. Medical facilities grew voluntarily both in number and capacity in keeping with the increasing demand for medical care.

## 1.  Medical Aid program

With the commencement of the Fourth Five-year Economic Development Plan (1977-1981), the Korean government had emphasized social development for the first time in its succession of five-year plans. As a part of this emphasis, the Medical Aid program for the indigent and low-income groups, including the elderly, was launched in January 1977 as a form of public assistance.

Under this program, which served about two million people, ambulatory care was made available free of charge to all clients in either of these groups. Inpatients of the indigent and the elderly categories were cared for free of charge, and the inpatients of the low-income group were required to pay back, eventually, 70 percent of the total cost of their medical care within two years without interest; the government assumed the remaining 30 percent of the cost. To implement the program, the government developed a health care delivery system which provided services in 56 regions throughout the country. The total national budget allocated for this program was the largest ever provided in Korea for a single health program.

As of 1985, a total of 3.3 million people, or about 8 percent of the entire population was being covered under this program. Beginning in 1986 the number of beneficiaries will be increased annually up to 15 percent. The budget for the Medical Aid program comes from the Ministry of Health and Social Affairs (about three-fourths) and local government (one-fourth). The central government allocates funds for the program in the annual budget and transfers the money to the local governement. Then the Medical Aid program is administered by the local city or county government.

Medical care is provided by the government at government-contracted private medical care facilities as well as at public medical care facilities. Medical institutions send the bill to the local government and are reimbursed by the latter. The demand for medical care, especially for chronic illnesses, has been increasing.

## 2.  Medical Insurance Scheme

Along with the Medical Aid program, a medical insurance scheme was launched in July 1977 in view of the improvement in the economy. Employees and dependents of employees of firms having 500 or more persons on their payroll were compulsorily insured. In 1979 this requirement was extended to firms with 300 or more employees. In 1981 it was further extended to include firms with 100 or more employees and in 1983, 16 or more. By 1985 about 12 million of those employed in firms and their dependents were insured.

These firms were required singly or as groups to organize nonprofit medical insurance societies (cooperatives) and 146 societies are now in existence. Premiums are around 3 percent of the monthly salary, half of the cost of which is deducted from the employee's pay. This scheme is centrally administered by the Federation of Medical Insurance Societies, which reviews bills, reimburses medical and hospital care fees, and provides other administrative support.

In 1979 a medical insurance program for government employees and teachers and staff of private educational institutions, from the elementary school level to the university level, was started. Half of the premium is paid by the employees and the other half is paid by the employer, regardless of whether it is the government or a private employer. This program, covering 4 million people including dependents of employees, is administered by the nonprofit corporation specifically set up to administer this medical insurance program.

The insurance benefits provided are similar under the two programs, covering sickness, injury, maternity care, and death. A coinsurance system was created to maintain a financially sound base for the insurance programs and to prevent unnecessary utilization and overutilization of insurance. It is anticipated that the use of this system will eventually lead successfully to saving insurance expenditures. Thirty percent of the patient's bill in clinics, 50 percent of it in the outpatient departments of hospitals, and 20 percent of it in inpatient care units of hospitals are paid by the patient. Certain expenses, such as those for cosmetic surgery and blood, are excluded from the benefits. However, coverage is rather wide and generous in general: there is no upper limit.

A third program of medical insurance, a regional health insurance plan, is in effect for those not covered by the above two schemes, that is, those in rural areas and those who are either self-employed or employed in small firms. This program was initiated in 1981 as a pilot project. Three rural counties were selected for the project originally, and two more counties and one city were added in 1982. It was hoped, of course, that this would at least light the way to a plan feasible and effective enough to be put into full-scale use for the benefit of this additional segment of the population, including rural people who have no regular cash income. The size of the premium is based on the income level of the household, and the payment of the entire amount is the sole responsibility of the insured; the government is responsible for the administrative costs.

At the beginning the premium collection rate was as low as 70 percent or less and a great financial deficit resulted in five out of six demonstration areas. However, in the ensuing three to four years the premium collection rate increased to more than 90 percent on the average except in the urban area. At first the public's view of regional medical insurance was negative, but it has changed. At present the government is planning to increase the number of persons participating in the regional insurance plan, year by year, at a rate that will mean that the entire population will be insured, at the latest, by the end of this decade.

Basically, regional medical insurance is administered by local societies, financially independent (although the government subsidizes them to the extent of covering administrative expenses), nonprofit cooperatives organized, one, in each county or city. Benefit coverage is the same as that in the two forgoing schemes. Review of the medical care bill is done by the Federation of Medical Insurance Societies.

## B. Public Health Care

Since the late 1950s the Korean government has emphasized the widespread establishment of public health services. The Korean War ended in 1953 and the country was in ruins in those early postwar days. Therefore, public health programs such as acute communicable disease control, vaccination, parasite eradication, etc., were urgently needed, while private medical care was needed, too.

The government established health centers, one in each county and city, totaling 200 in the early 1960s. The major functions of the centers were health education and the collection of vital statistics, environmental health and food sanitation, nutrition, the control of communicable diseases such as tuberculosis and venereal disease, maternal and child health, family planning, and general medical care. The director of each health center was a physician and primary medical care was provided.

Beginning in the early 1960s health subcenters were also built, in every township with a population of about 10,000. A practicing private physician was designated to serve as a public doctor in each township. He was free to practice privately at the health subcenter and the government gave him a monthly subsidy for his public services. A total of 1,300 health subcenters, one in each township, were placed in operation with three health workers stationed in each. One worker was responsible for tuberculosis control, another for maternal and child health, and the third for family planning. These subcenter health workers were nurses or nurses' aides. The government gave the health workers on-the-job training as well as regular refresher training.

This system continued in operation until the mid-1970s, when a new primary health care program was instituted as a result of the combined efforts of the government, private universities, and other groups in the private sector. The evolution of this system of public health care was a prominent feature of the 1970s because, as a result of the growth in the economy and an upgrading of the level of education, new demands for health care were created and the means for meeting the new demands, such as adequate manpower and governmental allocation of funds, were not available.

The current public health care system is planned and technically supervised by the Ministry of Health and Social Affairs, but the health centers and subcenters are, for all practical purposes, under the control of local (city or county) governments which are under the Ministry of Home Affairs. The Ministry of Health has no direct lower level administrative organizational structure in the periphery. This structure has been criticized by the health professionals since the supervision of the program by the Ministry of Health and the influence of the Ministry of Health on its operation cannot effectively enter into the functioning of the program. However, as yet no improvement has been made in the structure.

## IV.  PRIMARY HEALTH CARE

As mentioned in the previous section, the widespread establishment and maintenance of public health services have been emphasized since the late 1950s. Health centers were set up in both urban and rural areas. The urban health centers were mainly designed to provide public health services only, while rural health centers and subcenters were designed to provide both public health services and primary medical care. The focus of public health programs was on communicable disease control, maternal and child health, family planning, and tuberculosis control. Health services-quality-manpower drain was a serious problem in the 1960s in Korea, and the difficulty of recruiting physicians and nurses for public health work was one of the major constraints on the public health services program.

At the dawn of the 1970s, several community health projects were being developed by universities and other institutions, and the concept and philosophy of primary health care was finding favor. Even before the Alma-Ata declaration of the World Health Organization in 1978, the concept of primary health care was widely accepted among health professionals as well as the government officials in Korea.

It seemed to some of the health professionals that introducing the philosophy and principles of primary health care in the early 1970s in Korea would help to provide a solution to some of the aforementioned problems. During the 1970s a community health practitioners program was put into practice in some projects and was accepted by the government. The Special Act for Rural Health went into effect in December 1980 for this purpose. These community health practitioners were nurses or midwives who had received six months of training: eight weeks of theory, twelve weeks of clinical training, and four weeks of field practice. The program is continuing. A total of 1,600 community health practitioners have been trained and dispatched to community health posts, which are self-governing health facilities established in communities and supported by the government for grassroots-level care. This number will be increased up to two thousand by the end of 1986.

These posts are located far from the center of townships. One community health practitioner works in each community health post covering about 2,000 people and there are usually three village health workers, in addition, in every health post area. Each community health post is operated by a governing committee on which community leaders serve. The site for the community health post is donated by the community. The Ministry of Health and Social Affairs pays half of the salary of the community health practitioner and the local government the other half. Operating expenses are covered from the nominal charges to the clients under the control of the governing committee.

## V. NATIONAL HEALTH POLICY AND HEALTH CARE STRATEGY

To cope with the major health problems in Korea, the following objectives have been established for the health sector in the Fifth Five-Year Economic and Social Development Plan (1982-1986).

- First, the development and expansion of low cost health services for the urban poor and rural residents, and a more even geographical distribution of medical resources.
- Second, intensified public health measures, particularly in preventive care including disease control and maternal and child health.
- Third, better sanitation and water supply in rural areas and minimization of industrial pollution.
- Last, increased productivity of labor through the improvement of health.

To realize the above objectives, strategies such as expansion of preventive and promotive health care services by utilizing primary health care approaches, rational distribution of health resources, effective utilization and efficient training of health manpower, and improvement of health information systems are employed.

In line with the Korean government's emphasis on social justice and social welfare since the mid-1970s, the government health policy has laid stress on equality of opportunity, accessibility, and efficiency. In order to achieve health care for all, the government has been taking the following action, which will be strengthened in the immediate future.

First, health subcenter-level care is emphasized. Every physician is conscripted for service at a health subcenter as a public physician for a period of three years. (Physicians are not recruited for compulsory military service.) A total of 830 physicians were so employed under this provision in 1985. Most of them served as directors of health subcenters, seeing patients and supervising township health workers.

There is a total of 1,300 townships in Korea. At least one physician, public or private, had been made available in each township having a population of 7,000 to 10,000 by 1983. The number of public physicians will be further increased and the supply of physicians is adequate for this purpose. The government plans to give each new medical graduate one year of clinical training and then assign him to one of the township health subcenters. If this is done, the quality of medical care will be improved.

Second, even though a physician is available in every township, people who live in remote areas far from the center of townships still have limited access to health care facilities. In order to provide care for them, community health practitioners have been placed at community health posts in villages. This brings health care closer to them and, in fact, their rate of utilization of the posts is pretty high. The total number of posts planned is 2,000.

Third, establishing the health care delivery system is strongly emphasized. Since health care is given at the community level and primary medical care is available at the township level, provisions for offering secondary care are being considered. The government has encouraged the construction of at least 60 new community hospitals by introducing the possibility of obtaining a loan and receiving domestic funding in medically underserved areas. Therefore, secondary medical care has become readily available at or near the county level.

Primary health care is provided in connection with the availability of secondary care in community hospitals, and preventive care is offered at the township or village level. Thus, the concept of comprehensive health care becomes real.

In November 1985, one of the five rural regional medical insurance demonstration projects was designated for establishing a referral channel: the insured should be cared for at primary care facilities, but the community hospital cares for only those referred from the primary care facilities. The government is planning to establish a medical care referral system as soon as possible under the social security medical insurance system.

During the last one or two decades the Korean government has thought of health care in terms of accessibility, efficiency, and cost. Through the conscripting of physicians for public service and the assigning of them to every township, physician care is now available everywhere. Also, community health practitioners are serving in remote areas. Therefore, the needs for health care are being met a least quantatively. Since disease patterns and population structure have been changing, income is increasing, and the level of education climbing, health care demand has also changed. In order to meet the future demand effectively, several major strategies may be drawn from the experience.

First, since the geographical and financial accessibility of health care has been increased, a question as to the quality of health care should be raised.

Since economic growth is quite certain to continue and nearly 100 percent of the new generation is completing at least junior high school, the felt need or the demand for health care is changing. Management of a future program to meet this new demand remains a question.

Second, although physician manpower is evenly distributed, most public physicians, as opposed to private, physicians are those giving service only as a substitute for giving compulsory military service. Motivating them to serve conscientiously is a major task. If it cannot be done, it is a waste of manpower to conscript them for public health service.

Third, the major role of the community health practitioner is to give preventive and promotive service. However, it has been found that, in reality, curative services demand the major part of their time and effort, as had been anticipated by the health professionals. How to direct their time and energy to giving mainly preventive and promotive services is a challenging question.

Fourth, in connection with the social security medical insurance, it is quite natural for the insured to prefer to utilize private-clinic and private-hospital care since medical insurance pays the benefits for this. Finding a way to get the insured to use primary health care facilities is an important task to be done since the government is investing heavily in manpower and facilities for primary health care.

## SELECTED REFERENCES

Kim, I.S., Yu, S.H., Kim, H.J. et al. (1985). Impacts of countrywide government health insurance demonstration program on health utilization patterns of rural population in Kang Wha, Korea. Institute of Population and Health Services Research. Yonsei University, January.

Moon, O.R., and J.W. Hong. (1976). Study of mortality, morbidity, medical utilization and expenditure. Graduate School of Public Health, Seoul National University.

National Bureau of Statistics, Economic Planning Board. (1985). Social Indicators in Korea 1985. Republic of Korea.

Soh, C.T. (1980). Korea. A Geomedical Monograph of the Republic of Korea. Springer-Verlag, Berlin Heidelberg.

Yang, J.M., Kim, I.S., Yu, S.H., and Kim, H.J. (1983). Review of primary health care programme in Korea with policy recommendation. Institute of Population and Health Services Research. Yonsei University.

Yang, J.M., Yu, S.H., and Cho, W.H. (1984). Research fields and priority setting for health sciences in Korea. Institute of Population and Health Services Research, Yonsei University.

Yu, S.H. (1983). Study on hospital care services between insured and noninsured patients for selected diagnosis in Korea. *Yonsei Medical Journal,* 24(1):6-32.

Yu, S.H., Park, J.H., and Woo, K.H. (1984). Evaluation of community health practitioner's activities. *Yonsei Medical Journal,* 25:46-53.

# THE EVOLVING CHINESE RURAL HEALTH CARE SYSTEM

Carl E. Taylor, Robert L. Parker and Steven Jarrett

China has been uniquely successful in improving health care for one-quarter of the world's people. Since liberation in 1949, dramatic adjustments in national health policy have been based on pragmatic testing of alternative interventions and the courage to mobilize massive implementation of new approaches. The central motivation has been a consistent commitment to equity in improving the health of as many of its citizens as possible. Continuing progress has been made as the health system has adapted to major national social, political and economic developments as they have occurred.

In this report we will trace broad trends and review the major characteristics of the various periods of health care development in China. Our focus will be primarily on services for the 80 percent of the population who still live in villages. We will attempt to describe how previous developments have contributed to the present structure and function of the health system.

The sequence of health care developments in China falls naturally into the following periods:

Research in Human Capital Development, Vol. 5, pages 219-236.
Copyright © 1988 by JAI Press Inc.
All rights of reproduction in any form reserved.
ISBN: 0-89232-508-9

1. Preliberation;
2. Mass campaigns and increasing professionalization in the 1950s;
3. Quantitative expansion of coverage in the late 1950s, 1960s and 1970s—
   barefoot doctors, health cooperatives and antiepidemic services;
4. Modernization and qualitative improvement in the 1980s.

# I. PRELIBERATION

Health conditions in China before liberation were among the worst in the world. The extreme poverty of most of the people was reflected in gross malnutrition of children and recurrent severe famines in which millions of lives were lost. This situation was exacerbated by a high population density in spite of high mortality. Epidemics swept through the population with regularity, and multiple endemic diseases affected millions of people. The chronic fragility of the economy, political instability, internal and external exploitation of the poor, wars and almost constant civil strife heightened the other burdens the people had to bear.

China's ancient civilization has a distinguished tradition of health care. Historical developments over 3,500 years show both remarkable continuity and diversity. Unschuld has reveiwed the multiple subsytems in Chinese traditional medicine.[1] They include the coherent conceptual framework of "systematic correspondence" based on Yin-Yang duality and the five phases of regeneration and degeneration on which practices such as acupuncture are based. Herbal drug therapy steadily expanded, enriched by contacts with other cultures. An important underlying concept was that any educated person should learn about health care. As in most cultures numerous religious practices and folk healing methods based on beliefs in supernatural causation were part of the traditional society in China.

The introduction of Western medicine came mainly through missionaries, starting with the Jesuits in the seventeenth century followed by increased medical missionary activities in the nineteenth and twentieth centuries. They opened hospitals and started medical and nursing education. Medical colleges were also established, starting in the late nineteenth century. Western medicine, however, was accessible mainly to urban populations except for scattered rural mission efforts. Government health programs gradually took over, but the Ministry of Public Health at first focused mainly on epidemic control.

An important experiment in extending health care to rural areas, started in the 1930s, was the Ding Xian health program, part of the Rural Reconstruction and Mass Education Movement. The health activities were under the leadership of Dr. C.C. Chen and carried out in cooperation with Dr. J.B. Grant and the Peking Union Medical College (PUMC).[2] In this poor county in central Hebei, they showed that it was possible to provide health care at the low cost of 10 cents per capita per year. The Ding Xian experiment is frequently cited as the starting point for many similar demonstrations in other countries which helped provide the foundation for the current worldwide primary health care movement.

The directions of health care in China since 1949 were determined largely by experiences in the Liberated Areas during the 1940s. Of special importance in showing what could be achieved in health care was the remarkable effort of the People's Liberation Army (PLA) to provide health care to village people even when fighting an occupying army and a protracted civil war. Working out from referral and training medical facilities in centers such as Yanan, health care was organized for the Eighth Route Army, the new Fourth Army and the village people in the areas they controlled. Training of field staff was assisted by foreign volunteers, such as Dr. Norman Bethune and Dr. George Hatem (Ma Haide) working with Chinese colleagues. The network of health service for the armed forces was also extended to activities such as helping with harvests and reconstruction of war damage; this involvement proved a useful means of gaining the cooperation of the people. Since the PLA had few doctors, they trained young men and women volunteers who proved remarkably competent in providing basic health care. The schools that trained these volunteers laid the base for future developments in mobilizing and training vast numbers of paraprofessionals.

China also was one of the first developing countries in which UNICEF had a major program. From 1947 to 1949, under the leadership of Dr. Leo Eloesser, a remarkably effective program of training maternal and child health workers was evolved in the liberated areas. It was demonstrated that dramatic improvements could be made in the health of children and their mothers.

# MASS CAMPAIGNS AND EPIDEMIC PREVENTION SERVICES IN THE 1950s

With liberation, health for all the people became a high priority within the overall commitment to improve social conditions. Drastic political and social reforms were needed in turning from the urban orientation of the past to the systematic building of a broad new social order with special attention to rural areas. The party leadership recognized that health had to be improved not only because it was a social right, but also because all development efforts depend on healthy people. Chairman Mao enunciated four basic principles at the First National Congress in August 1950, less than one year after liberation:[3]

1. Medicine should serve the workers, peasants and soldiers;
2. Preventive medicine should take precedence over therapeutic medicine;
3. Chinese traditional medicine should be integrated with Western scientific medicine;
4. Health work should be combined with mass movements.

Each of these principles has had a profound impact. The first ensured broad access to health services. The second was implemented through the strong influence of the parallel structures of the health system and the Communist Party at all levels. Efforts to integrate traditional and scientific medicine were reinforced at the peripheral level because of the early scarcity of Western drugs, thus requiring health workers to grow, collect and formulate herbal medicines and to use acupuncture and other traditional treatments. In hospitals the two systems have tended to be provided as parallel and equally available services.

The education of health professionals was also a major achievement. The number of medical schools expanded rapidly, mostly following Soviet models. By 1965, more than 100,000 doctors, 170,000 middle level doctors, 185,000 nurses, 40,000 midwives and 100,000 pharmacists were trained.[3] The number of hospital beds increased from 84,000 to over 500,000. This expansion of professional services was, however, still focused largely in the cities.

Among the most publicized health efforts in the 1950s were the mass patriotic health campaigns. The mobilization of whole communities to join in specific tasks, such as destroying snails and other vectors of communicable diseases or working on environmental improvements, not only helped control disease but also had significant educational impact. Remarkable reductions of several epidemic and endemic diseases resulted. In implementing the "mass line" great stress was placed on trying to get people to understand why they were being asked to do specific tasks. The principle laid down was that local initiative, based on self-reliance, would solve many immediate problems once there was a thorough understanding of the nature of the problems. The high level of social mobilization and health awareness have significantly influenced the progress of health care delivery in China.

The First National Health Congress established a basic reorganization of health and medical care services, including measures to control and eradicate communicable diseases.[4] Health teams were sent to the countryside to establish epidemic prevention stations and work with the patriotic mass movements. Technical guidance from the epidemic prevention station channelled the mass mobilization of human energy, with leadership being provided by part-time health workers who had been trained for up to three months to assist with vaccination and surveillance against epidemic diseases. Mass vaccination was a principal tool in eradicating diseases such as smallpox; vector control was important in controlling endemic diseases; case identification and treatment were critical in eliminating contact diseases such as syphilis.

Epidemic prevention stations distributed supplies and vaccines for the mass campaigns, trained health workers and produced health education materials. They began to have an important role in environmental health and rural sanitation working along with village level committees and special groups.

Stations currently exist at provincial, prefectural, and county levels. The first six years from 1950-1955 saw the establishment of 315 stations. From 1955-1966, in one year alone, over 1,100 were established, as part of an intensified focus on rural health during the Great Leap Forward. By 1966, there were 2,513 stations but these were reduced to 1,480 by 1969, during the Cultural Revolution. Their important role in providing support and supervision to barefoot doctors was recognized once more and by 1972, the 1966 level had again been reached (2,558 stations). Since then, the number has grown steadily to 3,274 in 1983. Many epidemic prevention stations now have the laboratory infrastructure for surveillance of environmental conditions, water pollution, vaccine quality and food hygiene with facilities for bacteriology, virology, and chemistry.

Because of their dramatic quality, there has been a tendency to attribute the great improvement in health conditions that occurred in the 1950s and 1960s simply to the mass patriotic health campaigns. Much less mention has been made of the institutional role of epidemic prevention stations in facilitating mass mobilization by providing professional advice, health worker training, health education and appropriate supplies and equipment. Epidemic prevention stations are now primarily responsible for the very important national accelerated immunization (EPI) effort.

## III.  QUANTITIVE EXPANSION OF COVERAGE IN THE LATE 1950s, 1960s, AND 1970s

The physical infrastructure in the country as a whole has expanded greatly, with the number of health institutions of all types rising from 3,670 in 1949 to 196,017 in 1983. Of particular relevance to rural areas are the figures for MCH centers, which have risen from 9 to 2,649.

The deployment of human resources has been no less impressive, with total professional staff engaged in the provision of health services rising from 505,000 in 1949 to 3,344,000 in 1984.[5] In addition to these full-time health personnel are the part-time health staff which, in the early 1980s, came to about 1,500,000 barefoot or rural doctors, 29 percent of whom were women, a similar number of health aides and 540,000 rural midwives. The term "part-time" worker is relative since in some areas they seem to be working full-time. As early as 1980, data from a county survey show an average working day of seven hours for barefoot doctors during a one-week sample study.[6]

The township level constitutes the first level of referral, with some degree of specialization so that further referral is limited to severe cases. A major function of the township center is the continuous supervision and training of village doctors and aides, thereby coordinating the health work in the whole township. The county hospital typically accommodates a few hundred in-patients with a full range of specialties. County epidemic prevention centers and the MCH centers have the central role in initiating and supervising preventive health action in the whole county. There are over 2,500 counties in China, 75 percent of which have populations between 150,000 and 1,000,000 people. The county health school has a major role in training and supervision, but many county hospitals also are used for training students from the medical colleges.

Two innovations in mass health care in China which attracted special attention internationally were the barefoot doctor and health cooperatives. The impact and historical timing of these approaches are important in tracing the evolution of present services because they made health care accessible to all the people.

## A.   Barefoot Doctors

The Ding Xian experiment of the 1930s, demonstrated that ordinary village people who had received minimal education as part of the Mass Education Movement could specialize to become one of four types of "farmer scholars" with one of the four involving health activities. Services for health and family planning proved especially effective in gaining general community support.[7] These village health workers learned to apply simple, cheap and acceptable health measures which dramatically improved health conditions. In the liberated areas, these ideas were more widely extended with PLA medical assistants providing health care to the village people as part of a general program of tangible service.

During the Great Leap Forward in the late 1950s, Chairman Mao urged young doctors along with other college graduates to go to the villages. Large numbers responded to this call "to serve the people." An important result was the training of large numbers of primary health care workers. Out of this experience, the widespread use of "barefoot doctors" evolved. The term symbolized the notion that barefoot doctors were still community members involved in agricultural activities, but also trained to provide health care part-time. In addition to providing simple medical care, they became the main peripheral workers for preventive services. One of their more dramatic achievements now seems to have been that they contributed to lowering mortality from diarrhea by promoting oral rehydration with a salt and sugar solution.[8]

The Cultural Revolution from 1966 to 1976 refocused attention on the still-backward rural areas and promoted the universalization of health care coverage through increased national effort to train barefoot doctors. Urban hospitals and medical schools were closed and their personnel dispersed in small teams to serve village people and set up training programs for barefoot doctors. By the mid-1970s there were said to be about 1.8 million barefoot doctors providing health services.[3] Diversity in training and commitment makes generalization difficult, but they had a profound impact largely because in the villages most health needs required only simple and inexpensive interventions. Barefoot doctors were effective mainly because they were accessible.

The massive expansion of health care provided by the barefoot doctors was possible only because there was a simple social mechanism to pay for them. When communes, production brigades and production teams were established in the late 1950s, everyone's pay was based on work points, not money. Local units became responsible for their own health care, and health workers earned work points along with agricultural and other community activities.

## B.   Health Cooperatives

The evolution of rural health services in China following liberation created a three-tiered regionalized health service in most counties.[9] The basic units of these services were the health cooperatives which in 1980 financed care in 85 to 90 percent of production brigades (natural villages).[9,10] Most people relied for their primary health care on brigade level health cooperatives which were controlled and financed locally.[10,11] Above brigade level the commune health centers or small hospitals provided both referral care and supervision of preventive services. County hospitals, MCH centers, epidemic prevention stations and other county offices formed the third tier.[11] Staffing and financing of services at county and commune levels were the responsibility of county and commune governments. Moderate fees charged at these levels were normally paid by the local health cooperatives or the place of work.[12]

Brigade level health services generally were staffed by two to three barefoot doctors working out of a health station and serving a population of around 1,500. These barefoot doctors, with about three months initial training and periodic in-service training, provided basic curative care, MCH, family planning, sanitation and other preventive services. They were assisted by volunteer health aides attached to every 10 or more families. Barefoot doctors' part-time health activities were reimbursed through the brigade work point system. Funds for supplies and referral care at higher levels came from general brigade income and a small annnual contribution (premium) per person in the cooperative. In less wealthy cooperatives individuals usually paid for part of the referral costs out of their own pockets.[13]

An important concept in the cooperative health system was community control.[14] Mass organizations, such as for women and youth, were linked to the health services locally, the former usually taking the lead in MCH and family planning services. Leading groups were formed under the mass patriotic health campaigns to get people involved in preventive health activities, such as sanitation and infectious disease control. The direct control of the delivery of services was in the hands of a brigade medical care leading group who supervised the barefoot doctors in administrative matters. Technical supervision was provided by commune level health staff. Through training and frequent visits to the brigade, they maintained the focus on preventive programs.

The system functioned rather well in providing basic services throughout rural China. In spite of efforts to promote equity, however, the fact that local communities had to finance their own care, led to wide variation in the quantity and quality of care and its use.[15] Generally, preventive services were well supervised and implemented, but the quality of curative care depended heavily on the capacity of local barefoot doctors.[16] Improvement in capability was occurring, however, through a continuing effort to upgrade barefoot doctors by repeated short courses. In recent years, general economic and social changes have dramatically reduced the number of cooperative health systems.[9,10,17,18]

## IV.  MODERNIZATION AND QUALITATIVE IMPROVEMENT IN THE 1980s: FINANCING OF HEALTH CARE

The four modernizations (science and technology, agriculture, industry, and defence) have become the dominant theme in China's development plans for the 1980s. New economic polices are supported by wide public acceptance but they are producing an unforeseen shift in patterns of health care:

1.   The economic responsibility system returned most decision-making to individual families. Under contract with local authorities, each family was assigned land according to the number of available workers. They contract to sell to the State a fixed amount of produce from this land. Excess production can be sold in the free market. Agricultural production and rural family income have almost doubled in the last five years and the extra money is going mainly into consumer goods. Even though families have benefited financially, many social services which were previously communally-organized, are having to be reorganized to accommodate the new situation. Because of the success of the economic responsibility system in increasing agricultural production, incentive systems or private enterprise are now being encouraged in other production sectors and through sideline activities. In social services, however, development

and control still tend to be the responsibility of social groups, not individual families. Payment for health care depends on decisions of production units, which must take into account a growing diversity in the ability to pay as well as availability of services.

2.  To improve the quality of services, the term "barefoot doctor" which carried a denigrating tone was phased out. The new term "rural doctor" was applied to those who could pass standard qualifying examinations that led to formal certification as a mid-level practitioner.

3.  The one-child family program was started in 1979 to reduce the demographic ripple effect from the baby boom generation born in the 1950s and 1960s and will be maintained only for the next two decades. It is nevertheless, having a dramatic incidental impact on attitudes toward child care which may have long sequellae. People say that if they can have only one child, it must be a "perfect-child." Both parents and government agencies are devoting even greater attention to child care than before. This has led to greater awareness of the importance of effective maternal and child health services and new social patterns including more participation of fathers in child care.

4.  The "open-door policy" has increased international exchange. The basic principle of development through self-reliance has been modified to include the importation of technology from other countries as essential in the modernization drive. Hospitals, laboratories and all health facilities are being upgraded and improvement in the quality of health care is taking priority over further quantitative expansion.

The new economic responsibility system is having many repercussions on health conditions. With only about 2 percent of China's rural communes currently preserving collective farming, the cooperative health system has generally disappeared, except from educationally and economically-advanced areas where people have agreed to regular payments of premiums.[9,18,19] The underlying reason is the loss of cooperative mechanisms for paying rural doctors from brigade funds. Profits now flow to families through contracts and free markets. Equally important was the fact that rural doctors' salaries quickly fell behind the rapidly increasing incomes in most production sectors. Many barefoot doctors decided to revert to full-time agricultural and sideline work. A logical extension of the general pattern then was to permit rural doctors to shift to the responsibility system themselves which has meant charging fees for their services. Another increasing trend has been the by-passing of village level health care by villagers who prefer to use their increased income to pay for higher level services at township or county facilities.

In spite of the rapidity with which these changes appeared in the early 1980s, most rural communities were able to evolve mechanisms to provide and finance curative services. Fee-for-service care is now most common, with the rural doctors earning all or most of their income as private practitioners under the control of the local governing committees. Their income is often above the average for the area, and sometimes equals that of party cadres and officials.

Another mechanism has been to establish independent health provider groups who organize themselves in group practices. Fees collected by the group are used to pay the salaries of the doctors and staff working in the group. Some such groups have developed income generating activities such as growing and selling medicinal herbs to finance local services. Direct cash subsidies from higher government levels for poor communities in remote and minority areas is an important means of promoting equity.[9]

The decline of the health cooperatives had its greatest impact on preventive services. Some services, such as deliveries, quickly and successfully shifted to the fee system. Some immunization programs began to charge 10 fen (US $0.03) per immunization, but this has worked only in the communities where health education has produced demand. Other services, such as routine health monitoring of infants and children, have thus far had limited success in generating payments for rural health workers or evolving effective financing systems. In some areas, these services depend on a stipend or monthly payment from local government to rural doctors to assure implementation. Poorer areas have had to rely on the volunteer time of rural doctors as part of their being permitted to do private practice. The implementation of child health activities seem to have slowed down in recent years in less economically-advanced and remote areas, in spite of the genuine overall concern and policy statements which emphasize the importance of child health care. Since health care policy is highly decentralized, local financing arrangements vary greatly as each commune seeks to guarantee essential curative services and maintain preventive health programs.

## A.   Increasing Professionalism

Following the severe disruption of all organized activities during the Cultural Revolution when professionalism was condemned, the health professions have again reestablished their role in leading the drive towards modernization. Academic performance and admission standards have been reinstituted as criteria for selection for training. Curricula have been strengthened, training programs lengthened and graduate degree programs started again. The patterns of professionalization and specialization are similar to other countries.[3]

Rural primary health care depends on rural doctors who are upgraded barefoot doctors who have had special training and passed licensing exams. Those who do not qualify move to other activities or continue as part-time aides.[3] The training is to raise their competence to that of middle level doctors who are trained in county vocational schools and who staff township level health centers and hospitals.[9] The types of retraining include 6 to 12 months full-time courses in county vocational health schools or up to two years in part-time courses given through television lectures and examinations.[19] Innovative ways of supervising, monitoring and improving the performance of the new rural doctors are being introduced.[19]

These efforts to professionalize and upgrade rural doctors are also leading to more specialization and a greater emphasis on curative services. Both training and certification tend to focus on clinical knowledge and skills. Once certified, rural doctors get recognition and remuneration in their communities because of their curative work. Those who do not pass certifying exams frequently are not allowed to treat ill patients, and if they continue as health workers may be assigned only to preventive service.[19] In trying to balance priorities between curative and preventive activities, the main considerations are economic.

Since liberation, upgrading of maternal and child health (MCH) services throughout China has had high priority, especially since the start of the one child family program in 1979. China's accomplishments in reducing infant, child and maternal mortality are outstanding. Infant mortality has fallen from over 200 per 1,000 live births in 1949 to a reported nationwide average between 30 and 40 at present. Economically-advanced areas such as Shanghai report rates around 10 per 1,000,[20] but some remote areas still have rates over 100. MCH services need to be improved both in the quality of child development in areas that already have low mortality and quantitatively in extending essential child survival services to remote and needy populations.

The various components of MCH service have developed unevenly. Maternal care, particularly improved delivery services, has progressed more rapidly than routine child care. Some antenatal and postnatal visits are available to pregnant women in most parts of the country. Routine growth monitoring of children has, however, been introduced only in pilot projects.

MCH services in rural areas follow the three-tier structure of health services. MCH centers and county hospitals provide management, supervision and clinical referral services.[21,22] Township clinical facilities are supplemented by one or two full-time staff for MCH preventive activities spending up to two-thirds of their time supervising and assisting village MCH workers. At village level, both curative and preventive services are provided by rural doctors and village midwives. Although there is frequently a sharing of responsibility, often one or more doctors assume the main curative role while another, usually a female rural doctor or midwife, provides most of the maternal care. Preventive services for children such as EPI, may also be assumed by one village doctor.

One approach to implementing MCH services that seems promising is to develop special training for comprehensive MCH workers who can devote their total time to providing the full range of MCH services. This is working best where financial conditions and local awareness are sufficiently favorable so that these workers are paid good salaries from community funds. The problem is that, in less advanced areas where the needs are greatest, these MCH workers must do agricultural or other nonhealth work and charge for deliveries and curative care in order to support themselves. They will have little time for the preventive aspects of MCH work unless new financing mechanisms are developed.

## B.   Expanded Program for Immunization

Since 1949, China has stressed immunization against common infectious diseases. Following the principle of self-reliance in vaccine production, seven institutes were set up in different parts of the country. By 1985, production had reached a total of 480 million doses of vaccines for the expanded program of immunization (EPI) which included children up to 12 years of age. The quantity of vaccines seems to have kept pace with increasing demands, but the quality does not meet WHO standards. The institutes have out-dated buildings and equipment and inadequate cold storage facilities. Production is concentrated in favorable seasons when ambient temperatures do not cause inactivation of temperature-sensitive vaccines.

Organization of the world's largest national immunization effort makes use of all health facilities. County and township epidemic prevention stations serve the villages while hospitals, health centers, and antiepidemic stations provide coverage for the populations of towns and cities. Most of the immunizations are, however, done by the rural doctors who serve 80 percent of the people in villages. Due to lack of refrigeration, the vaccines have in the past been distributed in a rush-relay system going from the vaccine institute to end-use in three days. The rural doctor picked up vaccine by bicycle at the township or county center and rushed back to his village where he had arranged for the children to be waiting.

Even though vaccine production and immunization services have lacked modern technological methods, they have continuously produced noteworthy results in disease reduction. The reported incidences of notifiable EPI diseases was reduced from 1978 to 1984 per 100,000 population as follows: diphtheria 2.1 to 0.3; whooping cough 62 to 22; measles 114 to 62; and polio 1.0 to 0.1. As in many reporting systems, however, many more cases probably occurred that were not reported but the comparisons are valid because reporting has been improving. In China, relatively complete immunization records have been kept at the point of vaccination, but there has been little analysis and referral of information higher in the health system. The limited data on immunization coverage rates in 18 provinces in 1984 varied for BCG from 15 percent in Shanxi Province to 98 percent in Liaoning Province; for oral polio from 54 percent in Zhejiang Province to 96 percent in Shanghai Muncipality; for DPT from 17 percent in Gansu Province to 92 percent in Beijing Municipality; for measles from 53 percent in Guangdong Province to 94 percent in Beijing Municipality.

In 1985, the Government made the commitment to fully immunize 85 percent of children under one year of age in every province by 1988 and 85 percent in every county by 1990. These ambitious goals require reaching the most remote parts of the country and this means that more systematic approaches than the rush-relay system once or twice a year will be needed. To modernize immunization services for long-term sustainability, it was decided to:

1.  Provide national coverage with cold chain equipment to keep vaccines at appropriate temperatures from production through the various levels of distribution to use in the village.
2.  Introduce technological and managerial improvements in vaccine production to attain acceptable quality.
3.  Integrate MCH and epidemic prevention services to provide for eventual sustainability at the township and village levels as part of regular MCH services.
4.  Achieve social mobilization for childhood immunization and stimulate a high level of awareness among the population of the need for protecting children against the main childhood diseases. Innovative approaches will be particularly needed to increase acceptance among minority nationalities in the more remote regions.

In accordance with the general policy of decentralization, the provincial epidemic prevention stations will continue to be responsible for immunization services. Improved surveillance and monitoring of implementation are urgently needed to provide scientific evidence of local problems requiring corrective action as well as to document progress towards achieving the provincial and county goals. A computerized information system will permit nationwide consolidation of data. The financing of local immunization services will continue to be the responsibility of each level and unit of government, following the principle of self-reliance. The long-term challenge will be to maintain interest in and demand for routine child immunization in the face of increasing autonomy of families in choosing health services, the relatively low pay that rural doctors get for immunization services, and the decreasing incidence of the immunizable diseases.

## V.  LESSONS TO BE LEARNED FROM THE CHINESE EXPERIENCE

1.  Most impressive has been the flexible application of a learning process that admits mistakes and sanctions major changes. Even though the numerous abrupt changes have produced understandable public uncertainty at times, in general there is great awareness among the people that health status and the

quality of life have improved greatly. The mass campaigns mobilized the whole country and promoted self-reliance. The sending of massive numbers of doctors to the countryside refocused health care on rural areas. The emerging modern and professionalized health care system is geared to present patterns of family decision making even though this means that preventive measures now have to be based on health education rather than merely requiring people to follow mass directives.

2.    The health system in rural areas has consistently been based on unification of preventive and curative health services.

3.    The penetration of the rural health infrastructure guarantees convenient access to preventive and curative services by most of the people. This availability has been supplemented by mass publicity to create health awareness in the population. While the principle of self-reliance is applied to each level of the infrastructure, the flow between levels, both of case referral upwards and training and supervision downwards, has lent dynamism to the delivery of relevant and practical health services in rural areas. Flexible decision making has adapted higher policy directives to local needs.

4.    With the drive toward modernization, the quality of health care services in China will improve. The approximate doubling of family income means that people have more money to spend on health care; this, however, goes mainly into clinical services. MCH, nevertheless, is receiving renewed emphasis because people want the best possible care for their one child. On the other hand, the trend towards clinical specialization may well increase wage differentials and further contribute to greater emphasis on treatment rather than prevention.[3] With the responsibility system, the fee-for-service privatization of health care delivery by rural doctors increases the potential for separation of preventive and curative services and greater differences between care provided in rich and poor areas. The Government is aware of the risks in present trends. Even with growing economic differences, it will be important to maintain minimum acceptable standards of quality of life and health. For infant mortality (now about 40 per 1,000 live births) and life expectancy (about 68 years—1981) to improve further it will be necessary to concentrate efforts on poor and remote areas.

5.    Greater decentralization in recent years has created considerable provincial autonomy. National health planning has developed health policy and calculated aggregate provincial requirements. Differences in provincial health care systems seem to be emerging because of varying local conditions and needs. A major question is what should national health care funds subsidize what should be the balance between funding a minimal network of services in needy rural areas and the high quality urban centers for the most sophisticated referral care which are receiving increasing attention? As services increasingly respond to market demands for services, special attention will need to be given to maintaining health care for the poor.

6.  Financing of health care is becoming a major issue in current health care discussions in China, as in most countries of the world, because of rapidly increasing costs. As the new responsibility system has evolved, local communities struggle to find the most appropriate mechanisms to pay their staff, and simultaneously cope with rapidly escalating charges from township and county referral and hospital services. These institutions which previously had been heavily subsidized by their own levels of government have been given the "responsibility" to begin to recoup their costs through direct charges. Particularly important for public health is the issue that community-wide efforts in infectious disease control which effectively relied in the past on mass participation now must spend much more effort to convince individuals to take time from their own production activities to participate. To meet these challenges, multiple systems of fees, subsidies, salaries, incentives, etc., are currently being tried out across China.[9,10]

There is a particular need, therefore, for economic research on these diverse local experiments in financing. In many local units the same mistakes may be repeated and successes may go unnoticed. More importantly, the reasons for success or failure are often not explored. Straightforward analysis of the mulitiple local trials would accelerate finding appropriate solutions. Government has the responsibility to guarantee minimally-acceptable levels of health care and preventive services, especially for mothers and children. Services will probably continue to be based on integrated county health care because the county is the smallest government unit that can obtain revenues from taxation. The three-level health care system is already in place in most counties. Each county is establishing its own financing system, whether through taxation, health insurance, or other methods.

7.  Chinese health care is highly labor intensive, as indicated by the estimated one health worker to 160 population in rural areas. The situation in remote and poor areas is different since health workers are fewer and they have been less well paid. With the changed economic base of the responsibility system, staffing patterns in the health care system of China are rapidly changing. Rural, remote and poor areas may lose their health personnel more rapidly than more affluent areas. The challenge is to ensure that, as services become less labor intensive, they should become more efficient.

The changing patterns of health care suggest the need for scientific analysis of health manpower requirements both in numbers and type of function. A relevant methodology is functional analysis to help match needs to resources through more pragmatic role definitions and more relevant training. The five million health personnel in China have already shown great social responsibility and commitment, but this should be matched by increasing their effectiveness and efficiency, especially in delivering preventive services.

8.  Health education has been a dominant theme in the three decades since liberation. National policy was based on the conviction that ordinary people

could solve their health problems once they understood their nature and possible solutions.[23] Health awareness penetrated deeply through lectures, film shows, posters, blackboard signs and radio-talks. Group discussions, often using traditional Chinese sayings, internalized strong group consensus. Social mobilization and self-reliance went hand-in-hand. Collectively organized economic production units ensured people's participation in the management of local health services, through local revolutionary committees.[24] With the shift from collectives to household decision making under the responsibility system, previous channels of communication have become less tightly organized.[17] New methods of health education are being developed using mass media. High levels of literacy and the increasing availability of TV and radio provide new opportunities for informing the public. The mass organizations can continue to provide the organizing framework for health education activities. The health system will have to provide technical support and educational content.

9.   The current transition in health care will be greatly assisted by the systematic application of scientific management. In the past, policies were determined pragmatically and empirically. Now, with scientific modernization decision makers can use methods such as systems analysis and operations research and international experience in rationalizing planning. With decentralization the many local adaptations will enable China to compare, within its own borders, the relative advantages of different approaches, through well-designed epidemiological and evaluative research.[10] China may have the potential to rapidly develop its capacities for health systems research focusing on major questions concerning the organization, delivery and financing of health services.

10.   A health development network has been evolved in the maternal and child health model county project.[25] Starting in 1982, in cooperation between the Government and UNICEF, this project now includes 30 counties scattered over 17 provinces, with a total population of about 20 million. A medical college or a children's hospital has assumed responsibility to work with one to three model counties. The first emphasis was to strengthen services by careful planning and priority setting. A practical information system has been developed which includes: baseline and periodic surveys to identify priority problems; vital statistics; and surveillance for child growth and development and high risk pregnancy. A second major emphasis is to expand and strengthen training at all levels in each county. Workshops, training courses, and fellowships develop skills and expertise. Major changes are being implemented in the county health schools, which train most of the local personnel, because of their great need to shift from mostly didactic lectures to problem-solving and learning-by-doing methods. A third major emphasis is applied research which focuses on six priority diseases: pneumonia which is the greatest cause of death in children; diarrhea which causes much morbidity; perinatal mortality

associated with high risk pregnancies; anemia which is especially prevalent in rural Chinese children; rickets which still occurs throughout China but particularly in the North; and inadequate growth especially among children in rural areas and in the South. The latter may be due to the use of rice porridge as the main weaning food. In addition, a new range of research topics is being explored such as management issues, functional reallocation of workers' roles, and financing of rural doctors.

In summary, the Chinese experience shows the great value of concentrating first on rapid quantitive expansion of coverage with simple services and then moving on to improving quality. This sequence in China has taken three decades. Quantitative coverage was necessary to fulfill the egalitarian promises of the revolution. The commitment to equity to reach those in greatest need must now continue as the emphasis shifts to improving the quality of care.

## NOTES AND REFERENCES

1.   Unschuld, P.U. *Medical Ethics in Imperial China.* Berkeley: University of California Press, 1979.
2.   Chen, P.S.Y. *IIRR Founder Returns to China to Survey Rural Progress.* IIRR Report, Winter, 1986. International Institute of Rural Reconstruction, New York.
3.   Sidel, R., and V.W. Sidel. *The Health of China: Current Conflicts in Medical and Human Services for One Billion People.* Boston: Beacon Press, 1982.
4.   WHO. *Organization and Functioning of Health Services in China.* Geneva: World Health Organization.
5.   *Health Statistics.* People's Republic of China, 1984.
6.   Gong, Y.L., and L.M. Chao. "The Role of Barefoot Doctors."*American Journal of Public Health,* 1982, 72(Suppl):59-61.
7.   Seipp, C. (ed.). "Health Care for the Community: Selected Papers of Dr. John B. Grant." *The American Journal of Hygiene,* Monographic Series No. 21. Baltimore: The Johns Hopkins Press, 1963.
8.   Taylor, C.E., and Z.Y. Xu. "Oral Rehydration in China." *American Journal of Public Health,* 1986, 76:187-189.
9.   Chen, P.C., and C.H. Tuan. "Primary Health Care in Rural China: Post-1978 Development." *Soc. Sci. Med.,* 1983, 17:1411-1417.
10.   Jamison, D.T., J.R. Evans, T. King, et al. *China, the Health Sector-A World Bank Country Study.* Washington: The World Bank, 1984 pp. 94-104.
11.   Ye, X.F., D.Y. Hugan, A.R. Hinman, and R.L. Parker. "Introduction to Shanghai County." *Am. J. Public Health,* 1982, 72(Suppl):13-18.
12.   Hinman, A.R., and R.L. Parker. "Costs of Care." *Am. J. Public Health,* 1982, 72(Suppl):83-88.
13.   Chao, L.M., Y.L. Gong, and S.J. Gu. "Financing the Cooperative Medical System." *Am. J. Public Health,* 1982, 72(Suppl):78-80.
14.   *People's Involvement in and Management of Health Care.* (Report of Team No. 2.) Inter-Regional Seminar on Primary Health Care, Yexian County, Shandong Province, People's Republic of China, 13-26 June 1982. World Health Organization.

15.  Parker, R.L., and A.R. Hinman. "Use of Health Services," *Am. J. Public Health,* 1982, 72(Suppl):71-77.

16.  Hsu, R.C. "The Barefoot Doctors of the People's Republic of China—Some Problems." *N. Engl. J. Med.,* 1974, 291:124-127.

17.  Hsiao, W.C. "Transformation of Health Care in China." *N. Engl. J. Med.,* 1984, 310:932-936.

18.  Young, M.E.M. *A Study of Barefoot Doctors' Activities in China.* Doctoral Thesis, The Johns Hopkins University, School of Hygiene and Public Health, Baltimore, 1984.

19.  Koplan, J.P., A.R. Hinman, R.L. Parker, Y.L. Gong, and M.D. Yang. "The Barefoot Doctors: Shanghai County Revisited." *Am. J. Public Health,* 1985, 75:768-770.

20.  Gu, X.Y., and M.L. Chen. "Vital Statistics." *Am. J. Public Health,* 1982, 72(Suppl):19-23.

21.  Hu, X.J., S.Y. Zhu, and S.E. Xu. "Child Health Care." *Am. J. Public Health,* 1982, 72(Suppl):36-38.

22.  Hu, X.J., and B.J. Zhang. "Women's Health Care." *Am. J. Public Health,* 1982, 72 (suppl):33-35.

23.  Horn, J.S. *Away with All Pests: An English Surgeon in People's China, 1954-1969.* MR, New York, 1969.

24.  WHO. *Primary Health Care-The Chinese Experience. Report on an Inter-regional Seminar.* Geneva: World Health Organization, 1983.

25.  *MCH Model Counties (GR/84/001/001), Project Plan of Action, 1985-1989.* Government of the People's Republic of China and the United Nations Children's Fund (UNICEF), 1986.

# MORBIDITY COSTS:
## NATIONAL ESTIMATES AND
## ECONOMIC DETERMINANTS

David S. Salkever

## I.  INTRODUCTION

With the growing prominence of economic concerns in health policy discussions, increasing attention has been paid to the economic costs of illness. Cost-of-illness (COI) estimates are seen as potentially valuable guides to policy formulation.[1] Expert assessments of policies for confronting major health problems now routinely include consideration of illness costs.[2]

As COI estimates have gained wider significance, concerns about methods used to develop these estimates have also grown. In the absence of consensus as to methods, advocates of programs targeted at specific diseases may be tempted to devise methods that produce the largest COI estimates for the disease in which they are interested, and thereby buttress their claims for its significance. In addition, it has been noted that differences in methods among

**Research in Human Capital Development, Vol. 5, pages 237-288.**
**Copyright © 1988 by JAI Press Inc.**
**ISBN: 0-89232-508-9**

studies have produced large differences in cost estimates for the same health problems. To promote a standardization of methods, and thereby enhance the utility of COI studies for priority setting, a U.S. Public Health Service task force recently promulgated a set of methodological guidelines.[3]

It is to be expected, however, that further changes and refinements in methods will continue to occur. Major new approaches, such as the incidence or lifetime-costing method, have only recently appeared in the literature.[4] Important conceptual and practical issues, relating to such matters as the valuation of nonmarket work, and the use of consumer valuations (i.e., willingness-to-pay values) for reduced health risks, are still items of debate in the literature.[5]

Recent research has also raised substantive questions about the determinants of illness costs. The judicious interpretation and use of illness cost estimates requires some understanding of the factors that determine the magnitude of these costs. Evidence from many studies suggests that social and economic forces have an important influence on the incidence and prevalence of health problems. More recent research, however, indicates that economic factors also play a critical role in determining the indirect morbidity costs of these problems. In particular, these studies imply that the effects of health problems on individual labor supply and on the severity of self-reported work limitations due to poor health are strongly related to economic factors; thus, these factors become major determinants in the magnitude of indirect morbidity costs of illness.

The research presented in this paper addresses both methodological and substantive concerns relating to morbidity costs for noninstitutionalized adult working-age males. A substantial portion of this paper (Sections III-VI) provides new national cost estimates based on several alternative computational procedures. The methods used to develop these estimates differ from previous studies in several respects: (1) a more detailed classification of health problems was employed; (2) estimates of debility costs (one component of morbidity costs) are more complete; (3) information on education, residence, industry and occupation are incorporated into the estimation process; and (4) the impact on estimated costs of controlling for education, industry, and occupational characteristics is examined.

Section VII of the paper is a descriptive analysis of trends in disability and labor force participation for older working-age males. It addresses several substantive issues raised by recent empirical research including the hypothesis that the decline in male labor force participation *and* the increase in reported disability are both largely explained by more liberal disability benefit programs and other economic factors. Conclusions are summarized in Section VIII.

## II.  AN OVERVIEW OF PREVIOUS RESEARCH ON EARNINGS AND PRODUCTIVITY LOSSES DUE TO MORBIDITY

### A.  Introductory Comments

It is standard practice in COI studies to define and estimate three different components of illness costs: (1) "direct costs" of the resources used to treat an illness or ameliorate its consequences, (2) indirect costs due to premature mortality, and (3) indirect costs due to morbidity. The latter two components are intended to measure the lost productivity of illness victims due to premature deaths or morbidity. All empirical estimates of these productivity losses are based on earnings data; thus, they incorporate the assumption that earnings levels are equal to the value of workers' productivity, as would be true in a competitive economic system. These estimates also assume that observed prevailing wage levels are not affected by the incidence of health problems; thus, they ignore macroeconomic effects of illnesses that might change relative prices (of labor and other goods) in the economy.

As a framework for describing the COI component on which we shall focus, earnings and productivity losses due to morbidity, it is useful to divide these losses into two components: short-term and long-term losses. Short-term losses are the result of acute illness episodes or acute episodes of chronic illnesses. They may occur as temporary disruptions of individuals "normal" working schedules if time off from work is taken; alternatively, they may take the form of temporary declines from "normal" productivity while individuals are on the job but suffering from an acute illness episode. Thus, losses due to work-loss days (i.e., when one or more entire days of work are missed due to illness) are presumably a major component but not the entirety of these short-term losses.

Long-term losses are the result of chronic health problems. (Of course, these may result from acute illnesses; for example, permanent hearing loss can result from acute infections.) In any given time period, these losses are the difference between actual earnings of individuals with chronic problems and the amount these persons would have earned if they did not have chronic health problems. An expression for these losses is

$$N(p^H t^H w^H - p^I t^I w^I), \qquad (1)$$

where N is the number of persons with chronic health problems, the superscripts H and I (respectively) denote quantities that would have been observed if these persons had been healthy and actual observed quantities, p is the employment rate (i.e., fraction of persons working), t is "normal" scheduled work time, and w is earnings per unit of time. Formula (1) may be expanded to

$$N (p^H t^H w^H - p^I t^H w^H + p^I t^H w^H - p^I t^I w^I) =$$

$$(Np^H - Np^I) t^H w^H + Np^I (t^H w^H - t^I w^I). \qquad (2)$$

Note that $(Np^H - Np^I)$ equals the number of people who did not work at all because of a chronic health problem while $(t^H w^H - t^I w^I)$ equals the impact on average earnings of chronic health prolems for those who have such problems and still work. Thus, the right-hand side of Eq. 2 splits long-term earnings losses into two portions, (1) losses for people who do not work at all because of chronic health problems, and (2) losses in the form of lower average earnings for those with chronic health problems who do work. The latter portion is what is often referred to as "debility costs." These can be further decomposed as follows:

$$Np^I (t^H w^H - t^I w^I) = Np^I (t^H w^H - t^I w^H) + Np^I (t^I w^H - t^I w^I). \qquad (3)$$

Equation 3 breaks debility costs into two terms; the first right-hand side term is the earnings loss of shorter working hours (or fewer working days within the time interval), while the second term is the loss due to lower wages per unit of time. Conceptually, both of these terms are based on "normal" working hours and wages and do not include reductions in hours or earnings due to acute health problems.

In practice, estimates of these debility cost components (or of total debility costs) may in fact include some costs of acute problems. These estimates of debility costs are generally calculated as the difference between actual earnings of persons with chronic health problems $(t^I w^I)$ and the earnings of persons with similar characteristics but no chronic health problems $(t^H w^H)$. Both of these earnings figures may include short-term earnings losses due to acute illnesses if individuals are not fully covered by sick-leave provisions. In other words, empirical earnings measures will be $(t^I w^I - s^I)$ and $(t^H w^H - s^H)$ where $s^I$ and $s^H$ are the short-term earnings losses not covered by sick leave. If $s^I$ and $s^H$, then

$$t^H w^H - t^I w^I = (t^H w^H - s^H) - (t^I w^I - s^I) \qquad (4)$$

and using the right-hand side of Eq. 4 as the estimate of debility costs involves no double-counting. If $s^I > s^H$, however, the expression on the right-hand side of Eq. 4 exceeds $t^H w^H - t^I w^I$ by the amount $(s^I - s^H)$. This differential in short-term earnings losses (not covered by sick leave) will then be counted twice in *overall* morbidity cost estimates because it will also be included in short-term losses.[6]

## B.   Morbidity Cost Estimates from Comprehensive COI Studies

Empirical estimates of morbidity costs have been presented in comprehensive studies (that include all types of health problems and develop estimates for total morbidity costs) and in studies that focus on only one or several specific types of health problems. Among the first group of studies, the 1966 work by Rice has clearly been the most significant and influential.[7] Estimates of illness costs, including (1) direct costs, (2) mortality costs, (3) morbidity costs of institutionalized persons, and (4) morbidity costs for noninstitutionalized persons were developed for 1963. Separate estimates were presented for 19 illness categories defined on the basis of ICDA codes.[8] The fourth component, which is also the focus of our own study, included cost of work-loss days and losses for people unable to work or keep house. Debility costs, however, were not included in the estimates.

Costs of work-loss days were estimated from reported numbers of such days in the National Health Survey (the predecessor to the Health Interview Survey), and from Current Population Survey data on mean annual full-time earnings by age for males and estimated earnings by age figures for females. Annual earnings were converted to a daily basis by dividing them by 245. A further adjustment factor of 1.0776 was used to account for employer-paid fringe benefits.[9] Numbers of persons unable to work and unable to keep house were estimated from survey data reported by the Bureau of Labor Statistics and from the National Health Survey. After adjustment for labor force participation rates, annual earnings figures were used to estimate productivity losses for persons unable to work. The average earnings figure for domestic workers was used to value losses due to inability to keep house. In the present context, the results of principal interest in the Rice study relate to work-loss days of currently employed males and costs of earnings losses for noninstitutionalized males unable to work. These two figures are $7.2 billion and $4.8 billion in 1963 dollars respectively. About 44 percent of the work-loss day costs were accounted for by two diagnostic groups, diseases of the respiratory system and injuries. For persons unable to work, diseases of the circulatory system accounted for the largest share of morbidity costs (28.2 percent), with nervous system and sensory disorders, and mental disorders next in importance (accounting for 15.8 percent and 12.0 percent of costs respectively).

An update of this study by Cooper and Rice with 1972 data used a similar methodology.[10] While this study does not present detailed results for males separately, comparisons of the 1963 and 1972 cost estimates for both sexes are of some interest. These comparisons show that while 1963 work-loss day costs ($9.8 billion) were almost twice as large as losses due to inability to work of the noninstitutionalized population ($5.3 billion), by 1972 these two figures were nearly equal ($17.6 billion and $15.2 billion respectively). In terms of the relative importance of different disease categories, relatively little change was observed for work-loss day costs but in the costs of noninstitutionalized persons unable to work diseases of the circulatory system fell in importance (27.8 percent to 21.8 percent) while relative increases in cost percentages were observed for nervous system and sensory disorders (15.8 to 18.2 percent) and especially for musculoskeletal problems (9.2 to 18.8 percent). Furthermore,

more recent but less detailed results for 1975 reported by Berk et al.[11] show continued growth in the economic impact of musculoskeletal disorders; these problems accounted for 12.7 percent of total estimated morbidity costs (including both institutionalized and noninstitutionalized persons), up from the 12.1 percent in 1972 reported by Cooper and Rice.

An even more recent set of estimates for 1977 is presented by Hodgson.[5] He reports total costs, direct costs, and indirect costs for both sexes, and for males and females separately for the following broad problem categories: all neoplasms (and malignant neoplasms), heart disease, stroke, accidents, and all other problems. Following the approach of previous investigators, Hodgson presents estimates of three components of morbidity costs for the noninstitutionalilzed population: earnings losses of persons unable to work ($23 billion), work-loss day costs ($25.6 billion), and losses for women unable to keep house ($6.3 billion).

## C.  Empirical Evidence on Debility Costs

While the studies cited so far excluded debility costs from consideration, many other authors who have examined the impact of chronic health problems on earnings and labor supply have provided empirical evidence relating to these costs. For example, Luft's[12] work with the 1967 Survey of Economic Opportunity provides estimates of the two components of long-term morbidity costs shown in Eq. 2, that is, losses due to reductions in the number of people working and debility costs. Debility cost estimates are further decomposed, as in Eq. 3, into losses due to fewer weeks worked per year and due to lower earnings per week. Disability impacts on hourly wages and hours worked per week were also examined for wage and salary recipients. Note that Luft's estimate of the reduction in the number of people working is based on the coefficients for disability variables included in his labor force participation regressions; this differs from Rice's reliance on survey estimates of the numbers of persons reporting themselves unable to work which are then adjusted for labor force participation rates of the general population.

Luft did not analyze specific diagnostic or problem groups; his only reported estimates are for all disabilities combined. For noninstitutionalized males aged 18 to 64, his estimated earnings losses for 1966 due to reduction in the number of people working at all were $7.0 billion for whites and $0.9 billion for blacks. The sum of these figures is considerably larger than the $4.8 billion estimates by Rice for 1963.[13] The corresponding estimates of debility costs from Luft's study are $7.1 billion for whites and $0.6 billion for blacks; thus, debility costs are estimated to be roughly equal to the costs due to reduced numbers of people working at all. Moreover, Luft estimated that the two components of debility costs reflecting lower earnings per week and fewer weeks worked per year were about equal in magnitude.

In another recent study which applied a similar method of analysis to data on males aged 14-64 from the 1970 census public use samples, Fechter[14] found that disability caused a .31 reduction in the probability of working, but only a 17 percent reduction in the earnings of those who worked. This suggests that debility costs are sizable but somewhat smaller than earnings losses due to people not working at all. Analysis of the 1976 Survey of Income and Education (SIE) data by McNeil et al.[15] yielded an estimated reduction due to disability in the probability of working for males of 0.261 and a corresponding reduction in earnings for those who worked of about 35 percent.

Another recent study, by Mushkin and Landefeld,[16] also addressed the subject of debility costs but defined the term in a rather different way. Three categories of debility were identified: (1) temporary acute sickness which does not result in days lost from work, (2) temporary productivity declines of persons returning to work following a major illness, and (3) productivity losses of persons with "static disabilities or stabilized chronic conditions." Only item 3 corresponds to the definition of debility cost used in the present study. Items 1 and 2 correspond to our definition of short-term losses that do not result in work-loss days or time off from work.

In estimating the cost associated with item 3, the authors only considered reductions in earnings per hour, that is, $Np^I (t^I w^H — t^I w^I)$. It appears that they viewed earnings reductions due to less work time, $Np^I (t^H w^H — t^I w^I)$, as a component of work-loss days and did not consider the possibility that regular work schedules might be shorter because of chronic health problems. Furthermore, to compute their cost estimate they noted that Luft had found a reduction in earnings per hour due to disability of about 10 percent and they halved this to 5 percent.[17] This was then applied to an average annual earnings figure and a prevalence estimate of 4.4 million persons to yield a cost of $2.7 billion in 1975.[18] Because of presumed underreporting of mental illness in their data sources, the authors then added an additional $2.8 billion in debility costs of mental illness derived from a study of Conley et al.,[19] to arrive at a final total of $5.5 billion.

In contrast to this relatively small estimated cost for item 3, Mushkin and Landefeld estimated a cost figure nearly 10 times as great for the short-term losses included in their item 1. While this estimate was based on rather fragmentary data, it is interesting to note that it was about twice as large as their estimated cost of work-loss days. In other words, the costs of work-loss days were estimated to be less than one-third of the total short-term illness costs for persons at work.

Another group of empirical studies which supports the conclusion that debility costs are substantial is studies of disability impacts on labor supply.[20] While these studies do not estimate earnings impacts directly, they do generally find that disabled persons who work tend to work shorter hours and fewer weeks per year than nondisabled persons who work. Some researchers even suggest that these impacts are in fact much greater than disability impacts on earnings per hour, particularly for the severely disabled.[21]

## D.  Studies of Specific Health Problems

COI studies dealing with specific conditions or causes of health problems (e.g., smoking, motor vehicle accidents) are numerous and methodologically varied.[22] The general conceptual approach used by these studies is identical to that already described. The data sources often differ, however, with special surveys and longitudinal follow-up studies often drawn upon to compute morbidity costs. Even the most widely cited recent studies tend to rely on data about labor force status or inability to work in computing long-term morbidity costs, so that the debility component in these estimates tends to be minor or ignored altogether.[23] This largely reflects data limitations; information on hours of work and wages are often not available for reasonably large samples of individuals with a specific problem.

Some recent exceptions to this rule should be noted. Inman[24] has analyzed a recent survey of multiple sclerosis victims to determine direct and indirect costs. He finds that the negative impact on labor force participation is the most important morbidity cost component, but that negative impacts on wages per hour and hours worked for those who continue to work are significant.

The Commission for the Control of Epilepsy and Its Consequences[25] used information on average weekly earnings of epileptics in sheltered workshops and on occupational status of other employed epileptics to develop debility cost estimates (which they termed "underemployment costs"). In particular, they estimated that average weekly earnings for epileptics in regular employment were about 15 to 20 percent below the figure for the general work force while sheltered workshop earnings were only about one-eighth of the general work force level. Their debility cost estimate for 1975 ($517 million) was about exactly equal to their estimated earnings losses for noninstitutionalized epileptics who did not work at all.

One other problem category where the costs of reduced on-the-job productivity has received some attention is alcohol, drug abuse, and mental illness. A recent study by Cruze et al.[26] deals with this subject in considerable detail and reviews a number of previous studies. Several of the studies reviewed there focused on income or earnings differentials between problem drinkers and the general population, or between drug abusers and the general population. It is not clear from their description, however, whether the reported income or earnings differentials controlled for differences in employment rates. Cruze et al. also used prevalence data from the 1976 Survey of Income and Education (SIE) to estimate reduced productivity for the noninstitutionalized mentally ill, but their cost estimate involved an assumed 25 percent productivity differential rather than a differential computed from the earnings data actually reported in the SIE.

# III.  DATA AND METHODS USED IN THIS STUDY

The estimates developed in this study are for morbidity costs of noninstitutionalized males age 17 to 64 in the United States during 1974-1978. Three components of morbidity costs are estimated: earnings losses of persons unable to work, costs of work-loss days, and debility costs (i.e., earnings reductions, for people who work, caused by long-term health problems). Two sets of tasks were involved in the estimation process. First, numbers of persons unable to work, numbers of work-loss days, and number of working persons with long-term health problems had to be estimated in total and for specific problem categories. Second, earnings or productivity losses had to be estimated for each person unable to work, each work-loss day, and each working person with a long-term health problem, and aggregated to obtain total morbidity costs and costs for each problem category.

The data set employed for the first set of tasks was the Health Interview Survey (HIS) for the years 1974-1978. Individuals reporting themselves as unable to work because of a chronic health problem were identified on the HIS data tapes and the sum of their survey weights was used to obtain a national estimate of their numbers. These individuals were then arranged by the diagnostic code of the problem which was the primary cause of their inability to work and grouped into 61 problem categories based on these diagnostic codes. The process of grouping and the diagnostic codes included in each category are described in Appendix 1. Note that problems reported as a secondary cause of inability to work by persons with multiple problems were not considered in this grouping process.

Numbers of work-loss days were also reported by the HIS survey respondents and the survey weights were applied to obtain national estimates. The same 61 problem categories were used for grouping, although this resulted in a somewhat uneven distribution of work-loss days across groups. This occurred because acute conditions are the major causes of work-loss days but rarely are reported as long-term problems that prevent people from working. Moreover, diagnostic codes are generally not reported, on the HIS, for work-loss days due to chronic conditions which are not also reported by the respondent as causing some activity limitation. This amounted to about 20 percent of all work-loss days that could not be assigned to one of the 61 problem categories and were therefore treated as a residual group. Some adjustment was also required by the fact that several different conditions simultaneously caused an individual to miss work. Since there is no indication on the HIS data as to whether a condition is a primary or secondary cause of a work-loss day, a pro-rata adjustment was applied to avoid double-counting of days. This adjustment and other aspects of our methods for estimating numbers of work-loss days are described in Appendix 2.

All individuals who worked at all during the year and who suffer from long-term health problems should be included in an estimate of annual debility costs. Since the HIS data did not include information on work status for a 12-month recall period, a proxy indicator of whether or not someone worked at all in the past 12 months was used. More specifically, a respondent was presumed to have worked if he indicated that (1) working was his usual activity, (2) he had worked at all in the two weeks preceding the survey interview, or (3) he currently had a job. A test of this proxy was possible with the 1979 HIS data, which did include questions on weeks worked during the year; the test indicated that the proxy indicator was highly accurate, but probably resulted in a very slight underestimation of the number of people with long-term health problems who worked. A detailed discussion of this test of our estimation method is given in Appendix 3.

Estimation of dollar values of earnings or productivity losses required use of an additional data set, the 1976 Survey of Income and Education (SIE), since the HIS did not provide information on earnings or wage rates. For persons in the HIS reporting themselves as unable to work, these losses are equal to the income that we estimate they would have earned if they had not had a long-term health problem. This income figure was computed as the average earnings in 1975 by persons in the SIE data, without chronic health problems, classified by age group, education level, race, and region of residence. The specific computational procedures are described in Appendix 1. The productivity loss for each work-loss day reported in the HIS was based on a synthetic estimate of the respondent's hourly wage. This estimate was computed by inserting data on their personal characteristics into an hourly wage regression equation estimated with SIE data, and obtaining the predicted wage value based on the regression coefficients. Independent variables used in the regression pertained to age, education, race, presence or absence of a chronic health condition, region and urban or rural character of residence, industry where the person was employed, and average earnings for the occupation in which the person was employed. The procedures for obtaining the regression results, and the results themselves, are described in detail in Appendix 2.

For persons experiencing debility costs, the difference between the income that they could have earned if they had been free of health problems, and the income they actually earned is the earnings loss measure. Of course, neither of these income figures are on the HIS data, so synthetic regression estimates were again developed from the SIE data. The dependent variable in these regressions was annual earnings and the independent variables were similar to those used in the wage regression. Two regressions were estimated, one from data on persons reporting chronic health limitations and a second from data on persons without such limitations. A more detailed description of the regression methods and results is illustrated in Appendix 3.

Finally, alternative sets of earnings loss estimates for persons unable to work and for debility costs were developed; in these estimates variables such as education, occupation and industry were not used. Since these variables might themselves be affected by long-term health problems, their use in estimating earnings losses could understate the impacts of these problems. The use of our alternative set of estimates served to indicate the possible extent of understatement and, more generally, the sensitivity of our results to the inclusion or exclusion of these variables.

The general approach used in developing the alternative estimates was quite similar to that already described; more detail on the procedures is given in Section VI. Note also that an alternative hourly wage regression for valuing work-loss days was not estimated. Work-loss days represent short-term departures from regular working schedules due to acute illnesses or acute episodes of chronic problems; it is doubtful that the acute illnesses or episodes would have an impact on an individual's education, occupation, or industry, so the potential understatement alluded to above was not viewed as a serious problem in relation to work-loss days.

# IV.  FREQUENCY ESTIMATES

Table 1 presents selected results relating to our estimated annual average frequencies for the 1974-78 period. As indicated in the last line of this table, we estimate that in an average year among noninstitutionalized males age 17 to 64, 2.7 million persons were unable to work because of long-term health problems, 272 million work-loss days occurred, and 5.4 million persons who worked had long-term health problems that limited their activities. Note that the 2.7 million figure for men age 17-64 is well above the 1.8 million figure for all men in 1977 reported by Hodgson.[5] Presumably this difference arises from the use of two different data sources, the U.S. Labor Dept. data for Hodgson's estimates and the HIS for our own. On the other hand, Hodgson's estimate of work-loss days for males under age 65 (based on 1976 and 1977 HIS data and reported in a personal communication to the author) is extremely close to our own (264 million days per year).

Among the 61 problem categories, only 6 account for 100,000 or more persons unable to work: orthopedic impairments of the back and neck (Group 10), ill-defined heart trouble (Group 36), chronic ischemic heart disease (Group 30), emphysema (Group 45), nonspecific, nontraumatic arthritis (Group 56), and disc problems (Group 57). Groups 10 and 57 are also respectively first and third in importance as causes of limitations among persons who work (column 3 of Table 1). The two groups which are the most frequent reasons for inability to work (Groups 56 and 30) are also important causes of limitation among persons who worked.

*Table 1.*  Estimated Annual Frequencies (000's)

| Group No. | Problem Category | No. of Persons Unable to Work | No. of Work Loss Days | No. of Working Persons with Long-Term Health Problems |
|---|---|---|---|---|
| 1 | Blindness | 23.0 | 53.1 | 20.1 |
| 2 | Visual impairment, other | 17.3 | 246.0 | 134.2 |
| 3 | Other sensory impairment | 27.1 | 353.9 | 152.5 |
| 4 | Mental deficiency | 77.5 | 94.7 | 49.9 |
| 5 | Loss of more than 1 limb or digits | 31.7 | 515.5 | 89.5 |
| 6 | Loss of lung, kidney, bone, joint, muscle, extremity intact | 13.9 | 339.4 | 35.0 |
| 7 | Paralysis-upper or lower extremity, fingers or toes | 28.1 | 203.3 | 26.4 |
| 8 | Paralysis: para-, hemi-, quadriplegia | 28.8 | 76.2 | 13.9 |
| 9 | Cerebral palsy, partial paralysis, any site | 36.5 | 116.8 | 48.0 |
| 10 | Orthopedic impairment, neck, back/spine/vertebrae | 120.5 | 4043.9 | 521.1 |
| 11 | Orthopedic impairment, neck, arms/hands | 21.6 | 1317.7 | 147.7 |
| 12 | Orthopedic impariment, hip/pelvis w. any other site | 20.1 | 301.7 | 38.7 |
| 13 | Orthopedic impairment, knee, leg, ankle, foot | 73.2 | 2266.9 | 362.5 |
| 14 | Nonparalytic orthopedic impairment. Multiple sites (except as in Groups 10-13) ill-defined | 72.7 | 1875.6 | 146.9 |
| 15 | Deformity of limbs, trunk, back, NEC | 54.3 | 558.6 | 213.6 |
| 16 | Infective and parasitic diseases | 23.8 | 11119.1 | 33.8 |
| 17 | Neoplasms | 73.4 | 2044.1 | 69.9 |
| 18 | Endocrine, nutritional, metabolic and blood disorders | 26.6 | 1264.7 | 86.6 |
| 19 | Diabetes (mellitus) | 69.1 | 877.9 | 137.2 |
| 20 | Psychosis (schizophrenic) | 24.3 | 40.7 | 9.7 |
| 21 | Psychosis (nonschizophrenia) | 25.4 | 109.2 | 7.0 |
| 22 | Neurosis | 56.9 | 440.5 | 27.3 |
| 23 | Personality/other nonpsychotic disorders | 26.0 | 272.3 | 22.6 |
| 24 | Alcoholism and nonspecific nervous disorders | 91.4 | 1874.6 | 52.7 |
| 25 | Multiple sclerosis, paralysis agitans | 23.3 | 0 | 11.4 |
| 26 | Epilepsy | 47.9 | 91.2 | 49.3 |
| 27 | Other nervous system disorders | 47.1 | 1382.1 | 68.0 |
| 28 | Eye and ear diseases | 40.8 | 2200.0 | 128.2 |
| 29 | Chronic ischemic heart w. hypertension angina w. hypertension | 33.2 | 512.3 | 28.5 |

*Table 1.* (*continued*)

| Group No. | Problem Category | No. of Persons Unable to Work | No. of Work Loss Days | No. of Working Persons with Long-Term Health Problems |
|---|---|---|---|---|
| 30 | Chronic ischemic heart, w/o hypertension | 140.5 | 3265.7 | 198.6 |
| 31 | Acute myocardial infarction angina pectoris w/o hypertension | 37.1 | 881.2 | 66.1 |
| 32 | Any rheumatic condition | 18.5 | 333.3 | 43.7 |
| 33 | Heart-fibrillation/tachycardia/ arrhythmia | 20.3 | 366.4 | 36.4 |
| 34 | Heart-failure/stop/blockage | 20.3 | 160.4 | 18.0 |
| 35 | Heart disease, nos | 20.5 | 311.8 | 23.4 |
| 36 | Heart trouble, ill-defined | 132.6 | 2302.6 | 150.6 |
| 37 | Hypertensive heart disease, NEC, non-malig. | 52.2 | 178.2 | 42.9 |
| 38 | Hypertensive Disease, NEC | 74.5 | 915.3 | 165.3 |
| 39 | Cerebro-vascular disease w. benign hypertension | 18.7 | 170.0 | 5.7 |
| 40 | Cerebrovascular w. no hypertension, w. arteriosclerosis | 44.0 | 576.8 | 12.9 |
| 41 | Cerebrovascular disease, nos | 12.2 | 62.3 | 2.0 |
| 42 | Arterial disease | 21.4 | 57.9 | 24.5 |
| 43 | Venous disease | 20.5 | 1214.5 | 44.5 |
| 44 | General circulatory conditions | 23.5 | 1003.5 | 28.3 |
| 45 | Emphysema | 122.3 | 608.8 | 74.2 |
| 46 | Asthma | 30.7 | 819.2 | 196.0 |
| 47 | Other respiratory diseases | 61.3 | 66712.5 | 138.4 |
| 48 | Liver diseases | 21.5 | 2367.7 | 11.9 |
| 49 | Stomach-duodenal ulcer | 27.3 | 1614.8 | 73.3 |
| 50 | Abdominal cavity hernia | 23.7 | 2634.1 | 102.9 |
| 51 | Other diseases of digestive system nos | 26.4 | 6712.4 | 57.4 |
| 52 | Genito-urinary disorders | 20.1 | 2633.7 | 52.6 |
| 53 | Diseases of skin/subcutaneous tissue | 13.8 | 2427.0 | 57.1 |
| 54 | Rheumatoid arthritis and allied conditions | 24.3 | 217.2 | 33.1 |
| 55 | Traumatic and osteoarthritis | 32.8 | 382.0 | 60.9 |
| 56 | Nonspecific, nontraumatic arthritis | 155.2 | 2680.6 | 257.3 |
| 57 | Displacement intervertebral disc | 114.2 | 6024.3 | 338.7 |
| 58 | Other musculoskeletal, connective tissue diseases | 26.5 | 3777.7 | 91.3 |
| 59 | Congenital and ill-defined conditions | 64.9 | 7940.0 | 137.5 |
| 60 | Injuries | 20.2 | 60702.4 | 41.5 |
| 61 | Complications of surgical procedures | 17.3 | 1036.3 | 46.3 |

*Table 1.*   (*continued*)

| Group No. | Problem Category | No. of Persons Unable to Work | No. of Work Loss Days | No. of Working Persons with Long-Term Health Problems |
|---|---|---|---|---|
| 62 | Reported work-loss days on person's record, but no conditions data | 0 | 56456.3 | 0 |
| | Total | 2,709.1 | 272,035.0 | 5,416.1 |

Two other categories of orthopedic impairments (Group 13) and deformities (Group 15) were also frequent causes of limitations for working persons but were less important as reasons for inability to work.

The frequency distribition of work-loss days among the categories was very different and more uneven. Two categories, injuries (Group 60) and other respiratory diseases (Group 47) accounted for nearly one-half of all work-loss days.[27] Furthermore, about 20 percent of work-loss days could not be linked to a specific condition (Group 62), because the HIS does not generally retain data on chronic conditions unless these conditions are reported as a cause of activity limitation. If these conditions had been identified, obviously, the relative importance of some of the categories containing largely chronic conditions would have increased. Among the remaining groups, only infective and parasitic diseases (Group 16) accounted for more than 10,000 work-loss days.

## V.   COST ESTIMATES

Selected results pertaining to our estimates for each of the three components of morbidity costs under study here are presented in Table 2. Our estimates yield a total morbidity cost figure of $51.9 billion. More than half of this total consists of earnings losses for persons unable to work ($28.1 billion) while the costs of work-loss days are only $11.0 billion. The former figure is well above the $23 billion estimate for 1977 for both males and females reported by Hodgson, primarily because of our much higher prevalence estimate. In contrast, the latter figure is close to Hodgson's (unpublished) 1977 estimate of $16.77 billion once adjustment is made for the 24 percent increase in employee compensation between 1975 and 1977 and his inclusion of an additional 15.5 percent of costs to reflect fringe benefits.

Turning to the results for the individual problem categories, we observe that only seven categories account for more than $2 billion each in morbidity costs.

*Table 2.*   Estimated Annual Morbidity Costs in 1975 Dollars (000's)

| Group No. | Problem Category | Earnings Losses for Persons Unable to work | Productivity Losses Due to Work- Loss Days | Debility Costs | Total Morbidity Costs |
|---|---|---|---|---|---|
| 1 | Blindness | $ 223,977 | $ 2,215 | $ 54,914 | $ 281,106 |
| 2 | Visual, impairment, other | 169,447 | 10,470 | 283,934 | 463,851 |
| 3 | Other sensory impairment | 289,220 | 15,345 | 317,337 | 621,902 |
| 4 | Mental deficiency | 595,912 | 2,212 | 66,712 | 664,836 |
| 5 | Loss of more than 1 limb or digits | 309,147 | 19,580 | 205,826 | 534,553 |
| 6 | Loss of lung, kidney, bone, joint, muscle, extremity intact | 148,073 | 15,843 | 73,536 | 237,452 |
| 7 | Paralysis-upper or lower extremity, fingers or toes | 316,666 | 7,560 | 61,131 | 385,357 |
| 8 | Paralysis: para-, hemi-, quadriplegia | 307,005 | 2,905 | 36,046 | 345,956 |
| 9 | Cerebral palsy, partial paralysis, any site | 354,639 | 5,572 | 98,903 | 459,114 |
| 10 | Orthopedic impairment, neck, back/ spine/vertebrae | 1,203,663 | 148,545 | 1,254,460 | 2,606,668 |
| 11 | Orthopedic impairment neck, arms/ hands | 219,338 | 44,376 | 308,140 | 571,854 |
| 12 | Orthopedic impairment,hip/pelvis w. any any other site | 208,114 | 14,050 | 92,121 | 314,285 |
| 13 | Orthopedic impairment, knee, leg, ankle, foot | 717,156 | 84,044 | 747,325 | 1,548,525 |
| 14 | Nonparalytic orthopedic impairment. Mulitiple sites (except as in Groups 10-13) ill-defined | 747,004 | 69,599 | 336,349 | 1,152,952 |
| 15 | Deformity of limbs, trunk, back, NEC | 585,747 | 24,807 | 454,303 | 1,064,857 |
| 16 | Infective and parasitic diseases | 240,381 | 439,185 | 69,220 | 748,786 |
| 17 | Neoplasms | 831,454 | 92,305 | 181,498 | 1,105,257 |
| 18 | Endocrine, nutritional metabolic and blood disorders | 269,025 | 46,168 | 189,643 | 504,836 |

Table 2.   (continued)

| Group No. | Problem Category | Earnings Losses for Persons Unable to work | Productivity Losses Due to Work- Loss Days | Debility Costs | Total Morbidity Costs |
|---|---|---|---|---|---|
| 19 | Diabetes (mellitus) | 714,723 | 33,928 | 338,193 | 1,086,844 |
| 20 | Psychosis (schizophrenia) | 271,079 | 810 | 20,976 | 292,865 |
| 21 | Psychosis (non-schizophrenia) | 259,658 | 4,428 | 23,071 | 287,157 |
| 22 | Neurosis | 583,184 | 16,760 | 58,316 | 658,260 |
| 23 | Personality/other nonpsychotic disorders | 273,729 | 11,180 | 50,480 | 335,389 |
| 24 | Alcoholism and nonspecific nervous disorders | 941,385 | 74,695 | 122,406 | 1,138,486 |
| 25 | Multiple sclerosis, paralysis agitans | 292,577 | 0 | 26,147 | 318,724 |
| 26 | Epilepsy | 406,242 | 4,645 | 94,651 | 505,538 |
| 27 | Other nervous system disorders | 431,730 | 55,662 | 163,669 | 651,061 |
| 28 | Eye and ear diseases | 445,640 | 84,174 | 280,404 | 810,218 |
| 29 | Chronic ischemic heart w. hypertension, angina w. hypertension | 392,798 | 22,599 | 67,789 | 483,186 |
| 30 | Chronic ischemic heart, w/o hyper-tension | 1,704,124 | 156,877 | 540,775 | 2,401,776 |
| 31 | Acute myocardial infarction angina pectoris w/o hyper-tension | 424,593 | 42,242 | 168,664 | 635,499 |
| 32 | Any rheumatic conditions | 215,922 | 13,718 | 90,995 | 320,635 |
| 33 | Heart-fibrilation/ tachycardia/ar-rhythmia | 216,060 | 17,079 | 81,471 | 314,610 |
| 34 | Heart-failure stop/ blockage | 232,221 | 6,194 | 44,196 | 282,611 |
| 35 | Heart disease, nos | 226,886 | 11,901 | 62,217 | 301,004 |
| 36 | Heart trouble, ill-defined | 1,375,421 | 102,387 | 401,471 | 1,879,279 |
| 37 | Hypertensive heart disease, NEC, nonmailg. | 507,630 | 6,635 | 98,278 | 612,543 |
| 38 | Hypertensive Disease NEC | 758,773 | 38,908 | 437,726 | 1,235,407 |
| 39 | Cerebrovascular disease w. benign hypertension | 205,160 | 6,541 | 14,932 | 226,633 |

*Table 2.* (*continued*)

| Group No. | Problem Category | Earnings Losses for Persons Unable to work | Productivity Losses Due to Work- Loss Days | Debility Costs | Total Morbidity Costs |
|---|---|---|---|---|---|
| 40 | Cerebrovascular w. no hypertension, w. arteriosclerosis | 480,597 | 20,782 | 32,774 | 534,153 |
| 41 | Cerebrovascular disease, nos | 133,469 | 3,506 | 6,762 | 143,737 |
| 42 | Arterial disease | 250,707 | 2,443 | 62,233 | 315,383 |
| 43 | Venous disease | 221,475 | 60,713 | 115,605 | 397,793 |
| 44 | General circulatory conditions | 256,136 | 43,295 | 67,903 | 367,334 |
| 45 | Emphysema | 1,260,073 | 25,072 | 202,794 | 1,487,939 |
| 46 | Asthma | 288,184 | 28,277 | 36,111 | 677,572 |
| 47 | Other respiratory diseases | 581,666 | 2,771,879 | 301,476 | 3,655,021 |
| 48 | Liver diseases | 235,302 | 113,833 | 26,026 | 375,161 |
| 49 | Stomach-duodenal ulcer | 258,208 | 65,997 | 182,936 | 507,141 |
| 50 | Abdominal cavity hernia | 230,879 | 104,798 | 257,446 | 593,123 |
| 51 | Other diseses of diges- tive system nos | 275,769 | 254,459 | 150,493 | 680,721 |
| 52 | Genito-urinary dis- orders | 211,181 | 107,604 | 120,156 | 438,941 |
| 53 | Diseases of skin/sub- cutaneous tissue | 132,226 | 84,115 | 123,806 | 340,147 |
| 54 | Rheumatoid arthritis and allied conditions | 263,657 | 8,461 | 81,815 | 353,933 |
| 55 | Traumatic and osteo- arthritis | 351,544 | 15,120 | 146,086 | 512,750 |
| 56 | Nonspecific, non- traumatic arthritis | 1,580,109 | 100,751 | 691,399 | 2,372,259 |
| 57 | Displacement inter- vertebral disc | 1,218,092 | 249,832 | 1,035,127 | 2,503,051 |
| 58 | Other musculoskeletal connective tissue diseases | 288,957 | 153,031 | 224,657 | 666,645 |
| 59 | Congenital and ill- defined conditions | 631,023 | 312,226 | 291,117 | 1,234,366 |
| 60 | Injuries | 176,765 | 2,276,594 | 85,279 | 2,538,638 |
| 61 | Complications of surg- ical procedures | 184,697 | 47,581 | 113,207 | 345,485 |
| 62 | Reported work-loss days on persons record, but no condi- tions data | — | 2,439,915 | — | 2,439,915 |
|  | Total | $28,126,225 | $11,046,425 | $12,698,433 | $51,871,083 |

Three of these—other respiratory diseases (47), injuries (60), and the residual missing data category (62)—are primarily responsible for large costs of work-loss days. The remaining four—orthopedic impairments of the neck and back (10), chronic ischemic heart disease (30), nonspecific, nontraumatic arthritis (56), and disc problems (57)—are primarily responsible for costs due to inability to work and debility costs. Note also that all seven of these high-cost categories were noted above as resulting in high frequencies of health problems. In our estimates, frequency is more important than cost per person or per work-loss day in determining the significance of a problem catgory since the inter-category variation in the latter figure is small. Cost per person unable to work only ranged from $7,686 for category 4 (mental deficiency) to $12,531 for category 25 (multiple sclerosis). The range in debility cost per person was from $1,338 for category 4 to $3,321 for category 41 (cerebrovascular disease). The cost per work-loss day ranged form $19.85 for category 20 (schizophrenia) to $56.28 for category 41. Of course, the narrow ranges in estimated debility cost per person and cost per work-loss day are not surprising given our procedures. In particular, note that SIE data used to develop these figures did not allow us to estimate the impact of specific categories of problems on annual or daily earnings of persons with reported long-term health problems in the SIE data. Thus, intercategory variation in these cost figures is due solely to variation in the average socio-demographic and occupational characteristics of persons across the categories.

## VI.   REVISED MORBIDITY COST ESTIMATES AVERAGED ACROSS EDUCATION, INDUSTRY, AND OCCUPATION CATEGORIES

In estimating the two long-term components of morbidity costs (i.e., earnings losses of persons unable to work and debility costs), data on individuals' education level and (for debility costs) industry and occupation have been utilized. Thus, we have implicitly assumed that these individual characteristics are not themselves affected by the presence and nature of long-term health problems. In some instances, however, this assumption may be implausible; for example, it is doubtful that permanent mental deficiency at birth has no effect on the subsequent educational attainment, industry, or occupation of persons with this disorder. Therefore, it is clearly desirable to test the sensitivity of our estimates to this assumption. This section presents the methods and results of that sensitivity test.

### A.   Revised Earnings Loss Estimates for Persons Unable to Work

These estimates were computed by the methods described in Appendix 1 except that adjusted average earnings figures were averaged across education

*Table 3.* Estimated Annual Morbidity Costs in 1975 Dollars
with Endogenous Education, Industry, and Occupation (000's)

| Group No. | Problem Category | Earnings Losses for Persons Unable to work | Productivity Losses Due to Work-Loss Days | Debility Costs | Total Morbidity Costs |
|---|---|---|---|---|---|
| 1 | Blindness | $ 274,535 | $ 2,215 | $ 75,772 | $ 352,522 |
| 2 | Visual impairment, other | 206,889 | 10,470 | 457,913 | 675,272 |
| 3 | Other sensory impairment | 318,739 | 15,345 | 530,935 | 865,019 |
| 4 | Mental deficiency | 797,782 | 2,212 | 104,560 | 904,554 |
| 5 | Loss of more than 1 limb or digits | 359,148 | 19,580 | 323,661 | 702,389 |
| 6 | Loss of lung, kidney, bone, joint, muscle, extremity intact | 171,732 | 15,843 | 124,997 | 312,572 |
| 7 | Paralysis-upper or lower extremity fingers or toes | 359,968 | 7,560 | 101,698 | 469,226 |
| 8 | Paralyisis: para-, hemi-, quadri-plegia | 348,091 | 2,905 | 57,085 | 408,081 |
| 9 | Cerebral palsy, partial paralysis, any site | 423,510 | 5,572 | 166,848 | 595,930 |
| 10 | Orthopedic impairment, neck/back/spine/vertebrae | 1,449,244 | 148,545 | 1,952,531 | 3,550,320 |
| 11 | Orthopedic impairment, neck, arms/hands | 258,718 | 44,376 | 516,336 | 819,430 |
| 12 | Orthopedic impairment, hip/pelvis w. any other site | 238,461 | 14,050 | 135,502 | 388,013 |
| 13 | Orthopedic impairment, knee, leg, ankle, foot | 854,989 | 84,044 | 1,238,300 | 2,177,333 |
| 14 | Nonparalytic orthopedic impairment. Multiple sites (except as in Groups 10-13) ill-defined | 875,074 | 69,599 | 588,365 | 1,503,038 |

*Table 3.* (*continued*)

| Group No. | Problem Category | Earnings Losses for Persons Unable to work | Productivity Losses Due to Work-Loss Days | Debility Costs | Total Morbidity Costs |
|---|---|---|---|---|---|
| 15 | Deformity of limbs, trunk, back, NEC | 691,573 | 24,807 | 708,565 | 1,424,945 |
| 16 | Infective & parasitic diseases | 286,614 | 439,185 | 122,979 | 848,778 |
| 17 | Neoplasms | 916,257 | 92,305 | 288,551 | 1,297,113 |
| 18 | Endocrine, nutritional, metabolic and blood disorders | 316,052 | 46,168 | 324,497 | 686,717 |
| 19 | Diabetes(mellitus) | 847,630 | 33,928 | 534,835 | 1,416,393 |
| 20 | Psychosis (schizophrenia) | 271,675 | 810 | 28,387 | 300,872 |
| 21 | Psychosis (nonschizophrenic) | 287,143 | 4,428 | 29,089 | 320,660 |
| 22 | Neurosis | 650,949 | 16,760 | 96,473 | 764,182 |
| 23 | Personality/other nonpsychotic disorders | 316,690 | 11,180 | 81,136 | 409,006 |
| 24 | Alcoholism and nonspecific nervous disorders | 1,090,236 | 74,695 | 196,973 | 1,361,904 |
| 25 | Multiple sclerosis, paralysis agitans | 311,485 | 0 | 41,741 | 353,226 |
| 26 | Epilepsy | 501,092 | 4,645 | 154,928 | 660,665 |
| 27 | Other nervous system disorders | 483,892 | 55,662 | 265,158 | 804,712 |
| 28 | Eye and ear diseases | 503,724 | 84,174 | 439,987 | 1,027,885 |
| 29 | Chronic ischemic heart w. hypertension, angina w. hypertension | 438,714 | 22,599 | 109,364 | 570,677 |
| 30 | Chronic ischemic heart, w/o hypertension | 1,873,660 | 156,877 | 841,107 | 2,871,644 |
| 31 | Acute myocardial infarction angia pectoris w/o hypertension | 496,622 | 42,242 | 265,291 | 804,155 |
| 32 | Any rheumatic condition | 251,423 | 13,718 | 153,622 | 418,763 |
| 33 | Heart-fibrillation/ tachycardia/arrhythmia | 258,484 | 17,079 | 124,551 | 400,114 |

*Table 3.* (*continued*)

| Group No. | Problem Category | Earnings Losses for Persons Unable to work | Productivity Losses Due to Work-Loss Days | Debility Costs | Total Morbidity Costs |
|---|---|---|---|---|---|
| 34 | Heart-failure/stop /blockage | 257,794 | 6,194 | 76,491 | 340,479 |
| 35 | Heart disease, nos | 261,096 | 11,901 | 97,361 | 370,358 |
| 36 | Heart trouble, ill-defined | 1,644,271 | 102,387 | 590,870 | 2,337,528 |
| 37 | Hypertensive heart disease, NEC, nonmalig. | 605,117 | 6,635 | 171,167 | 782,919 |
| 38 | Hypertensive Disease, NEC | 881,561 | 38,908 | 656,669 | 1,577,138 |
| 39 | Cerebro-vascular disease w. benign hypertension | 227,857 | 6,541 | 22,725 | 257,123 |
| 40 | Cerebrovasular w. no hypertension, w.arteriosclerosis | 550,246 | 20,782 | 48,212 | 619,240 |
| 41 | Cerebrovascular disease, nos | 149,813 | 3,506 | 8,307 | 161,626 |
| 42 | Arterial disease | 286,227 | 2,443 | 104,001 | 392,671 |
| 43 | Venous disease | 269,473 | 60,713 | 181,280 | 511,466 |
| 44 | General circulatory conditions | 304,673 | 43,295 | 106,716 | 454,684 |
| 45 | Emphysema | 1,573,160 | 25,072 | 296,968 | 1,895,200 |
| 46 | Asthma | 353,748 | 28,277 | 542,835 | 924,860 |
| 47 | Other respiratory diseases | 753,892 | 2,771,879 | 451,702 | 3,977,473 |
| 48 | Liver diseases | 277,194 | 113,833 | 44,034 | 435,061 |
| 49 | Stomach-duodenal ulcer | 318,354 | 65,997 | 283,951 | 668,302 |
| 50 | Abdominal cavity hernia | 279,078 | 104,798 | 396,936 | 780,812 |
| 51 | Other diseases of digestive system nos | 324,231 | 254,459 | 205,768 | 784,458 |
| 52 | Genito-urinary disorders | 241,062 | 107,604 | 188,729 | 537,395 |
| 53 | Diseases of skin/ subcutaneous tissue | 165,520 | 84,115 | 188,607 | 438,242 |
| 54 | Rheumatoid arthritis and allied conditions | 309,936 | 8,461 | 137,215 | 455,612 |
| 55 | Traumatic and osteoarthritis | 420,136 | 15,120 | 247,204 | 682,460 |

*Table 3.*   (*continued*)

| Group No. | Problem Category | Earnings Losses for Persons Unable to work | Productivity Losses Due to Work-Loss Days | Debility Costs | Total Morbidity Costs |
|---|---|---|---|---|---|
| 56 | Nonspecific, non-traumatic arthritis | 1,914,389 | 100,751 | 1,033,723 | 3,049,313 |
| 57 | Displacement in-tervertebral disc | 1,458,055 | 249,832 | 1,591,673 | 3,299,560 |
| 58 | Other musculo-skeletal, connec-tive tissue diseases | 343,715 | 153,031 | 323,424 | 820,170 |
| 59 | Congenital and ill-defined conditions | 757,127 | 312,226 | 459,371 | 1,528,724 |
| 60 | Injuries | 212,169 | 2,276,594 | 137,413 | 2,626,176 |
| 61 | Complications of surgical pro-cedures | 216,626 | 47,581 | 184,121 | 448,328 |
| 62 | Reported work-loss days on persons record, but no condi-ditions data | — | 2,439,915 | — | 2,439,915 |
| | Total | $33,073,114 | $11,046,425 | $19,929,213 | $64,048,752 |

categories. This yielded a new set of earnings figures based on residence, race, and age.[28]

Aggregating across individuals on the basis of our 61 categories of health problems yielded the cost estimates shown in the first column of Table 3. In total, our estimate rose from $28.1 billion to $33.1 billion. This increase is consistent with the fact that reported educational attainment is lower for persons unable to work than for nondisabled persons. With regard to results for the individual problem categories, we observe the largest relative increase (33.9 percent) for mental deficiency (Group 3) and the smallest (0.2 percent) for schizophrenia (Group 20).

## B.   Revised Debility Cost Estimates

Revision of the debility cost estimates involved reestimation of the regressions in Table 1 of Appendix 3 excluding the education, industry, and mean occupation earnings variables. (The latter was excluded since it was based in part on the occupation codes reported by the individuals.) Additional dummy variables for geographic location were also added, including dummies for each of 18 large SMSAs and for 47 of the 48 contiguous states and the District of Columbia. (California was the omitted reference category.) The estimated regressions are shown in Appendix 3, Table 2.

For persons on the HIS files with missing geographical data, earnings predictions were based on race and age and were derived from a cross-tabulation of predicted earnings by race and age for persons on the HIS file with complete data (Appendix 3, Table 3).

The revised debility cost estimates are presented in column 3 of Table 3. In comparison with the earlier results in Table 2, we observe that total debility costs have increased by 56.9 percent, from $12.7 billion ot $19.9 billion. While there is some variation across the 61 categories in the corresponding percentage increase, debility costs rose by less than 40 percent in only a few categories (20, 21, 41, and 51).

To explain this large increase in debility costs, we first note that the cost for each disabled individual can be expressed as $Y_N(E_N,O_N) - Y_L(E_L,O_L)$ where $Y_L,E_L$ and $O_L$ denote their actual earnings, education level, and occupational classification while $Y_N,E_N,O_N$ denote the predicted values of these variables for the individual if he were not disabled. This differential can be decomposed into $\{Y_N(E_N,O_N) - Y_N(E_L,O_L)\} + \{Y_N(E_L,O_L) - Y_L(E_L,O_L)\}$. The second bracketed term represents the debility costs holding education and occupational status constant and corresponds to the cost estimates shown in Table 2; the first bracketed term represents the costs due to lower educational attainment and occupational status.

Simple computations with the SIE data used in the regressions in Tables 1 and 2 of Appendix 3 and the regression coefficients were used to get a rough idea of the relative magnitude of these two bracketed terms. First, we multiplied the mean values for the education variables from the SIE sample with health limitations by the education coefficients in Table 1 and compared the result with that obtained when the mean value for healthy SIE individuals was used. This yielded a decline of 0.0458 in the predicted logarithm of earnings. Next we computed the mean value of the occupational earnings variable, based on the earnings data for healthy SIE individuals and the occupational classifications for SIE individuals with health limitations ($10,161) and compared this result with the mean value based on the occupational classifications for healthy individuals ($11,009). The difference in logarithms of these two figures multiplied by the regression coefficient for the occupational earnings variable in Table 1 (0.7214) implies a further decline of 0.0577 in the predicted logarithm of earnings. Using the mean value of the logarithm of earnings for healthy individuals in the SIE sample (8.9136) to calculate $Y_N(E_N,O_N)$, and subtracting 0.1035 (=0.0458 + 0.0577) from this figure to calculate the logarithm of $Y_N(E_L,O_L)$ yields a differential of $730 (=$7432-$6702). Similarly, if the mean value of the logarithm of earnings of persons with health limitations in the SIE (8.6359) is used to calculate $Y_L(E_L,O_L) =$

$5630, we obtain $Y_N$ ($E_L,O_L$) — $Y_L$ ($E_L,O_L$) = $6702 -$5630 = $1072. Thus, adding the $730 value of $Y_N(E_N,O_N)$ — $Y_N(E_L,O_L)$ increases our original debility cost estimate ($1,072) by 68.1 percent according to these calculations. Since the increase in debility cost shown in Table 3 relative to Table 2 is about 57 percent, it appears from our calculations that this increase is more than accounted for by the differences in educational attainment and occupational status between persons with and without chronic health problems. Another implication is that changes in regression results for other variables (industry, race, location, and age), with differences in the distributions of these other variables between the healthy and disabled groups, tended to offset the increases in our debility cost estimate related to the education and occupation variables.

## C.  Summary

Allowing for health problem impacts on education, industry, and occupation of persons unable to work and persons with debility costs results in a substantial increase in estimated morbidity costs from $51.9 to $64.0 billion. The seven highest-costs problem categories in Table 2 are still the largest categories in Table 3, but the increase for the categories whose costs arise mainly from work-loss days (47, 60, and 62) is obviously smaller since the work-loss day cost estimates were not revised. Moreover, two additional categories (13 and 36) have costs in excess of $2 billion with the revised estimates.

Our analysis of the differences between the two sets of estimates indicated that differences in occupation and education between persons with and without long-term health problems account for the increase in the revised estimates. In effect, these estimates attribute the entirety of these differences to the impact of health problems. In some cases, where the onset of a problem occurs early in life (e.g., mental retardation), this may be appropriate. In other cases, the causation may actually run the other way, that is, from low education and occupation status to higher exposure to health hazards, to a higher prevalence of health problems. In this event, the revised estimate of Table 3 will overstate the true impact of the health problems.

## VII.   TRENDS IN DISABILITY AND LABOR FORCE PARTICIPATION: DATA FROM THE HEALTH INTERVIEW SURVEY

The cost estimates in the preceding sections are based on estimates of the prevalence and severity of disabilities developed from responses to household interviews. A number of recent studies have suggested, however, that these prevalence and severity estimates are themselves influenced by economic conditions. For example, it has been argued that liberalized disability benefit and retirement programs and increases in unemployment rates have encouraged people to define themselves as disabled and to apply for benefits. This response to changing economic conditions will directly affect our estimates of morbidity costs.

In this section, we briefly review selected recent literature on economic factors and trends in disability and labor force participation. We then examine evidence from the HIS concerning trends in disability and in labor force participation for males age 45-64. One specific issue to be addressed is the extent to which the observed trends reflect actual differences in prevalence of health problems rather than individuals' responses to changing economic conditions. We also compare the magnitude of the labor force and disability trends to assess the importance of disability as a factor in declining labor force participation.

## A.   Previous Research

The most forceful proponent of the view that self-reported disability is strongly affected by economic incentives is Donald Parsons.[29] In a cross-sectional analysis of males age 48-62, based on 1969 data from the National Longitudinal Surveys, he examined dichotomous dependent variables indicating that an individual (1) reported his health status as poor, and (2) that a health problem limited the amount or kind of work the individual could do. Independent variables included age, a mortality index based on the individual's survival experience in the 1969-76 period, and three variables relating to economic incentives. These three variables were the fraction of the year the person was unemployed in 1966, general assistance plus AFDC payments per family in the state in 1969 divided by the individual's 1966 hourly wage rate, and the ratio of an estimated potential Social Security disability benefit to the individual's 1966 hourly wage. Regression results indicated a positive and significant coefficient for the unemployment variable and the Social Security benefit variable and were interpreted by Parsons as confirming his hypothesis that self-reported health measures are strongly affected by economic incentives. In an alternative specification, he replaced the economic variables with a predicted probability of nonparticipation in the labor force developed from a regression including these economic variables, their interactions with the mortality index, and other sociodemographic variables. The predicted probability of nonparticipation has a significant positive coefficient which is consistent with Parsons' hypothesis; it is also included in an interaction with the mortality index where its coefficient is negative and significant. This seems to indicate the odd result that economic factors are more likely to cause healthier people to report poor health; Parsons, however, interprets this as "reflecting double counting" of the effects of the mortality and predicted participation variables. It is not clear what is meant by this, but it may also be an indicator of collinearity between the interaction and its two components.

Based on these results, Parsons further argued that models estimating the effect of disablity benefit programs on labor force participation should exclude self-reported health status measures since these measures are themselves strongly affected by the disability benefit programs. Furthermore, when he used cross-sectional labor force participation models to simulate the decline in male labor force participation since 1956 in the U.S., he found that models that excluded self-reported health status measures did a much better job of explaining this decline than did a model including these variables.

The factors influencing self-reports of work limitations due to health problems were also studied by Chirikos and Nestel in a cross-sectional analysis of 1976 data from the same National Longitudinal Survey.[30] As an explanatory variable intended to control for health status, they include an "impairment status" index which was derived by factor analysis from self-reported data on the presence and severity of eleven specific functional limitations (e.g., difficulty in walking) and on the occurrence of seven signs or symptoms (e.g., shortness of breath). Other explanatory variables in their regression analysis were age, race, marital status, south vs. nonsouth location, education, dummy variables for job characteristics of the current or last job, and other family income. The authors give the following summary of their regression results:

> Even though impairment status is a statistically significant predictor of the probability of reporting a work-limiting health problem, almost two-thirds of the variance in this dependent variable is left unexplained by the model. This clearly suggests that the alternative health measures do not capture the same underlying phenomena, nor can they necessarily be mapped onto each other very easily. It also implies that a number of factors impinge on such self-reports beyond matters relating to physiological or psychological functioning per se. We find that the probability of reporting a health problem is higher for men who are older, less well educated, who live in the south, are self-employed, and have higher "other family income." The magnitude of the other income variable, however, is not as great as the recent literature seems to suggest (page 109).

Though references to the "recent literature" are not cited here, it appears that they are referring to Parsons' findings about disability benefit programs (discussed above).

While both of these studies provide some support for the contention that self-reported work disability is influenced by economic incentives, the strength of this influence is open to question for a number of reasons. Their explanatory variables pertaining to health status probably omit important dimensions of ill health, as is suggested by the limited explanatory power of the regression models. Moreover, in the Parsons study the main economic incentive variable (the ratio of disability benefits to wages) is probably strongly and negatively correlated with wages (which are omitted from his model.)[31] Since wages will be negatively correlated with ill health, omitted dimensions of ill health will tend to produce an upward bias in the estimated coefficient of the ratio of benefits to wages, thereby exaggerating the apparent impact of economic incentives on self-reported disability. Wolfe has criticized the specification of this ratio variable as confounding wage and disability benefit effects, and has pointed out other possible biases in Parsons' specification and estimation procedure.[32] Finally, since both of these studies used the same survey data base which included only about 3,500 respondents, they obviously can not provide a firm foundation for general conclusions about the strengths of economic incentives. In summary, evidence on the proposition that self-reported work disability is primarily a description of labor-market behavior, rather than health status, is far from conclusive.

### B. Labor Force Participation Trends of Males Age 45-64, 1969-80.

In this section, we present and discuss trends in labor force participation rates from the HIS data for the 1969-80 period. Labor force participation in the HIS is defined in response to questions about the individual's activity in the 2-week period preceding the interview. In particular, the labor force is defined to include all persons who reported that they (1) worked in the past two weeks, (2) did not work but had a job (including persons on layoff), or (3) did not work and had no job but were looking for work or on layoff.

HIS labor force participation rates by race and age for males age 45 to 64 in the civilian noninstitutionalized population are reported in Table 4. For whites, the rate for age 45-54 moved downward through most of the 1970-1978 period but then rose from 1978 to 1980. The rate for age 55-64 declined

*Table 4.* Labor Force Participation of Males Age 45 to 64

| Year | White | | Nonwhite | |
|------|-------|-------|----------|-------|
| | *45-54* | *55-64* | *45-54* | *55-64* |
| 1969 | .9401 | .8459 | .8898 | .8081 |
| 1970 | .9429 | .8336 | .8994 | .7921 |
| 1971 | .9372 | .8198 | .8713 | .7617 |
| 1972 | .9288 | .8168 | .8408 | .7579 |
| 1973 | .9282 | .7882 | .8587 | .7442 |
| 1974 | .9249 | .7887 | .8653 | .6901 |
| 1975 | .9208 | .7644 | .8498 | .6939 |
| 1976 | .9213 | .7599 | .8136 | .6675 |
| 1977 | .9156 | .7345 | .8240 | .6568 |
| 1978 | .9132 | .7547 | .8773 | .6635 |
| 1979 | .9186 | .7326 | .8541 | .6261 |
| 1980 | .9221 | .7357 | .8081 | .6054 |

fairly steadily from 1969 to 1977 and then fluctuated. For nonwhites, the sharp and persistent decline in the rate for older males (age 55-64) is especially striking. The decline for males age 45-54 from 1969 to 1976 was also rapid but followed by a sharp increase to a peak in 1978 and then another sharp decline.

## C.  Trends in Reported Activity Limitations

Activity limitations due to chronic health problems are reported on the HIS in three categories: limitations that prevent a person from working, limitations on the amount or kind of work a person can do, and limitations on activities outside of work. Since these data are self-reported, several concerns about their use may be raised. First, one may question their validity in the absence of clinical verification. Second, the studies reviewed above suggest that they may be influenced by a variety of socioeconomic factors. In particular, if a person is a Social Security Disability Insurance (SSDI) recipient or applicant, he may be more likely to report that a health problem prevents him from working since receipt of these benefits is conditional on the inability to work. If so, trends in the percent of persons reporting inability to work may be influenced by changes in the benefits, eligibility provisions, and administration of the SSDI program. This same observation applies to other disability benefit programs that are conditional on ability to work.[33]

In spite of these problems, the HIS activity limitation data may still be a useful indicator of trends in disability rates in the population; these data have in fact been used in this way in a variety of official reports from the U.S. Dept. of Health and Human Services and by other nongovernmental experts.[34] It is also pertinent to note that reporting of limitations in outside activities should be less positively influenced by more liberal disability program provisions when these programs offer benefits that are conditional on inability to work or on limitations in working abilities. Indeed, increased liberality of programs may have a negative impact on reported limitations in outside activities since individuals have a stronger financial incentive to claim that these limitations inhibit their ability to work. (This would not, of course, apply to programs like veteran's benefits which are not conditional on work limitations.)

Rates of activity limitations for the 1969-80 period are reported in Table 5 for males age 45-54.[35] For whites, increasing prevalence of limitations that prevent work and of limitations in outside activities are seen up through the mid-1970s. For nonwhites, the prevalence of limitations that prevent work moved upward erratically, resulting in a substantial increase over the entire period. Limitations in amount or kind of work, in contrast, increased through the mid-1970s and then declined. In the 55-64 age group (Table 6), limitations that prevent work increased for whites to a peak in 1977 and then held fairly steady while limitations in outside activities rose until 1974 and then fluctuated;

*Table 5.* Percent Distribution by Activity Limitation for Males Aged 45-54

| | White | | | | Nonwhite | | | |
|---|---|---|---|---|---|---|---|---|
| Year | Cannot Perform Usual Activity | Limited In Usual Activity | Limited In Outside Activity | Not Limited | Cannot Perform Usual Activity | Limited In Usual Activity | Limited In Outside Activity | Not Limited |
| 1969 | .0405 | .0954 | .0302 | .8340 | .0938 | .0759 | .0199 | .8105 |
| 1970 | .0394 | .0753 | .0447 | .8406 | .0930 | .0861 | .0236 | .7973 |
| 1971 | .0406 | .0872 | .0481 | .8241 | .1025 | .0746 | .0187 | .8042 |
| 1972 | .0413 | .0868 | .0477 | .8243 | .1216 | .0830 | .0256 | .7698 |
| 1973 | .0474 | .0852 | .0569 | .8105 | .1060 | .1108 | .0213 | .7619 |
| 1974 | .0533 | .0865 | .0542 | .8060 | .0937 | .0908 | .0356 | .7799 |
| 1975 | .0503 | .0781 | .0451 | .8266 | .0945 | .1015 | .0359 | .7682 |
| 1976 | .0551 | .0852 | .0512 | .8085 | .1301 | .0902 | .0385 | .7413 |
| 1977 | .0565 | .0733 | .0488 | .8214 | .1261 | .0648 | .0301 | .7789 |
| 1978 | .0541 | .0836 | .0445 | .8177 | .0841 | .0839 | .0328 | .7992 |
| 1979 | .0525 | .0821 | .0514 | .8140 | .1182 | .0760 | .0470 | .7588 |
| 1980 | .0563 | .0753 | .0540 | .8145 | .1429 | .0498 | .0317 | .7756 |

*Table 6.* Percent Distribution by Activity Limitation for Males Aged 55-64

| | White | | | | Nonwhite | | | |
|---|---|---|---|---|---|---|---|---|
| Year | Cannot Perform Usual Activity | Limited In Usual Activity | Limited In Outside Activity | Not Limited | Cannot Perform Usual Activity | Limited In Usual Activity | Limited In Outside Activity | Not Limited |
| 1969 | .1012 | .1201 | .0348 | .7440 | .1578 | .0853 | .0216 | .7353 |
| 1970 | .1079 | .1215 | .0478 | .7228 | .1659 | .1220 | .0215 | .6906 |
| 1971 | .1061 | .1153 | .0457 | .7329 | .1848 | .1095 | .0233 | .6824 |
| 1972 | .1036 | .1241 | .0488 | .7235 | .1800 | .1035 | .0343 | .6822 |
| 1973 | .1212 | .1247 | .0520 | .7021 | .1893 | .1322 | .0340 | .6441 |
| 1974 | .1284 | .1255 | .0599 | .6862 | .2426 | .1365 | .0305 | .5904 |
| 1975 | .1341 | .1155 | .0531 | .6973 | .2200 | .1258 | .0224 | .6323 |
| 1976 | .1345 | .1218 | .0547 | .6890 | .2215 | .0956 | .0313 | .6516 |
| 1977 | .1501 | .1207 | .0449 | .6843 | .2265 | .1144 | .0317 | .6274 |
| 1978 | .1420 | .1098 | .0493 | .6989 | .2428 | .1180 | .0380 | .6012 |
| 1979 | .1487 | .1028 | .0569 | .6916 | .2849 | .0960 | .0367 | .5824 |
| 1980 | .1468 | .1181 | .0521 | .6831 | .2265 | .0959 | .0377 | .6399 |

limitations in amount or kind of work were slightly lower in 1978 and 1979 but generally showed no trend. For nonwhites, limitations that prevent work and limitations in outside activities rose sharply through the early 1970s, leveled off, and then tended upward later in the period; limitations in the amount or kind of work also moved upward until 1974 and then declined.

*Table 7.*  Change in Labor Force Participation and
Disability Percentages for Older Working-Age Males

|  | 1969-1976 | 1969-1978 | 1969-1980 | 1970-1976 | 1970-1978 | 1970-1980 |
|---|---|---|---|---|---|---|
| *White, 45-54* | | | | | | |
| • Labor Force | | | | | | |
| Participation | -1.88 | -2.69 | -1.80 | -2.16 | -2.97 | -2.08 |
| • Unable to Work | +1.46 | +1.36 | +1.58 | +1.57 | +1.47 | +1.69 |
| • Any Reported | | | | | | |
| Disability | +2.55 | +1.63 | +1.95 | +3.21 | +2.29 | +2.61 |
| *Nonwhite, 45-54* | | | | | | |
| • Labor Force | | | | | | |
| Participation | -7.62 | -1.25 | -8.17 | -8.58 | -2.21 | -9.13 |
| • Unable to Work | +3.63 | -0.97 | +4.91 | +3.71 | -0.89 | -4.99 |
| • Any Reported | | | | | | |
| Disability | +6.92 | +1.13 | +3.49 | +5.60 | -0.19 | +2.17 |
| *White, 55-64* | | | | | | |
| • Labor Force | | | | | | |
| Participation | -8.60 | -9.12 | -10.02 | -7.37 | -7.89 | -9.79 |
| • Unable to Work | +3.33 | +4.08 | +4.56 | +2.66 | +3.41 | +3.89 |
| • Any Reported | | | | | | |
| Disability | +5.50 | +4.51 | +6.09 | +3.38 | +2.39 | +3.97 |
| *Nonwhite, 55-64* | | | | | | |
| • Labor Force | | | | | | |
| Participation | -14.06 | -14.46 | -20.27 | -12.46 | -12.86 | -18.67 |
| • Unable to Work | +6.37 | +8.50 | +6.87 | +5.56 | +7.69 | +6.06 |
| • Any Reported | | | | | | |
| Disability | +8.37 | +13.41 | +9.54 | +3.90 | +8.94 | +5.07 |

While our data show roughly parallel disability and labor force participation
trends, two questions should be considered. First, is the increase in the
prevalence of disability large enough to account, in an arithmetic sense, for
the decline in labor force participation? Second, is the increase in prevalence
largely the result of changes in economic incentives, as suggested by Parsons?

To answer the first question, one can compare the overall changes in the
labor force and disability measures. These comparisons are presented in Table
7 using several different end points. Except for whites age 45-54, these
comparisons clearly indicate that the increase in disability prevalence does not
fully account for the decline in labor force participation and thus they suggest
that other important causes of this decline were operative.

Confirmation of this is seen in Table 8, which shows trends in retirement
status for older working-age males. For both white and nonwhite men age 55-
64 over the 1970-1980 period, the increase in the percent retired for reasons
other than poor health was nearly as great as the increase in the percent retired

*Table 8.*   Percent Retired for Health or Other Reasons, Males Age 45-64

| | White | | | | Nonwhite | | | |
|---|---|---|---|---|---|---|---|---|
| | 45-54 | | 55-64 | | 45-54 | | 55-64 | |
| Year | Retired for Health | Retired for Other | Retired for Health | Retired for Other | Retired for Health | Retired for Other | Retired for Health | Retired for Other |
| 1970 | .0202 | .0038 | .0861 | .0514 | .0423 | 0 | .1051 | .0326 |
| 1971 | .0203 | .0042 | .0833 | .0572 | .0483 | .0026 | .1325 | .0410 |
| 1972 | .0242 | .0068 | .0811 | .0600 | .0422 | .0016 | .1010 | .0480 |
| 1973 | .0268 | .0050 | .0996 | .0726 | .0497 | 0 | .1331 | .0381 |
| 1974 | .0308 | .0062 | .1035 | .0777 | .0483 | .0058 | .1498 | .0468 |
| 1975 | .0289 | .0075 | .1069 | .0827 | .0428 | .0080 | .1338 | .0543 |
| 1976 | .0296 | .0091 | .1102 | .0985 | .0655 | .0186 | .1570 | .0418 |
| 1977 | .0343 | .0111 | .1263 | .1069 | .0469 | .0114 | .1599 | .0713 |
| 1978 | .0335 | .0096 | .1177 | .0949 | .0457 | .0072 | .1713 | .0757 |
| 1979 | .0334 | .0098 | .1248 | .1055 | .0471 | .0186 | .2131 | .0655 |
| 1980 | .0325 | .0117 | .1270 | .1083 | .0615 | .0074 | .1840 | .0927 |

for health reasons. This presumably reflects the influence of more generous retirement and Social Security benefits rather than the impact of more liberal disability benefits per se. For whites in the 45-54 age group, the same pattern is observed; for nonwhites age 45-54 the increase in retirement for nonhealth reasons is somewhat smaller and the figures seem to show more year-to-year sampling variability.[36]

The second question, concerning the reasons for the increased prevalance of disability, cannot be answered definitively without more detailed and rigorous statistical modelling. Within the limits of our descriptive analysis, however, several pertinent observations can be made. We have already suggested that the economic incentives of disability benefit programs are likely to influence the reported level of disability, as well as the reporting of any disability *at all.* Thus, we would expect to see a shift in this level as a behavioral response. In particular, if programs encouraged people to report more severe work limitations to qualify for benefits, a shift in the distribution of disabled persons toward the most severe level (i.e., unable to work) should be observed. The data for older males presented above (Tables 5 and 6) do not clearly confirm this hypothesis. From 1969 to the mid-1970s, prevalence rates for the least severe category (limited in outside activity) rose at least as fast (in relative terms) as rates for the most severe category (unable to work); rates for the intermediate category, however, only rose sharply for nonwhites age 55-64. In the latter portion of the study period, a shift of the distribution toward the most severe level and away from the intermediate and least severe levels was perceptible.

*Table 9.*   Prevalence per 1,000 Persons of Selected
Chronic Conditions and Impairments, Males Age 45-64

| Impairments | 1971 | 1977 |
|---|---|---|
| Severe Visual | 6.0 | 6.1 |
| Paralysis | 12.0 | 13.0 |
| Absence of Major Extremity | 5.3 | 5.3 |
| Orthopedic | | |
| • Back or Spine | 68.2 | 67.6 |
| • Upper Extremity and Shoulder | 25.3 | 23.1 |
| • Lower Extremity or Hip | 50.7 | 45.9 |
| • Other and Multiple, NEC, and Ill-Defined | 11.5 | 11.6 |
| | | |
| *Digestive Conditions* | *1968* | *1975* |
| Ulcer of Stomach and Duodenum | 45.0 | 39.2 |
| Abdominal Hernia | 34.0 | 38.2 |
| Liver Conditions | 2.2 | 5.7 |
| Stomach Trouble NOS | 5.3 | 3.1 |
| | | |
| *Musculoskeletal Conditions* | *1969* | *1976* |
| Arthiritis NEC | 148.0 | 197.1 |
| Rheumatism | 11.2 | 6.7 |
| Bone Diseases | 7.0 | 12.6 |
| Displaced Disc | 21.2 | 31.6 |
| Gout | 17.0 | 25.4 |

*Sources:*   U.S. National Center for Health Statistics, Vital and Health Statistics, Series 10, Numbers 83, 123,
99, 134, 92, and 124.

Additional evidence on this point comes from published HIS data concerning the prevalence of chronic conditions and impairments. These data are based upon individuals' responses to questions about ever having had specified conditions rather than to questions about whether they are limited in their activities by health problems. Thus, prevalence data of this type should be less affected by behavioral responses to economic incentives.[37]

The published data appropriate to our time frame are limited to three categories of chronic conditions: impairments, digestive conditions, and musculoskeletal conditions. Prevalence rates for selected conditions from these groups are shown in Table 9.[38] For impairments and digestive conditions, there is no clear pattern of change over time. For musculoskeletal conditions, however, the *relative* increase in prevalence was large for all conditions except rheumatism.

Since these conditions vary widely in their severity and the obstacles to working which they pose, simply adding up these rates to get an idea of the overall change in prevalence rates would not be meaningful. Therefore, to derive a more useful overall measure, we multiplied each prevalence rate by the percent of cases in which that condition caused reported activity limitation

*Table 10.* Severity-Weighted Changes in Prevalence
Rates for Selected Conditions and Impairments

| | (1) % of Reported Conditions Causing Activity Limitations 1975-1977 | (2) 1968-1971 Prevalence Rate x Col. (1)/100 | (3) Change in Prevalence Rate | (4) Col. (1) x Col. (3) /100 |
|---|---|---|---|---|
| *Impairments* | | | | |
| Severe Visual | 37.0 | 2.220 | +0.1 | .037 |
| Paralysis | 58.4 | 7.008 | +1.0 | .584 |
| Absence of Majority Extremity | 65.9 | 3.493 | 0 | 0 |
| Orthopedic | | | | |
| • Back or Spine | 25.5 | 17.391 | -0.6 | -.153 |
| • Upper Extremity & Shoulder | 21.4 | 5.414 | -2.2 | -.471 |
| • Lower Extremity or Hip | 26.6 | 13.486 | -4.8 | -1.277 |
| • Other | 54.8 | 6.302 | +0.1 | .055 |
| Total Impairments | | 55.314 | | -1.225 |
| *Digestive Conditions* | | | | |
| Ulcer of Stomach & Duodenum | 13.5 | 6.075 | -5.8 | -.783 |
| Abdominal Hernia | 17.6 | 5.984 | +4.2 | .739 |
| Liver Condition | 27.3 | .601 | +3.5 | .956 |
| Stomach Trouble NOS | 13.2 | .700 | -2.2 | -.290 |
| Total Digestive Conditions | | 13.360 | | +.622 |
| *Musculoskeletal Conditions* | | | | |
| Arthritis | 20.3 | 30.044 | +49.1 | +9.967 |
| Rheumatism | 9.7 | 1.086 | -4.5 | .437 |
| Bone diseases | 18.2 | 1.274 | +5.6 | 1.019 |
| Displaced Disc | 49.0 | 10.388 | +10.4 | 5.096 |
| Gout | 19.4 | 3.298 | +8.4 | 1.630 |
| Total Musculoskeletal Conditions | | 46.090 | | +17.275 |
| Overall Total | | 114.764 | | +16.872 |

in the most recent year for which data were published. These percentages are
shown in the first column of Table 10.[39] In the second column these percentages
are multiplied by the prevalence rate from the first column of Table 9. They
may be interpreted as prevalence rates of activity limitations due to the specified
condition. Column (3) in Table 10 is the algebraic difference between the two

rates shown in Table 9, while column (4) is the estimated change in the prevalence rate of activity limitations caused by the condition using the column (1) percentages.[40] Finally, the within group and overall totals are obtained simply by summing over the specific conditions. This produces a slight upward bias in the prevalence rates (because of persons with mulitiple conditions) which will presumably have a negligible effect on conclusions about relative increases in prevalence over time.

The last column of Table 10 again confirms that virtually all of the increase in prevalence is in the musculoskeletal conditions and that this increase is a very substantial 37.5 percent ($100 \times 17.275/46.090$). This increase is the main component of the overall total increase of 14.7 percent ($100 \times 16.872/114.764$). The latter figure is somewhat smaller than the percent increase from 1969 to 1976 in the prevalence rate for all activity limitations for all males age 45-64 (20.5 percent) but at least comparable in magnitude.

The conclusion which emerges from these calculations is that the rise in reported prevalence of chronic conditions is an important source of increase in the reported prevalence of activity limitations.[41] If the former is less sensitive to changing economic incentives, as we have argued, this implies that additional factors which account for the rise in prevalence of chronic conditions must be viewed as important causes of the increase in reported activity limitations and of the decline in labor force participation. Identification of these additional factors is an important task for future research. These factors might be demographic in nature (e.g., changes in the age distribution of the population) or they may correspond to increasing risk factors in our environment, society, or life styles. Of course, it is also possible that increases in *reported* prevalence exceed increases in actual prevalance of chronic conditions because of improvements in diagnostic techniques, increased use of the medical system in general by high-risk population groups, or increasing public awareness.

Finally, two potentially important qualifications to our argument should be noted. First, our assumption that changes in economic incentives have little effect on reported prevalance rates of chronic conditions may be wrong. Even if the direct effect of these changes is modest, there may also be indirect effects working, for example, through increased general awareness of disability programs. Second, we have been generalizing here from data on three sets of conditions about increases in prevalence; to support such generalizations, data on other important groups of conditions (e.g., respiratory and cardiovascular conditions) must also be assembled.

## VIII.   CONCLUDING COMMENTS

The major findings of our research on morbidity cost estimates (Sections II-VI) may be summarized in the following way:

1.  Although it has been omitted from most comprehensive COI studies, debility cost is a major component of morbidity costs for noninstitutionalized males age 17-64. We estimate that these costs are at least as large and probably larger than the costs of work-loss days.
2.  Earnings loss estimates for persons unable to work based on the HIS prevalence data are considerably larger than earnings loss estimates based on U.S. Labor Dept. prevalence data.
3.  Allowing for health problem impacts on education and occupation increased morbidity costs for noninstitutionalized males age 17-64 by about 25 percent. Most of this increase is in the debility cost component, which rose by almost 60 percent. Our findings also suggest that this increase in debility costs is relatively greater for nonwhites.
4.  Of the 61 health problem categories defined in this study, the six highest cost categories (Groups 10, 30, 47, 56, 57, and 60) account for about 25 percent of total morbidity costs.[42]
5.  Our results for the individual problem categories would not be changed substantially by alternative methods for allocating the costs of work-loss days or disabilities with multiple causes, though increases in costs for several categories such as arthritis (Groups 54-56) and hypertensive disease (Group 36) might be fairly substantial.
6.  Because of procedures for recording data on the HIS tape files, more than 20 percent of both work-loss days and costs for these days could not be assigned to specific problem categories.
7.  The use of a more detailed problem grouping scheme based on long-term disabilities resulted in a very uneven distribution of work-loss day costs among groups since these costs are mainly the result of acute conditions. Increasing the number of groups to deal with this problem will increase the variability in the estimates of our other two cost components for groups with small numbers of persons with long-term disabilities. Additional years of data may therefore be required to deal with this problem.

The methods used in the study have a variety of limitations and possible biases which should also be noted. First, in the assessment of costs of short-term illnesses, note that lost productivity or time off from work due to illness is not captured here unless a work-loss day is reported. Mushkin and Landefeld[16] suggest that the omitted costs of short-term illness may in fact be larger than the costs of work-loss days. Second, there is a possibility of double counting some portion of work-loss day costs as debility costs, although our data suggest that this is a very minor problem. Third, we may in fact have overestimated work-loss day costs for persons who typically work less than eight hours a day since we assessed these costs on the assumption of an eight-hour day. Conversely, for people working more than an eight-hour day our procedure causes an underestimate. Fourth, our estimates of costs for individual problem categories are not based on actual earnings data for people who report problems in these categories. As a result, the frequency of disabilities or work-loss days caused by each category of problems becomes the major determinant of its costs. Better data on actual earnings for people with specific problems, as might be obtained by adding earnings questions to the HIS, are needed to remedy this situation. Fifth, because HIS data do not typically indicate whether or not a person worked at all during the year, let alone how many weeks or hours they worked, a proxy indicator of working was developed. This probably resulted in a slight understatement of debility costs. (See Appendix 3). Finally, there is a more general problem relating to cost estimates for debility and for persons unable to work based on cross-sectional comparisons with people with no reported health problems. If the occurrence of long-term health problems is correlated with personal characteristics not captured in our earnings-prediction model, and if these personal characteristics also influence earnings, our earnings predictions will be biased. The direction of the bias cannot be determined a priori; however, the use of longitudinal data sets to generate earnings predictions would mitigate this problem substantially.

In terms of directions for future research, our own results point-up several issues worthy of further investigation. First, the differences between HIS and Labor Department data on numbers of persons unable to work should be investigated since these differences have a substantial impact on estimated morbidity cost. Second, the impact of health problems on education and occupation should be examined in more detail. This would help to determine whether or not to control for education in estimating morbidity costs for specific types of problems. The possibility of racial differences in these impacts (as noted in Appendix 3) should also be examined more closely.

The descriptive data analysis from the HIS (Section VII) supports the following conclusions:

1. The HIS labor force participation data for the 1969-80 period indicate a decline in the labor force participation rates for older working age males. This decline is largest for nonwhites.
2. The magnitude of the increase in disability prevalence leaves an important portion of the labor force participation decline "unexplained."
3. HIS data on reasons for retirement among older males confirm that reasons other than poor health have been important causes of declining labor force participation.
4. The increase in the prevalence of low-severity disabilities in the period from 1969 to the mid-1970s for older males, along with the absence of a clear shift in the disability distribution toward more severe levels over this period suggest that the increased overall rates of disability were not due solely to a response to changing economic incentives. HIS

prevalence data on selected chronic conditions and impairments (rather than disabilities) support this contention; this is particularly true for data on musculoskeletal conditions.

5.  The evidence of a shift in the disability distribution (among severity levels) in the latter part of the study period, however, along with the much weaker evidence of such a shift in the period from 1969 to the mid-1970s is consistent with the hypothesis that changes in economic incentives do have some impact on reported disability data and hence on national morbidity cost estimates based on these data.

## ACKNOWLEDGMENTS

Thanks are due to Alison Jones and Valerie Waudby for their substantial efforts in the many tasks required to complete this project (programming, proofreading, editing, manuscript preparation, etc.).

Financial support under Grant No. HS-4369 from the U.S. Center for Health Services Research is also gratefully acknowledged.

## NOTES AND REFERENCES

1. H.G. Tolpin and J.D. Bentkover, "Economic Cost of Illness: Decision-Making Applications and Practical Considerations," in R. Scheffler and L. Rossiter (eds.), *Advances in Health Economics and Health Services Research,* vol. 4 (1983); D.P. Rice, J.J. Feldman, and K.L. White, *The Current Burden of Illness in the United States,* an Occasional Paper of the Institute of Medicine, National Academy of Sciences, 1976; D.W. Dunlop, "Returns to Biomedical Research in Chronic Diseases: A Case Study of Resource Allocation," paper presented at the Conference on Functional Health Status and Medical Technology, Georgetown University, Sept. 1977.

2. See, for example, Commission for the Control of Epilepsy and its Consequences, *Plan for Nationwide Action on Epilepsy* (HEW Publication No. HIH-78-276) and *Report to the President from the President's Commission on Mental Health* (Washington: U.S. Government Printing Office, 1978).

3. T.A. Hodgson and M.R. Meiners, "Cost of Illness Methodology: A Guide to Current Practices and Procedures," *Milbank Memorial Fund Quarterly,* Vol. 60, No. 3 (Summer 1982).

4. N.S. Hartunian, C.N. Smart, and M.S. Thompson, *The Incidence and Economic Cost of Major Health Impairments* (Lexington, Mass.: Lexington, Books, 1981).

5. T.A. Hodgson, "The State of the Art of Cost-of-Illness Estimates," in R. Scheffler and L. Rossiter (eds.) op. cit.

6. If there were no sick leave coverage, so that all short-term losses took the form of reduced earnings to the individual (rather than simply reduced output for the employer,), this double counting could be eliminated simply by using $s^H$ as the per person estimate of short-term losses for persons both with and without chronic health problems. Since this is not the case, correction of the double counting becomes much more difficult.

7. D.P. Rice, *Estimating the Cost of Illness.* Public Health Service Pub. No. 947-6, May 1966.

8. These 19 major categories (ICDA codes in parentheses) are: infective and parasitic diseases (002-138); neoplasms (140-239); allergic, endocrine, metabolic and nutritional disorders (240-289);

diseases of the blood and blood-forming organs (290-299); mental disorders (300-329); nervous system and sensory disorders (330-398); diseases of the circulatory system (400-468); diseases of the respiratory system (470-527); diseases of the digestive system (530-587); diseases of the genito-urinary system (590-637); maternity care (640-689); diseases of the skin and cellular tissue (690-716); diseases of the bones and organs of movement (720-749); congenital malformations (750-759); certain diseases of early infancy (760-776); symptoms, senility, and ill-defined conditions (780-795); injuries (800-999); special conditions and examinations (Y00-Y18); and miscellaneous. Within the first of these categories, Rice also reported results separately for tuberculosis and for all other conditions.

9.    This factor was based on data reported in the July, 1964 *Survey of Current Business;* of course, a comparable factor based on more recent data would be much higher.

10.    B.S. Cooper and D.P. Rice, "The Economic Cost of Illness Revisited," *Social Security Bulletin,* Feb. 1976.

11.    A. Berk, L. Paringer, and S.J. Mushkin, " The Economic Cost of Illness: Fiscal 1975," *Medical Care,* Sept. 1978.

12.    H.S. Luft, *Poverty and Health* (Cambridge, Mass.: Ballinger, 1978).

13.    Increases in productivity and inflation between 1963 and 1966 could only account for a small part of the difference in these estimates. Over this period, the average weekly earnings of private, nonagricultural production workers only rose by 11.7 percent.

14.    A.E Fechter, "Imputation of Measures of Severity of Disability to the Low-Income Disabled File: Methods and Findings," Urban Institute Working Paper 977-07, June 1976 (revised).

15.    J. McNeil, F. Slade, and D. Sater, "Work Disability, Labor Force Participation, and Earnings: Data from the 1976 Survey of Income and Education," *Proceedings of the Social Statistics Section,* American Statistical Association Annual Meeting, 1980.

16.    S.J. Mushkin and J.S. Landefeld, *Biomedical Research: Costs and Benefits* (Cambridge, Mass.: Ballinger, 1979), chapter 10.

17.    An explanation for the use of 5 percent rather than 10 percent was not given.

18.    In deriving the 4.4 million prevalance estimate from the Health Interview Survey data, only persons reporting their usual activity as working were included and some categories of impairments and chronic diseases were excluded, presumably on the grounds that their earnings impact was small and because the authors explicitly sought to derive "conservative" estimates.

19.    R.W. Conley, M. Conwell, and S.G. Willner, *The Cost of Mental Illness, 1968.*NIMH Statistical Note 30, 1970.

20.    W.Y. Oi, "Three Paths from Disability to Poverty," report to the U.S. Dept. of Labor under contract No. J-9-M-5-0119; D.O. Parsons,"Health, Family Structure, and Labor Supply," in D.O. Parsons, B.M. Fleisher, and H.P. Marvel *Economic Responses to Poor Health in Older Males* (Columbus, Ohio: Ohio State University Research Foundation, March 1980); and R.M. Scheffler and G. Iden, "The Effect of Disability on Labor Supply," *Industrial and Labor Relations Review,* Vol.28, No.1 (October 1974);

21.    Oi, op. cit.

22.    For a recent overview and citations to numerous studies, see T.W. Hu and F.M. Sandifer, "Synthesis of Cost of Illness Methodology," report to the U.S National Center for Health Services Research on Contract No. 233-79-3010, February 1981.

23.    For example, Hartunian et al., op. cit.; and G. Oster, G.A. Colditz, and N.L. Kelly, *The Economic Costs of Smoking and the Benefits of Quitting* (Lexington, Mass.: Lexington Books, 1984).

24.    R.P. Inman, "The Consumption Losses with Debilitating Illness: The Case of Multiple Sclerosis," University of Pennsylvania, in progress.

25.    Op. cit., Vol. IV.

26.    A.M. Cruze, H.J. Harwood, P.L. Kristiansen, J.J. Collins, and D.C. Jones, "Economic Costs to Society of Alcohol and Drug Abuse and Mental Illness—1977," report to the U.S. Alcohol, Drug Abuse, and Mental Health Administration on Contract No. 283-79-001.

27.   Note that injuries (Group 60) as coded in the HIS refers primarily to acute problems such as sprains, fractures, and lacerations with no residual health limitations. Thus, many conditions listed in other categories in our data may have been the result of an accident or injury; for example, an accident causing permanent impairment would be coded in the HIS as an impairment (e.g., Group 10) rather than as an injury (Group 62).

28.   For the 96 records on the HIS file which could not be linked to the SIE region-residence codes, the process described in Appendix 1 for the three HIS records with missing education data and no geographic link to SIE codes was again employed to assign an earnings figure.

29.   D.O. Parsons, "The Male Labor Force Participation Decision: Health, Reported Health, and Economic Incentives," in D.O. Parsons, B.M. Fleisher, and H.P. Marvel,*Economic Responses to Poor Health in Older Males* (Columbus, Ohio: Ohio State University Research Foundation, March 1980).

30.   T.N. Chirikos and G. Nestel, "Impairment and Labor Market Outcomes: A Cross-Sectional and Longitudinal Analysis," in H.S. Parnes (ed.), *Work and Retirement: A Longitudinal Study of Mean* (Cambridge, Mass.: The MIT Press, 1981).

31.   B.L. Wolfe, "Economics of Disability Transfer Policies," paper presented at the American Public Health Association annual meeting, Nov. 14, 1983.

32.   *Op. cit.*

33.   Examples are the civil service disability program and the Black Lung program. For further information on various programs and their eligibility provisions, see *Disability Compensation: Current Issues and Options for Change,* U.S. Congressional Budget Office, June 1982.

34.   See, for example, U.S. Dept. of Health and Human Services, *Health–United States and Prevention Profile: 1983*DHHS Pub. No. (PHS) 84-1232, Dec. 1983.

35.   The term "usual activity" in our tables refers to working; "outside activities" are activities other than working.

36.   The connection between private and Social Security retirement benefits and the declining labor-force participation of older males has been studied by several researchers. See, in particular, V.R. Fuchs, "Self-Employment and Labor Force Participation of Older Males," *Journal of Human Resources,* Summer 1982 and "Though Much is Taken: Reflections on Aging, Health and Medical Care," *Milbank Memorial Fund Quarterly/Health and Society,* Spring 1984.

37.   Of course, economic incentives may have *some* effect on reported prevalence of chronic conditions. Other "psychosocial" factors, such as respondents' knowledge and changes in lay terminology may also impact on these rates. For evidence on this, see L.M. Verbrugge, "Prevalence of Chronic Conditions in National Health Surveys," Paper presented at the Public Health Conference on Records and Statistics, August 1983, Washington, D.C.

38.   Published data for other chronic conditions in these groups are not considered here because the conditions were unimportant as causes of activity limitations.

39.   Note that these rates apply to all persons rather than males age 45-64.

40.   The column (1) percentages are applied to prevalence rates in both years to control for changes over time in the likelihood of reporting activity limitations in response to economic incentives.

41.   Another way to support this argument is to compute, for each condition in Table 9, RxP, R'x P', and R'x P where R is the reported prevalence rate in the first year shown in the Table, P is the reported percent of conditions causing activity limitations in that year, and R' and P' are the corresponding figures for the second year shown in the table. Then $X = (R'P'/RP) - 1$ is the overall estimated percent increase in prevalence of activity limitations caused by the conditions and $Y = (R'P/RP) - 1$ is the percent increase caused by increased prevalence of the condition itself. Similarly $X = (R'P'/RP) - 1$ and $Y = (R'P'/R'P) - 1$ can be computed by summing over conditions within or across the three categories shown in the table. The result of these calculations summing across all categories is $X = .2801$ while $Y = .1303$. Thus, 46.5 percent ( $= 100 \times .1303/.2801$) of the overall increase in the estimated prevalence of activity limitations

caused by the conditions shown in Table 9 is attributable to increased prevalence of the conditions rather than an increased rate of reported activity limitations among persons who have the conditions.

42.   This calculation excludes from total morbidity cost the costs of work-loss days which could not be attributed to specific conditions (Group 62).

## APPENDIX 1:   METHODS FOR ESTIMATING EARNINGS LOSSES

Our predicted earnings figure for each individual in the HIS who is unable to work is the average earnings reported in the SIE for persons with the same sociodemographic characteristics, but with no reported chronic health problems. The sociodemographic characteristics used in this calculation included age, race, education and location (geographic region and urban vs. rural residence). In order to eliminate income that includes returns on capital which would not be a measure of human productivity, farm and self-employment income were excluded in calculating the average earnings figures.

Because farm and self-employment income were excluded, it was necessary to compute an adjusted average earnings figure ($A^*$) which is based on the assumption that nondisabled persons who report farm or self-employment income earn, on average, the same labor income as their nondisabled counterparts, who reported labor income but not farm or self-employment income. Where $A_w$ is the average earnings figure for nondisabled working males (excluding those with farm or self-employment income), $W =$ the number of working males, and $N =$ the number of nonworking males (i.e., those with no reported earnings, farm income or self-employment income), the average predicted earnings figure for nondisabled individuals based on the assumption that all people who report farm or self-employment income earn a labor income of $A_w$ is given by $A^* = A_w \times (W + F)/(W + N + F)$, where $F =$ the number of males reporting farm or self-employment income.

Values of $A^*$ were calculated from the SIE data based on 9 geographic region codes, 3 urban-rural residence codes (metro, nonmetro, undisclosed), 3 race codes, 7 education classes, and 5 age groups. Education classes were defined as follows: 0-7 years, 8 years, 9-11 years, 12 years, 13-15 years, 16 years, 17+ years. The age categories were 17 to 24 years, 25 to 34 years, 35-44 years, 45-54 years, and 55-64 years. The race categories were white, black, and other. Since this classification scheme results in a 2835-cell matrix and many cells would contain very small numbers, it was decided to combine geographic locations defined by region and urban-rural residence codes for each race based on similar wage patterns. To do this, we calculated average adjusted earnings ($A^*$) from the SIE data by race, geographic region, and residence codes, and ranked the locations in ascending order of $A^*$ for each of the 3 races. Based on these results, we identified 5 geographical groupings for each race. By using these groupings instead of the original region and urban-rural residence codes, we reduced the number of cells in our classification scheme to 525. Even with this reduced number of cells, some were quite small (N less than 10) and therefore were combined with adjacent cells by taking a weighted average.

There were a number of additional calculations and modifications that had to be made in computing the earnings figures for some of the records in the file. Two HIS records in region 3 fell into cells that were empty in the SIE data. The adjusted SIE earnings figures for these two records were taken from adjacent region 4, for the same residence codes and age and education groups.

Another difficulty concerned the 184 nonworking males in the HIS data who had education codes of 12 or 13 (unknown/not reported). For these records, a weighted average of region, residence, race, and age cells from the SIE data was computed across all seven education codes.

Ninety-three records on the HIS file could not be linked to SIE region-residence codes. Their adjusted predicted earnings estimates were calculated as the average predicted earnings figures for all other nonworking males on the HIS file classified by one of the four region codes on the HIS file, SMSA/ non-SMSA residence, and the education, age, and race categories defined above.

Finally, three HIS records could not be linked to the SIE region-residence codes and also had missing education data. For these records, we assigned earnings figures obtained by taking the weighted average of the average earnings figures described in the preceding paragraph across education categories.

Earnings-loss estimates for each of the adult males unable to work were aggregated to national figures by applying the HIS weights and grouping individuals by the diagnostic classifications available on the HIS files. These classifications are based on a modified 4-digit ICDA coding scheme. We formed groups by first examining frequencies of each four-digit code in our data, and frequencies of each three-digit recode (HIS recode #1).[1] When the unweighted frequency for a single 4-digit code exceeded 50, it was generally treated as a separate group in our analysis; however, exceptions to this rule occurred when the three-digit ICDA code or HIS recode containing the four-digit code contained few other cases (i.e., cases with other four-digit codes), and when these few other cases could not be logically grouped with cases with different three-digit codes. Similarly, a three-digit code was usually treated as a separate group when its unweighted frequency exceeded 50, except in a few instances where other less frequent three-digit codes could only be logically combined with this code. This grouping process resulted in the creation of 61 groupings.

Persons with multiple conditions were assigned to groups based on their report of the condition which was the major cause of their limitation. Of the 7,167 persons on our data file, 3,097 (or 43.2 percent) reported at least one other condition as a secondary cause of their activity limitations. The five most frequent categories of conditions reported as secondary causes, in descending order of frequency, were: arthritis NEC (212), diabetes (90), hypertensive disease NEC (133), emphysema (152), and heart trouble NOS or ill-defined (130). (Numbers in parentheses are the HIS Recode #1 codes for these categories.) These five categories accounted for roughly 20 percent of all reported secondary conditions.[2,3]

# NOTES

1.  The coding schemes are described in the following NCHS documents: *National Health Interview Survey, 1977: Diagnostic Recodes* (NTIS PB 80-203987) and *Health Interview Survey Medical Coding Manual and the Short Index* (NTIS PB 281-130).
2.  One possible source of potential bias in the prevalence data should be noted. In the years 1975 - 1978, some selected condition checklists were used as part of the HIS Interviews to identify persons with selected conditions but who do not report disability, work-loss, or medical care use for these conditions. While the inclusion of such a list should not, in principle, affect our data on prevalence of disabilities, it is possible that inclusion of such a list may encourage people to report disabilities for conditions on the list. Since lists for circulatory or respiratory conditions were not used in those years, it is possible that we have understated slightly the relative economic significance of these types of conditions.
3.  For further details on the methods described here and in Appendixes 2-3 below, see David S. Salkever, "Morbidity Costs: National Estimates and Economic Determinants." Final Report on Grant No. HS 4369, U.S. National Center for Health Services Research, September 1984.

# APPENDIX 2:   METHODS FOR ESTIMATING COSTS OF WORK-LOSS DAYS

In order to estimate the economic cost of work-loss days due to illness, all males in the Health Interview Survey between the ages of 17 and 64 who reported work-loss days due to some health condition within the two weeks preceding the interview were identified. Males who were not in the work force, were known to be laid off during the two-week recall period, or were unable to perform their usual activity because of a chronic condition were excluded.

All acute or chronic conditions for which work loss days were reported were assigned to one of the 61 diagnostic groups. In the HIS, a condition being the cause of work-loss days, and the number of such days, is indicated by individuals' response(s) to questions regarding that condition. However, more than one condition may be reported as the cause of the individual's work-loss days and no distinctions between primary and secondary causes is made.

The HIS also contains data on the total work-loss days due to all conditions (PWLD) for an individual in a two-week period on the person record in the HIS file. The work-loss days on the person record will not always equal the sum of the work-loss days on that individuals' condition records (CWLD). The sum of CWLD may be less than work-loss days on the persons record because some reported conditions are not retained in the HIS data. (In particular, reported chronic conditions that did not cause any degree of activity limitation were not retained unless they were reported in response to interviewer questions pertaining to a checklist of selected conditions. This checklist varied from year to year and included approximately 20 specific conditions in each of the years 1975, 1976 and 1977. In 1974, there was no checklist; in 1978 there were six different checklists (though still only one checklist per respondent), each containing approximately 20 conditions. Since only conditions with work-loss days greater than zero were assigned to diagnostic groups 1-61, the difference between the person work-loss days (PWLD) and the sum of the conditions work-loss days (CWLD) was assigned to a residual category, group 62.

The sum of CWLD can also be greater than the PWLD when work-loss days were due to more than one condition. For example, if the individual had 10 work-loss days attributed jointly to three conditions, the number 10 would be recorded on each condition record, resulting in a total of 30 condition work-loss days. Since this would involve double counting, the condition work-loss figures were adjusted as follows:

$$CWLD_i = PWLD \times CWLD_i / \sum_{j=1}^{+} CWLD_j$$

where PWLD = each person's total work-loss days, $CWLD_i$ = the person's work-loss days due to the ith condition, and t = total number of conditions with work-loss days for the individual.

A comparison of the adjusted and unadjusted days identified the groups of conditions reported by persons for whom $\sum_j CWLD_j$ often exceeds PWLD. In percentage terms, Arterial Disease (group 42) showed the greatest differential between the adjusted and unadjusted figures (57.9 vs. 171.1 thousand days annually) presumably because people reporting this condition have a number of other related health problems. Thus, judgments about the relative importance of costs due to work-loss days for this group of conditions is somewhat dependent upon our allocation procedure. In absolute terms, the greatest differential between adjusted and unadjusted work-loss days (about 23 million annually) is in Group 60 (Injuries).

The economic cost of each work-loss day was calculated as eight times the predicted hourly wage figure for each individual. In order to calculate a predicted wage figure, an OLS regression was run using a 10 percent sample of all males 17 to 64 in the SIE. The dependent variable was the logarithm of the SIE hourly earnings figure (annual labor earnings divided by the product of weeks worked and usual working hours per week).

The 10 percent sample drawn from the SIE was all males age 17 to 64 whose labor earnings were greater than zero and who had no farm or self-employment income. Every tenth record was drawn. This process yielded a sample of 11,181 individuals to be included in the regression.

Independent variables in the regression included dichotomous indicators for race, education, age, health status, region of residence, and industry in which the person was employed. The industry codes included in the SIE were the 3-digit 1970 Census Codes. These were grouped into 10 categories:

1.  Agriculture/Forestry/Fisheries
2.  Mining
3.  Construction
4.  Manufacturing
5.  Transportation and Public Utilities
6.  Wholesale and Retail Trade
7.  Finance, Insurance, and Real Estate
8.  Services and Miscellaneous
9.  Public Administration
10. Unknown

The last of these categories was used as the reference category for the regression. Other reference category characteristics were other race, age 55-64, more than 16 completed years of education, residence in the Pacific region, and metropolitan vs. non-metropolitan residence not disclosed.

An additional independent variable was included to capture hourly wage variations among occupations. This variable was calculated as the mean hourly earnings of all males age 17 to 64 in the SIE who worked more than 49 weeks per year and more than 34 hours per week, had no farm or self-employment income, and who were within the same occupation based on the 3-digit Census occupation code reported in the SIE. It was included in the regression analysis in logarithmic form. (This necessitated dropping individuals with zero or blank SIE occupation codes so the regression sample size was reduced to 10,840.)

Results of the regression analysis are reported in Table 1. While the mean occupational wage was overwhelmingly important (explaining almost 22 percent of the dependent variable variance), most other regression coefficients are highly significant and have the expected signs. The pattern of the coefficients for the education dummies shows a consistent increase in hourly wages as education increases. The age coefficients show a rapid rise in wages over the 17-34 age range and a continued rise to peak in the 45-54 age range with a drop in the (omitted) 55-64 age category. This inverted U-shape is commonly observed in age-earnings profiles. The health limitation coefficient implies that on average hourly wages are about 10 percent lower for persons with such health limitations.

*Table 1.* Regression—Earnings Per Hour for All Males Age 17 to 64 From the 1976 Survey of Income and Education

| Variable | Coefficient | F |
|---|---|---|
| Mean Hourly Earnings by Occupational Category | 0.6366 | 977.067 |
| White | 0.0975 | 7.924 |
| Black | -0.0025 | 0.004 |
| 0 to 7 Years Education | -0.3702 | 114.353 |
| 8 Years Education | -0.2905 | 86.700 |
| 9 to 11 Years Education | -0.2567 | 107.853 |
| 12 Years Education | -0.1308 | 36.199 |
| 13 to 15 Years Education | -0.1011 | 20.073 |
| 16 Years Education | -0.0446 | 3.276 |
| | | |
| Health Limitations on Ability to Work Present | -0.1086 | 32.483 |
| 17 to 24 Years of Age | -0.5610 | 838.642 |
| 25 to 34 Years of Age | -0.1571 | 71.818 |
| 35 to 44 Years of Age | 0.0305 | 2.488 |
| 45 to 54 Years of Age | 0.0553 | 8.318 |
| | | |
| Metropolitan Area | 0.0828 | 34.389 |
| Non Metropolitan Area | -0.0208 | 1.781 |
| New England | -0.1024 | 20.927 |
| Middle Atlantic Region | -0.0199 | 0.660 |
| East North Central Region | -0.0518 | 5.515 |
| West North Central Region | -0.1389 | 37.734 |
| South Atlantic Region | -0.1134 | 23.438 |
| East South Central Region | -0.2253 | 50.591 |
| West South Central Region | -0.1950 | 49.011 |
| Mountain Region | -0.1132 | 27.610 |
| | | |
| Mining | 0.1839 | 18.753 |
| Construction | 0.1133 | 21.848 |
| Manufacturing | 0.0586 | 7.870 |
| Communications, Utilities, Transportation | 0.0858 | 6.764 |
| | | |
| Wholesale Trade | -0.0395 | 1.703 |
| Retail Trade | -0.1309 | 33.714 |
| Finance, Insurance, Real Estate | -0.0585 | 3.198 |
| Services | -0.1348 | 37.302 |
| Public Administration | 0.0357 | 1.719 |
| Constant | 0.7300 | |
| $R^2$ | 0.3504 | |

For each individual in the HIS with work-loss days, the regression coefficients shown in Table 1 were combined with relevant data on the independent variables from the HIS to generate their predicted hourly wage. A small number of persons in the HIS could not have an hourly wage assigned from Table 1 because a mean wage for their occupation code could not be computed from the SIE data and/or values for other variables (such as education) were missing. To assign an hourly wage to these persons, we computed the average predicted hourly wage by age and race for the HIS records where the coefficients in Table 1 could be used. These means were then assigned to all persons with missing predicted wages since data on race and age were reported for all these persons.

# APPENDIX 3:
## METHODS FOR ESTIMATING DEBILITY COSTS

Debility costs are defined as the difference between predicted annual earnings in the absence of chronic illness and actual annual earnings of individuals with chronic illnesses. Note that this definition excludes on-the-job productivity losses of persons with no chronic illnesses who experience acute illness but do not miss work. Productivity losses of persons with chronic illness that are not reflected in reduced earnings are also excluded from our estimates. There is also a possibility of double counting between the estimates presented here and the costs of work-loss days if work-loss days exceed sick-leave provisions, and earnings are thereby reduced, more frequently for disabled than nondisabled persons. Since our calculations are restricted, however, to persons with chronic illnesses, it is likely that the great bulk of the estimated costs represent lower earnings per hour and shorter work schedules on a regular basis. Thus, adding the estimated debility costs to the costs of work-loss days should result in a relatively modest degree of double counting.

To verify that the double-counting is indeed small, we used the SIE data to compute the mean weeks worked per year by males age 17 to 64 who worked at all, as well as their mean earnings per hour and earnings per year. A comparison of these figures, for men with and without health limitations showed an average differential of $2,112 (23.9 percent of disabled men's earnings). More than half (51.3 percent) of this differential derives from differences in earnings per hour which can be presumed to measure long-term productivity differences.[1] Moreover, note that the 23.9 percent differential in annual earnings greatly exceeds the percent difference in working hours minus sick time. Data from the 1979 HIS on males age 17 to 64 show that mean work-loss days in a two-week period for the non-disabled were 0.15 while the corresponding mean for the disabled (excluding persons unable to work because of their disability) was 0.46 days. Even with no sick-leave provisions, this difference in work-loss days could only account for a small fraction of the earnings differential.

In principle, our debility cost estimates should be developed for all males age 17-64 in the 1974-78 HIS data who suffered from activity limitations due to chronic illness and who worked at all during the survey year. (Of course, it is possible that some persons with chronic conditions but no reported activity limitations experienced debility costs. These individuals can not be identified in the HIS data however.)

In practice, persons with chronic conditions who worked at all in the survey year cannot be identified with certainty in the HIS since annual hours of work are not reported. Therefore, we identified individuals who presumably worked based on reported work status information in the HIS. Individuals who reported working as their usual activity, that they had worked in the past two weeks, or that they currently had a job were assumed to have worked in the survey year. This includes all persons defined on the HIS as being in the labor force except for those who did not work in the past two weeks, did not report working as their usual activity, had no job at the time of the survey but were looking for work or on layoff.

As a check on our assumption we examined data for the one year of the HIS in which weeks and hours of work were reported, namely, 1979. We computed (1) the percentage of persons who reported at least one week of work in the previous year and who would be classified as having worked under our assumptions, and (2) the corresponding percentage for persons who would be classified as not having worked under our assumptions. (Persons with unknown weeks of work were excluded as were persons who reported themselves as unable to work or having no chronic disability.) Our computations showed that only about one half of one percent of persons in the first group (18 out of 2,818) reported zero weeks worked while about 60 percent of persons in the second group (212 of 357) reported zero weeks worked. This indicated that our assumption is reasonably good but that we may be understating debility costs by assuming that individuals in the second group did not work at all.

Since earnings data are not reported in the HIS, it was necessary to estimate *both* predicted annual earnings in the absence of chronic illness and actual earnings from the SIE data. This estimation was based on separate annual earnings regressions for males age 17 to 64 with and without health limitations. The regression of men without health limitations was estimated from the same 10 percent sample of the SIE data file used for the wage regression analysis in Appendix 2. The regression for men with health limitations used data from the entire SIE data file. In both cases, only persons with positive reported wage earnings and zero farm and self-employment income were included. In both cases, the first step in the estimation process was to calculate the average annual earnings figure for each 1970 census 3-digit occupation category found in the data. This calculation used the entire SIE file of men age 17 to 64 with positive

*Table 1.*   Regression Of Annual Earnings For Males Age 17 to 64

| Variable | Males With No Health Limitations | | Males with Health Limitations | |
|---|---|---|---|---|
| | Coeff | F | Coeff | F |
| Mean Annual Earnings by | | | | |
| Occupations Category | 0.7214 | 1344.82 | 0.8594 | 1027.36 |
| White | 0.1792 | 13.089 | 0.0155 | 0.047 |
| Black | 0.0077 | 0.018 | -0.1475 | 3.339 |
| 0 to 7 Years Education | -0.3500 | 47.363 | -0.6321 | 91.078 |
| 8 Years Education | -0.3050 | 45.834 | -0.3011 | 22.011 |
| 9 to 11 Years Education | -0.3443 | 97.130 | -0.3188 | 29.803 |
| 12 Years Education | -0.0826 | 7.455 | -0.1216 | 4.776 |
| 13 to 15 Years Education | -0.1269 | 16.215 | -0.0938 | 2.661 |
| 16 Years Education | -0.0704 | 4.224 | -0.0215 | 0.108 |
| 17 to 24 Years of Age | -1.1155 | 1542.03 | -0.9743 | 761.572 |
| 25 to 34 Years of Age | -0.1831 | 46.370 | -0.1430 | 18.753 |
| 35 to 44 Years of Age | 0.0825 | 8.645 | 0.0091 | 0.072 |
| 45 to 54 Years of Age | 0.0889 | 9.932 | 0.0893 | 9.356 |
| Metropolitian Area | 0.0136 | 2.212 | 0.0927 | 11.311 |
| Non-Metropolitan Area | -0.0386 | 3.018 | 0.0171 | 0.304 |
| New England | -0.1688 | 28.346 | -0.0580 | 1.628 |
| Middle Atlantic Region | -0.0859 | 6.129 | -0.0051 | 0.011 |
| East North Central Region | -0.0734 | 5.493 | -0.0093 | 0.045 |
| West North Central Region | -0.0795 | 6.141 | -0.0892 | 3.744 |
| South Atlantic Region | -0.1132 | 11.597 | -0.0849 | 3.342 |
| East South Central Region | -0.2372 | 27.492 | -0.2172 | 13.134 |
| West South Central Region | -0.1452 | 13.294 | -0.1838 | 12.028 |
| Mountain Region | -0.0978 | 10.201 | -0.0672 | 2.496 |
| Mining | 0.1408 | 5.409 | 0.3405 | 15.626 |
| Construction | -0.0738 | 4.746 | 0.0441 | 0.855 |
| Manufacturing | 0.0065 | 0.050 | 0.1294 | 9.793 |
| Communication, Utilities, Transportation | 0.0228 | 0.243 | 0.2498 | 11.884 |
| Wholesale Trade | -0.0614 | 2.107 | 0.0686 | 1.179 |
| Retail Trade | -0.1606 | 25.563 | -0.0475 | 1.105 |
| Finance, Insurance, Real Estate | -0.1294 | 7.974 | -0.0814 | 1.477 |
| Services | -0.2416 | 60.154 | -0.1693 | 15.157 |
| Public Administration | -0.0450 | 1.393 | 0.1496 | 8.445 |
| Constant | 2.7472 | | 1.2717 | |
| $R^2$ | 0.4772 | | 0.3537 | |
| n | 11,271 | | 8,633 | |

wage earnings and no farm or self-employment income. Separate averages were computed for men with and without health limitations. The logarithm of this average for the relevant occupation category and health limitation status was then added to each individual's record and used as an independent variable. (Individuals with missing occupation codes were dropped from the analysis.)

Other independent variables related to race, age, education, region of residence, and industry group (defined as in Appendix 2).[2] The dependent variable was the logarithm of annual wage earnings.

Results of the regression analysis for males with no health limitations are shown in Table 1 (Columns 1 and 2). Most independent variables are highly significant and the explanatory power of the regression is high ($R^2 = 0.48$). Results conform to prior expectations in that earnings peak in the 45-54 age group, and are much lower for blacks. The education dummies show a marked earnings differential between high school graduates and persons with less education. Earnings of college graduates (16 years of education) are only slightly higher than for high school graduates, while persons with 13 to 15 years of education earn less than both high school and college graduates. Not surprisingly, persons with post-graduate education (the omitted category) earn significantly more. The very high explanatory power of the mean earnings variable is not unexpected since individuals in the 10 percent sample were also part of the full sample on which the means were computed, but it does support previous research findings on the explanatory power of the census occupation grouping scheme.[3]

The analogous regression for males with health limitations is shown in columns 3 and 4. The pattern of results is generally similar. The education coefficients, however, show a weaker positive effect of higher education and a much stronger differential between persons completing eighth grade and those who do not. It is possible that the failure to complete eighth grade is serving as a proxy in this regression for impaired mental capacity or other aspects of severity of disabilities which interfere with education.

The process for merging predicted earnings figures in the absence of disability was analogous to the procedures described in Appendix 2. For individuals whose predicted earnings could not be computed from the regressions due to missing data, we again assigned mean values based on age and race, computed from the HIS records with complete data.

Finally, for each individual we subtracted predicted earnings from predicted earnings in the absence of disability, and then weighted and aggregated these figures over the 61 condition categories defined previously.[4]

As noted above (Section VI.B), we re-estimated the regressions in Table 1 excluding the education, industry, and mean occupation earnings variables. Dummy variables were also added for each of 18 large SMSAs and for 47 of the 48 contigous states and the District of Columbia. (California was the omitted reference category.) The estimated regressions are shown in Table 2. Note that race coefficients are somewhat larger and more significant (except for the coefficient for blacks without health limitations). The pattern of the age coefficients is similar to the previous results but the positive effect of age on earnings up to 54 years of age is more pronounced than before.

*Table 2.*　Regressions of Annual Earnings for Males Age 17 to 64

| Variable | Males With No Health Limitations | | Males with Health Limitations | |
|---|---|---|---|---|
| | Coeff | F | Coeff | F |
| White | 0.4215 | 52.683 | 0.2786 | 10.643 |
| Black | -0.0108 | 0.026 | -0.2025 | 4.462 |
| 17 to 24 Years of Age | -1.4023 | 2421.373 | -1.2652 | 1226.911 |
| 25 to 34 Years of Age | -0.1229 | 18.560 | -0.0947 | 7.160 |
| 35 to 44 Years of Age | 0.1760 | 33.398 | 0.0675 | 3.259 |
| 45 to 54 Years of Age | 0.1557 | 25.336 | 0.1297 | 15.967 |
| Metropolitan Area Except 18 Large SMSA's | 0.1196 | 8.386 | 0.2902 | 25.705 |
| Nonmetropolitan Area | 0.0513 | 1.151 | 0.1987 | 8.862 |
| Los Angeles | -0.1973 | 4.252 | -0.0442 | 0.102 |
| San Francisco | 0.0965 | 0.495 | -0.1672 | 0.668 |
| Miami | 0.1471 | 0.663 | 0.7672 | 6.711 |
| Atlanta | 0.0633 | 0.127 | 1.0439 | 20.856 |
| Chicago | 0.0869 | 0.637 | 0.7652 | 23.938 |
| St. Louis | 0.1004 | 0.670 | 0.5441 | 9.822 |
| New Orleans | 0.3091 | 3.250 | 0.4517 | 3.489 |
| Baltimore | 0.4131 | 7.872 | 0.3388 | 2.628 |
| District of Columbia (SMSA) | 0.4798 | 14.678 | 0.4295 | 5.107 |
| Boston | 0.0873 | 0.619 | 0.3745 | 4.913 |
| Detroit | 0.3013 | 8.585 | 0.4948 | 11.693 |
| Minneapolis | 0.3365 | 8.501 | 0.6022 | 13.813 |
| New York (SMSA) | 0.2815 | 6.461 | 0.4046 | 4.405 |
| Buffalo | 0.0210 | 0.012 | 0.2932 | 1.072 |
| Cleveland | 0.1888 | 2.431 | 0.6432 | 15.911 |
| Philadelphia | 0.2614 | 7.540 | 0.4810 | 12.281 |
| Pittsburgh | 0.1990 | 2.522 | 0.1823 | 1.258 |
| Houston | 0.6622 | 23.438 | 0.8800 | 23.636 |
| Dallas | 0.4531 | 9.379 | 0.2055 | 0.856 |
| Maine | -0.4430 | 24.315 | -0.1910 | 2.190 |
| New Hampshire | -0.2986 | 16.168 | -0.0724 | 0.427 |
| Vermont | -0.4075 | 28.047 | -0.5715 | 24.317 |
| Massachusetts | -0.3373 | 16.761 | -0.1599 | 1.549 |
| Rhode Island | -0.2784 | 12.698 | -0.1172 | 1.054 |
| Connecticut | -0.2635 | 17.630 | -0.1922 | 3.873 |
| New York | -0.3224 | 14.636 | -0.2612 | 3.771 |
| New Jersey | -0.2881 | 20.278 | -0.0971 | 1.030 |
| Pennsylvania | -0.2871 | 14.056 | -0.2678 | 5.756 |
| Ohio | -0.1502 | 4.916 | -0.2587 | 6.809 |
| Indiana | -0.2493 | 14.144 | -0.2109 | 4.689 |
| Illinois | -0.2839 | 9.405 | -0.4701 | 12.178 |
| Michigan | -0.2901 | 14.426 | -0.2382 | 4.327 |
| Wisconsin | -0.2850 | 17.016 | -0.3141 | 9.235 |
| Minnesota | -0.3281 | 14.296 | -0.3987 | 9.004 |
| Iowa | -0.2402 | 12.691 | -0.3582 | 11.642 |
| Missouri | -0.2860 | 8.848 | -0.4477 | 9.526 |

*Table 2.* (*continued*)

| Variable | Males With No Health Limitations | | Males with Health Limitations | |
|---|---|---|---|---|
| | Coeff | F | Coeff | F |
| North Dakota | -0.1580 | 3.740 | -0.0508 | 0.160 |
| South Dakota | -0.2302 | 5.699 | -0.2304 | 2.682 |
| Nebraska | -0.2776 | 12.709 | -0.0595 | 0.243 |
| Kansas | -0.1547 | 4.150 | -0.1713 | 2.055 |
| Delaware | -0.1101 | 1.679 | -0.0344 | 0.074 |
| Maryland | -0.3600 | 7.926 | -0.1738 | 0.903 |
| District of Columbia | -0.5754 | 12.813 | -0.1404 | 0.354 |
| Virginia | -0.4514 | 26.943 | -0.4630 | 14.357 |
| West Virginia | -0.3500 | 15.065 | -0.4662 | 15.106 |
| North Carolina | -0.3984 | 17.627 | -0.4246 | 10.687 |
| South Carolina | -0.2358 | 5.763 | -0.3016 | 4.588 |
| Georgia | -0.3727 | 10.150 | -0.5289 | 15.862 |
| Florida | -0.3549 | 15.527 | -0.6273 | 23.657 |
| Kentucky | -0.4998 | 26.284 | -0.4030 | 9.002 |
| Tennessee | -0.4914 | 28.647 | -0.4496 | 12.832 |
| Alabama | -0.3207 | 12.183 | -0.3440 | 7.706 |
| Mississippi | -0.3714 | 13.696 | -0.4831 | 11.789 |
| Arkansas | -0.3901 | 14.206 | -0.4383 | 10.764 |
| Louisiana | -0.2925 | 8.222 | -0.4801 | 13.164 |
| Oklahoma | -0.2544 | 7.787 | -0.3095 | 6.739 |
| Texas | -0.4614 | 34.868 | -0.6247 | 30.613 |
| Montana | -0.1831 | 4.962 | -0.0951 | 0.705 |
| Idaho | -0.2471 | 11.203 | -0.1429 | 1.730 |
| Wyoming | -0.2161 | 9.482 | -0.1730 | 2.661 |
| Colorado | -0.2715 | 14.043 | -0.2558 | 5.545 |
| New Mexico | -0.5773 | 51.729 | -0.3724 | 9.515 |
| Arizona | -0.3603 | 18.788 | -0.4531 | 15.483 |
| Utah | -0.2674 | 16.376 | -0.1536 | 2.663 |
| Nevada | -0.0914 | 1.444 | -0.0468 | 0.179 |
| Washington | -0.1321 | 3.461 | -0.1118 | 1.197 |
| Oregon | -0.3534 | 27.866 | -0.2129 | 4.657 |
| Constant | 9.0629 | | 8.6238 | |
| $R^2$ | .37262 | | .20427 | |
| n | 11,271 | | 8,633 | |

Predicted earnings by race and age for persons on the HIS file with complete data based on Tables 1 and 2 are shown in Table 3. Comparing predicted logarithms of disabled and nondisabled earnings within the cells of this table, we see that exclusion of education, industry and occupation increased the average within-cell difference for whites from 0.305 to 0.407; for blacks and others the respective increases were 0.317 to 0.476 and 0.122 to 0.274. Thus, it appears that the increase in estimated debility costs (reported in Section VI.B) was especially large for nonwhites.

*Table 3.*   Logarithm of Predicted Annual Earnings for Males Age 17 to 64

| Age | | White | | Black | | Other | |
|---|---|---|---|---|---|---|---|
| | | Disabled | Non-Disabled | Disabled | Non-Disabled | Disabled | Non-Disabled |
| 17-24 | A | 7.6534 | 7.9253 | 7.1369 | 7.4964 | 7.5419 | 7.6596 |
| | B | 7.538 | 7.9179 | 7.4040 | 7.6101 | 7.6081 | 7.6272 |
| 25-34 | A | 8.8304 | 9.2133 | 8.3437 | 8.7778 | 8.6458 | 8.8970 |
| | B | 8.9258 | 9.1536 | 8.5282 | 8.7842 | 8.8371 | 8.9553 |
| 35-44 | A | 8.9758 | 9.5034 | 8.4796 | 9.0707 | 8.7753 | 9.1570 |
| | B | 9.0942 | 9.4405 | 8.6003 | 8.9786 | 9.0381 | 9.2943 |
| 45-54 | A | 9.0360 | 9.4765 | 8.5364 | 9.0537 | 8.8598 | 9.2117 |
| | B | 9.1387 | 9.4197 | 8.6656 | 8.9692 | 9.0979 | 9.1726 |
| 55-64 | A | 8.9011 | 9.3152 | 8.4134 | 8.8913 | 8.7927 | 9.0584 |
| | B | 8.9861 | 9.2743 | 8.3860 | 8.8258 | 9.0852 | 9.2249 |

A - Based on regressions in Table 2
B - Based on regressions in Table 1

# NOTES

1.   One could argue that this differential overstates long-term productivity differences due to disability because it does not control for socioeconomic and demographic characteristics that are correlated with disability. However, our coefficient estimate for health limitations in Appendix 2, Table 1 implies a similar differential in earnings per hour (about 10 percent) even when other individual characteristics are statistically controlled.

2.   The reference category characteristics in these regressions were: race = other, industry = unknown, age = 55-64, education= 16+ years, region = Pacific, and metropolitan vs. non-metropolitan residence = not disclosed.

3.   Finis Welch and Iva MacKennan, *The Census Occupational Taxonomy: How Much Information Does It Contain?* Rand Corporation Report R-1849, Sept. 1976.

4.   As in the analysis in Appendix 2, persons with multiple conditions were assigned to problem groups based on the reported primary cause of their limitation. Of the 14,338 persons on the HIS data file used for the estimates reported here, only 2,507 (or 17.5 percent) reported at least one other condition as a secondary cause. The four most frequent secondary causes (using the HIS Diagnostic Recode No. 1 coding scheme), in descending order of frequency, were: arthritis NEC (code 212), hypertensive disease NEC (code 133), diabetes (code 090), and blindness in one eye (code X02). These four accounted for 24.9 percent of all reported secondary causes.

# AUTHOR INDEX

# Research in Human Capital and Development

Edited by
**Ismail Sirageldin**
*Departments of Population Dynamics
and Political Economy
The Johns Hopkins University*

Research in Human Capital and Development brings together theoretical and empirical developments in the field of human capital formation that are relevant to developmental issues including education, manpower training, fertility behavior, health, and the important triangle of equity, efficiency and development.

**Volume 1,** 1979, 258 pp.                    $63.50
ISBN 0-89232-019-2

J A I   P R E S S

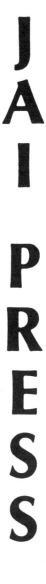

Alamgir, Bangladesh Institute of Developmental Studies. **Barriers to Educational Development in Underdeveloped Countries: With Special Relevance to Venezuela,** *Kristin Tornes, University of Bergen.* **Manpower Planning and the Choice of Technology,** *S.C. Kelley, Center for Human Resource Research, Ohio State.* **The Growth of Professional Occupations in U.S. Manufacturing: 1900-1973,** *Carmel Ullman Chiswick, University of Illinois, Chicago Circle.* **Summary and Discussion,** *Alan Sorkin, University of Maryland.* **PART III: DISTRIBUTION AND EQUITY. Equity Social Striving, and Rural Fertility,** *Ismail Sirageldin and John Kantner, The Johns Hopkins University.* **Index.**

**Volume 2, Equity, Human Capital and Development**
1981, 224 pp.                                    $63.50
ISBN 0-89232-098-2

Edited by **Ali Khan** and **Ismail Sirageldin,** *The Johns Hopkins University*

**CONTENTS: Introduction and Summary,** *Ali Khan and Ismail Sirageldin, The Johns Hopkins University.* **PART I: MEASURES AND PARADOXES. Measures of Poverty and their Policy Implications,** *Koichi Hamada and Noriyuki Takayama, University of Tokyo.* **Paradoxes of Work and Consumption in Late 20th Century America,** *Nathan Keyfitz, Harvard University.* **PART II: THEORETICAL ISSUES. A Model of Economic Growth with Investment in Human Capital,** *Ronald Findlay and Carlos A. Rodriguez, Columbia University.* **The Influence of Nonhuman Wealth on the Accumulation of Human Capital,** *John Graham, University of Illinois.* **The Changing Role of Breastfeeding in Economic Development: A Theoretical Exposition,** *William P. Butz, The Rand Corporation.* **PART III: CASE STUDIES. The Effects of Income Maintenance on School Performance and Educational Attainment in the U.S.A.,** *Charles D. Mallar and Rebecca A. Maynard, Mathematica Policy Research.* **An Analysis of Education, Employment and Income Distribution Using an Economic Demographic Model of the Philippines,** *G.B. Rodgers, International Labour Organization.* **The Welfare Implications of Relative Price Distortions and Inflation: An Analysis of the Recent Argentine Experience,** *Ke-young Chu and Andrew Feltenstein, International Monetary Fund.* **Index.**

# JAI PRESS

**Supplement 1, Manpower Planning in the Oil Countries**
1981, 276 pp.                                              $63.50
ISBN 0-89232-129-6

Edited by **Naiem A. Sherbiny,** *The Work Bank*

REVIEW: "This book constitutes an attempt at *pioneering* on several *fronts* simultaneously. To begin with it tackles a new complex of problems, which may be characterized as "planning for development in a situation of *manpower scarcity*"... The novelty of the subject means, to begin with, that, for the countries concerned, the *goals*of development have to be reformulated."

— *Jan Tingergen, Chapter 1*

Volume 3, Health and Development
1983, 364 pp.                                    $63.50
ISBN 0-89232-166-0

Edited by **Ismail Sirageldin** and **David Salkever**, *The Johns Hopkins University* and **Alan Sorkin**, *University of Maryland.*

CONTENTS: PART I: CONCEPTS AND MEASURES. A Conceptual Model of Health, *Hector Correa, University of Pittsburgh.* A Conceptual Framework for the Planning of Medicine in Developing Countries, *Peter Newman, The Johns Hopkins University.* Health and Development: A Discussion of Some Issues, *Oscar Gish, University of Michigan.* PART II: HEALTH IN HUMAN CAPITAL FORMATION. Adolescent Health, Family Background, and Preventive Medical Care, *Linda Edwards and Michael Grossman, National Bureau of Economic Research.* An Economic Analysis of the Diet, Growth and Health of Young Children in the United States, *Dov Chernichovsky, Ben-Gurion University and NBER and Douglas Coate, Rutgers University.* The Demand for Prenatal Care and the Production of Healthy Infants, *Eugene M. Lewit, New Jersey Medical School.* Life Environments and Adult Health: A Policy Perspective, *Anthony E. Boardman, University of British Columbia and Robert Inman, University of Pennsylvania.* Summary and Discussion, Part II, *David Salkever, The Johns Hopkins University.* PART III: HEALTH IN DEVELOPMENT. Correlates of Life Expectancy in Less Developed Countries, *Robert N. Grosse and Barbara H. Perry, University of Michigan.* The Power of Health, *Wilfred Malenbaum, University of Pennsylvania.* Health Planning in the Sudan, *Ronald J. Vogel, University of Arizona and Nancy T. Greenspan, Health Care Financing Administration.* Health Expenditure in a Racially Segregated Society—A Case Study in South Africa, *M.D. McGrath, University of Natal, Durban.* Analytical Review of the World Health Organization's Health Manpower Development Program 1948-1978, *W.A. Reinke, The Johns Hopkins University and T. Fulop, WHO.* Summary and Discussion, Part III, *Alan Sorkin, University of Maryland.*

# JAI PRESS

**Volume 4, Migration, Human Capital and Development**
1986, 185 pp.             $63.50
ISBN 0-89232-416-3

Edited by **Oded Stark,** *Havard University and Bar-lian University*

This compliation of original articles edited by Harvard economist Oded Stark focuses on an innovative approaches to recent migration phenomona. In spite of discernible variance with regard to many variables, several features stand out. First, migrants from a given origin are not randomly or evenly spread across the absorbing economy nor are they all concentrated in one single labor market or location. Migrants tend to form clusters. Second, in comparison with the absorbing population, migrants constitute a relatively small group. Third, recent migrants are assisted by established migrants; there is heavy reliance upon and usage by the new migrants of "network and kindship capital." Fourth, migrants have traits distinguishing them from members of the economy they join. Quite often this is concurrent with a statistical or economic discrimination against the migrants. Fifth, some after their arrival at the receiving economy, migrants out-perform the native born. This is manifested when the wage curve of migrants intersects that of the non-migrants—a relation that tends to hold even after allowance is made for the standard controls. The contributors to this volume, all leading scholars in the field, have many years of experience in theory and practice. This provides the papers in this volume to have a special depth and insight on migration issues.

**J A I P R E S S**